D1231471

WOUND CARE

Fourth Edition

Cathy Thomas Hess, RN, BSN, CWOCN
President
Wound Care Strategies, Inc.
Harrisburg, Pa.

SPRINGHOUSE
Springhouse, Pennsylvania

STAFF

Publisher
Judith A. Schilling McCann, RN, MSN

Creative Director
Jake Smith

Clinical Director
Joan M. Robinson, RN, MSN, CCRN

Editorial Director
H. Nancy Holmes

Clinical Editor
Jana Sciarra, RN, MSN, CRNP

Editors
Jennifer P. Kowalak (senior associate editor), Naina D. Chohan, Peter H. Johnson, Liz Schaeffer, Ingrid Schaefer Sprague, Teresa P. Sussman

Copy Editors
Jaime Stockslager (supervisor), Richard H. Adin, Catherine B. Cramer, Joy Epstein, Celia McCoy

Designers
Arlene Putterman (senior art director), Joseph John Clark, Linda Franklin, Diane Frederick, Donna S. Morris, Susan Sheridan

Electronic Production Services
Diane Paluba (manager), Joyce Rossi Biletz

Manufacturing
Patricia K. Dorshaw (manager), Beth Janae Orr (book production manager)

Editorial Assistants
Danielle Jan Barsky, Beverly Lane, Linda Ruhf

Indexer
Barbara E. Hodgson

Cover
Four-color photographs of ulcers ©Wound Care Strategies, Inc., 2001

For information, write Lippincott Williams & Wilkins, 323 Norristown Road, Suite 200, Ambler, PA 19002.

Printed in the United States of America.
CGWC4 - D N O S A J J M A M
05 04   12 11 10 9 8 7 6 5

Library of Congress Cataloging-in-Publication Data

Hess, Cathy Thomas, 1961-
    Wound care / Cathy Thomas Hess.— 4th ed.
        p. ; cm. — (Clinical guide)
    Includes bibliographical references and index.
    ISBN 1-58255-169-3 (alk. paper)
Wounds and injuries—Nursing—Handbooks, manuals, etc. 2. Wound
    Healing—Handbooks, manuals, etc. I. Title. II. Series.
    [DNLM: 1. Wounds and Injuries- -nursing—
Handbooks. 2. Decubitus
    Ulcer—nursing—Handbooks. WY 49 H586w 2002]
RD95 .H47 2002
617.1'4—dc21   2001048357

Contents

Contributors and consultants

CONTRIBUTORS

Nancy Collins, PhD, RD, LD/N
Consultant Dietitian
Private Practice
Pembroke Pines, Fla.

Anna Falabella, MD
Assistant Professor of Dermatology
Department of Dermatology and Cutaneous Surgery
University of Miami School of Medicine
Miami, Fla.

Elizabeth E. Hogue, JD
Attorney
Private Practice
Burtonsville, Md.

Kathleen D. Schaum, MS
Director
Strategic Business Development
Wound Care Strategies, Inc.
Lake Worth, Fla.

N. Blair Wall, MHS, PT, CWS
Director
FMH Advanced Skin & Wound Care Center
Frederick Memorial Hospital
Frederick, Md.

CONSULTANTS

David Armstrong, DPM
Department of Surgery
Southern Arizona Veterans Affairs Medical Center
Tucson, Ariz.

Elizabeth A. Ayello, PhD, RN, CS, CWOCN
Clinical Associate Professor
New York University
New York, N.Y.

Morris D. Kerstein, MD, FACS
Professor of Surgery
Vice Chair, Department of Surgery
Mt. Sinai Hospital School of Medicine
New York, N.Y.

Robert S. Kirsner, MD
Associate Professor
Department of Dermatology and Cutaneous Surgery
Department of Epidemiology and Public Health
University of Miami School of Medicine
Miami, Fla.

Foreword

Patient-tailored care is a cornerstone of effective wound manage-ment, which promotes hemostasis and healing, reduces transmis-sion of infection and further injury, and maintains skin viability. Ample consideration must be given to both the patient and the wound in an attempt to achieve a positive outcome.

Clinical Guide: Wound Care, Fourth Edition, concisely inte-grates wound care principles and practices appropriate for all types of wounds. This comprehensive guide offers wound care profes-sionals the tools they need to provide individualized care for a person with a wound. The guide addresses proper wound as-sessment, dressing selection, and management, and emphasizes infection prevention and control during wound care procedures.

Part I begins with the fundamentals of wound healing in chap-ter 1, which gives the reader a concise yet comprehensive overview of the basic anatomic, physiologic, and etiologic principles need-ed in the clinical application of wound care. It also covers the prin-ciples for establishing a wound management system and serves as a practical how-to guide, with a step-by-step pathway to treatment options.

Chapter 2 on nutrition prompts the reader to consider the im-portance of intrinsic metabolic factors linked to the promotion of an organized wound-healing process.

Chapters 3, 4, and 5 provide a comprehensive guide to the management of, respectively, pressure ulcers, venous and arterial ulcers, and diabetic foot ulcers.

Chapter 6 focuses on wound assessment, documentation, and outcome management. It also reviews recognized assessment tools and evaluation techniques for chronic wounds.

Chapter 7 offers a timely discussion of legal and payment and accountability issues facing wound care providers. This section covers the contemporary, must-know, administrative issues, in-cluding a menu for billing and reimbursement.

Part II is a practical, quick reference to a comprehensive array of the most up-to-date and widely used wound care products. Profiles of more than 280 wound care products used as primary or secondary dressings are arranged by category. Each product category section begins with a category description, including the action, indications, advantages, and disadvantages of the product type, and the Health Care Financing Administration Common Procedure Coding System (HCPCS) billing codes now in effect.

Each product profile describes the product in detail, including the forms, available sizes, action, indications, contraindications, and application and removal instructions. Where appropriate, precautions and adverse reactions are included, and photographs of the product have been included whenever possible. Product information and photographs were provided by the product manufacturers themselves. Every attempt has been made to accurately document the information contained in each profile. However, every health care professional should review the package insert information for each product before using it to identify product changes that may have occurred.

Part III provides a concise look at additional dressings and products, from compression stockings and cohesive wraps to wound cleansers and deodorizers.

The appendices cover a range of issues, from treatment guidelines for various wound types to a wound classification tool and risk assessment tools for arterial, diabetic, venous, and pressure ulcers. Finally, a manufacturer resource guide provides contact information for the products listed.

Clinical Guide: Wound Care, Fourth Edition, is a must for all members of the multidisciplinary wound care team—from the basic to the advanced—as well as for students of medicine, nursing, and physical therapy. I view the new edition as the "desk reference" for wound care.

Richard "Sal" Salcido, MD
Chairman
Department of Rehabilitation Medicine
The University of Pennsylvania Health System
Philadelphia

Part One

WOUND CARE AND PREVENTION

1

Fundamentals of wound healing

Health care professionals are strategically building state-of-the-art skin and wound care systems that best support clinical practices spanning care settings and patient populations. Structuring these systems requires careful thought and consideration to support both the art and science of wound care. *Art* refers to the skill and application technique a team member uses when applying the preferred management modality for the wound care patient. *Science* refers to the team member's knowledge and understanding of the disease process and the preferred modality used in managing the patient. *Art* and *science*, the basic components of wound healing, directly impact the patient's clinical and financial outcomes.

The superficial wounds we all experience, such as a paper cut or a scraped knee, usually heal in a few days without complications. However, acute and chronic wounds may require additional interdisciplinary care and specific protocols. An understanding of the anatomy and physiology of the skin, the phases of the healing process, and the types of wounds and wound repair are fundamental to recognizing factors that may complicate or delay wound healing. Each of these considerations plays a key role in the art and science of managing wounds. (See *Wound identification key*, pages 4 and 5.)

Anatomy and physiology of the skin

Knowledge of skin anatomy and physiology is essential to classifying wounds when the health care professional uses a system such as staging to assess and document tissue destruction.

ANATOMY OF THE SKIN

The skin is made up of two major layers—the epidermis and the dermis. Each layer is composed of different types of tissue and has different functions. (See *Layers of the skin,* page 6.)

The epidermis, the outermost layer of the skin, is thin and avascular; it normally regenerates every 4 to 6 weeks. Its primary functions are to maintain skin integrity and to act as a physical barrier. Layered with epidermal cells, the epidermis consists of five sublayers—the outermost stratum corneum, the stratum lucidum, the stratum granulosum, the stratum spinosum, and the innermost stratum germinativum, or basal cell layer. The stratum germinativum anchors the epidermis to the second and thicker layer of the skin, the dermis.

The function of the dermis is to provide strength, support, blood, and oxygen to the skin. This layer contains blood vessels, hair follicles, lymphatic vessels, sebaceous glands, and sweat glands. The dermis is composed of fibroblasts, collagen, and elastic fibers. Fibroblasts are responsible for the formation of collagen, ground substance, and elastin proteins. Collagen gives skin its strength, and elastin is responsible for skin recoil. Thick bundles of collagen anchor the dermis to the subcutaneous tissue and underlying supporting structures, such as fascia, muscle, and bone.

The subcutaneous tissue is composed of adipose and connective tissue as well as major blood vessels, nerves, and lymphatic vessels. The thickness of the epidermis, dermis, and subcutaneous tissue varies from person to person and from one part of the body to another.

PHYSIOLOGY OF THE SKIN

The skin is the largest organ of the body, constituting about 10% of the body's weight. It's exposed to physical and mechanical assaults daily, which may or may not have permanent physical consequences.

Wound identification key

TYPE	DESCRIPTION
Wounds	
Acute wound	Caused by trauma or surgery and usually requiring limited local care
Chronic wound	Takes longer than usual to heal because of underlying conditions, such as pressure, diabetes mellitus, poor circulation, poor nutritional state, immunodeficiencies, or infection
Full-thickness wound	Tissue destruction extending through the dermis to involve subcutaneous tissue and possibly muscle or bone; tissue can appear snowy white, gray, or brown, with a firm leathery texture
Laceration	Torn or jagged wound
Partial-thickness wound	Tissue destruction through the epidermis extending into, but not through, the dermis
Ulcers	
Arterial ulcer	Caused by ischemia; related to the presence of arterial occlusive disease; symptoms include pain and tissue loss
Diabetic ulcer	Caused by trauma or pressure secondary to neuropathy or vascular disease related to diabetes mellitus
Pressure ulcer	Caused by ischemia from pressure; this localized tissue damage is also called a decubitus ulcer, bedsore, or pressure sore
Venous ulcer	Local losses of epidermis and various levels of dermis and subcutaneous tissue, occurring over or near the malleoli of the distal lower extremities; caused by edema and other sequellae of impaired venous return

Wound identification key *(continued)*	
TYPE	**DESCRIPTION**
Burns	
Superficial (first-degree burn)	Damage limited to the epidermis characterized by erythema, hyperemia, tenderness, and pain
Partial-thickness (second-degree burn)	Superficial to deep partial-thickness wound characterized by large blisters, edema, pain, and wet, weeping, and shiny surface
Full-thickness (third-degree burn)	Full-thickness wound characterized by deep-red, black, or white appearance; edema; painless nerve ending damage; and exposed subcutaneous fat layer

The six functions of the skin are:

- *Protection.* Skin acts as a physical barrier to microorganisms and other foreign matter and protects against infection and excessive loss of fluids.
- *Sensation.* Nerve endings in the skin allow a person to feel pain, pressure, heat, and cold.
- *Thermoregulation.* Skin regulates body temperature through vasoconstriction, vasodilation, and sweating.
- *Excretion.* Skin assists in thermoregulation by excreting certain waste products, such as electrolytes and water.
- *Metabolism.* Synthesis of vitamin D in skin exposed to sunlight, for example, activates the metabolism of calcium and phosphate, minerals that play an important role in bone formation.
- *Body image.* Skin details our appearance, uniquely identifying each individual.

Phases of wound healing

When skin integrity is altered and a wound results, the healing process begins. The first phase is the inflammatory phase (defensive or reaction phase), followed by the proliferative phase (fi-

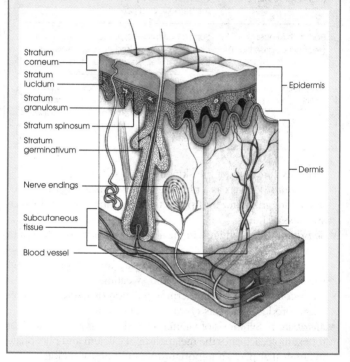

Layers of the skin

The skin is composed of two fused layers — the epidermis and dermis. As this illustration shows, the epidermis has five strata — the stratum corneum, stratum lucidum, stratum granulosum, stratum spinosum, and stratum germinativum. Subcutaneous tissue, found beneath the dermis, is a loose connective tissue that attaches the skin to underlying structures.

Stratum corneum
Stratum lucidum
Stratum granulosum
Stratum spinosum
Stratum germinativum
Nerve endings
Subcutaneous tissue
Blood vessel

Epidermis
Dermis

broblastic, regeneration, or connective tissue phase). The final phase is the maturation or remodeling phase. (See *Cascade of wound-healing events.*) Patients without compromising conditions usually heal throughout these phases without difficulty.

INFLAMMATORY PHASE

The inflammatory phase — characterized by edema, erythema, heat, and pain — begins at the time of injury and typically lasts 4 to 6

Cascade of wound-healing events

This diagram shows the cascade of events that occurs during the wound-healing process.

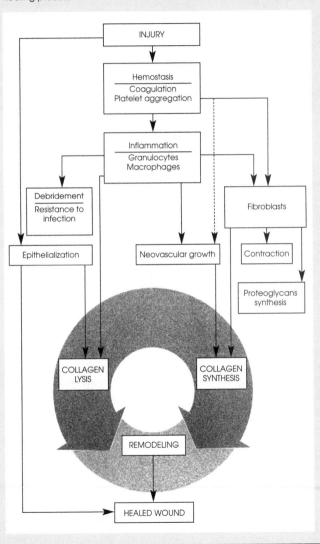

days. Bleeding is controlled by hemostasis, and any present bacteria are destroyed by granulocytic leukocytes, particularly the polymorphonuclear neutrophils. About 4 days after the injury, macrophages, specialized cells derived from monocytes, migrate to the area, destroy bacteria, and clean the wound site of cellular debris. Macrophages replace the leukocytes and produce chemoattractants and growth factors, which attract the cells needed for tissue repair. Macrophages also convert macromolecules into the amino acids and sugars necessary for wound healing.

PROLIFERATIVE PHASE

The proliferative phase typically lasts 4 to 24 days. In an open wound, granulation tissue is generated, producing red, beefy, shiny tissue with a granular appearance. Granulation tissue consists of macrophages, fibroblasts, immature collagen, blood vessels, and ground substance. As this type of tissue proliferates, fibroblasts stimulate the production of collagen, which gives tissue its tensile strength and, ultimately, its structure.

As the wound site fills with granulation tissue, its margins contract, or pull together, decreasing the wound's surface. During epithelialization, the final step of this phase, cells migrate from the wound margins, divide and, ultimately, touch one another, sealing the wound from the external environment. Epithelialization can only occur in the presence of viable, vascular tissue. When epithelialization is complete, a scar results.

MATURATION PHASE

During the maturation phase, which can last from 21 days to 2 years, the collagen fibers reorganize, remodel, and mature, gaining tensile strength. This process continues until the scar tissue has regained about 80% of the skin's original strength. This tissue will always be at risk for breakdown because its tensile strength is less than that of uninjured skin.

Types of wound repair

Once the skin is impaired and a wound is created, the health care professional decides how to repair the wound. The three types of wound repair are primary intention, secondary intention, and tertiary intention. Each type depends on the wound and how it's managed.

Many acute wounds such as surgical wounds are closed by primary intention with the skin edges approximating. Such wounds have a lower risk of infection, involve little tissue loss, and heal with minimal scarring after 4 to 14 days.

Chronic wounds such as pressure ulcers heal by secondary intention with the skin edges not approximating. Chronic wounds involve greater tissue loss, a higher risk of infection, and longer healing time.

Surgical wounds that are left open for 3 to 5 days to allow edema or infection to resolve or exudate to drain, then closed with sutures, staples, or adhesive skin closures heal by tertiary intention, or delayed primary intention. Risks of infection and tissue loss are higher during the days that the wound is left open.

Factors that impede wound healing

Various factors may delay or impede healing. Local factors occur directly within the wound, whereas systemic factors occur throughout the body.

LOCAL FACTORS

Local factors that may impede wound healing include pressure, a dry environment, trauma, edema, infection, necrosis, and incontinence.

Pressure

When a wound site sustains excessive pressure or continuous pressure, the blood supply to the capillary network may be disrupted, impeding blood flow to the surrounding tissues and delaying healing.

Dry environment

Wounds heal three to five times faster and less painfully in a moist environment than in a dry one. Typically, in a dry environment, cells dehydrate at the wound site and cell death occurs. This causes a scab or crust to form over the wound site, which impedes healing. Keeping the wound hydrated with a moisture-retentive dressing enhances epidermal cell migration and encourages ep-ithelialization.

Trauma and edema

Wounds heal slowly or perhaps not at all in an environment in which the wounds are repeatedly traumatized or deprived of lo-cal blood supply by edema. Edema interferes with the transportation of oxygen and cellular nutrition to the wound.

Infection

A systemic or local infection may delay or impede healing. Presence of an infection—as evidenced by purulent drainage or exudate, induration, erythema, or fever—necessitates a wound culture. When a pressure ulcer or full-thickness wound that extends to the bone fails to heal, the patient should be assessed for osteomyelitis. Any abnormal cultures or other test results may require antibiotics to manage the infection.

Necrosis

Dead, devitalized (necrotic) tissue can impede healing. Two types of necrotic tissue may appear in a wound: slough and eschar. Slough is hydrated, loose, stringy necrotic tissue that is typically yellow. Eschar, which appears as dehydrated, thick, leathery tis-sue, may be black. Necrotic tissue is an impediment to the heal-ing process and must be removed before repair and healing can occur.

Incontinence

Urinary and fecal incontinence can alter skin integrity. Providing proper skin care is essential for successful skin and wound man-agement.

SYSTEMIC FACTORS

Systemic factors include age, body build, chronic diseases, nutri-tional status, vascular insufficiencies, immunosuppression, and ra-diation therapy.

Age

Wounds in the geriatric population tend to heal more slowly than those in younger patients, and the healing may also be impaired.

Over time, elderly patients may have inadequate nutritional intake; compromised immune, circulatory, and respiratory systems; and poor hydration. These factors increase the risk of skin breakdown and delay wound healing.

Body build
Body build may also affect wound healing. In an obese patient, wound healing may be compromised because adipose tissue has a poor blood supply. Conversely, in an emaciated patient, the lack of oxygen and nutritional stores may interfere with or delay wound healing.

Chronic diseases
Examples of chronic diseases that affect wound healing are coronary artery disease, peripheral vascular disease, cancer, and diabetes mellitus. In the insulin-dependent diabetic population, chronic wounds typically heal slowly. Because granulation tissue production depends on insulin, an insufficient amount of insulin can delay granulation tissue formation. Therefore, the health care professional should monitor the diabetic patient's serum glucose level and watch for signs and symptoms of wound infection.

Nutritional status
Wound healing requires ongoing nutritional assessment because the visual appearance of the patient or the wound isn't a reliable indicator of whether the patient is receiving the proper amount of nutrients. Laboratory values—such as serum albumin level, total lymphocyte count, and transferrin level—are indicators that must be assessed and monitored regularly. (See Chapter 2, Nutrition assessment and therapy.)

Vascular insufficiencies
Various wounds or ulcers, such as arterial, venous, diabetic, and pressure ulcers, can affect the lower extremities. Common causes of these ulcers are decreased or impaired blood supply or pressure. Selecting the appropriate topical and supportive therapies depends on properly identifying the type of ulcer. (See Chapter 4, Venous and arterial ulcers.)

Immunosuppression and radiation therapy
Suppression of the immune system by disease or medication may delay wound healing. Radiation therapy can cause ulcerations or changes in the skin either immediately after treatment or sometime later.

WOUND-HEALING COMPLICATIONS
The most common complications of healing include:

- *infection*—drainage of purulent material and inflamed wound edges that, if uncontrolled, may lead to osteomyelitis, bacteremia, and sepsis
- *hemorrhage*—internal (hematoma) or external bleeding
- *dehiscence*—separation of skin and tissue layers that commonly occurs 3 to 11 days after injury
- *evisceration*—protrusion of visceral organs through a wound opening
- *fistula*—abnormal passage between two organs or between an organ and the surface of the body.

Wound care and procedures

Achieving successful wound healing depends on carefully fulfilling every step in wound management, including critical assessment, planning, implementation, evaluation, and documentation. The responsibilities of the health care professional include assessing the patient's skin, wounds, and dressings; implementing the wound care plan; selecting and changing dressings; and preventing infection during procedures.

Clinical interventions vary, depending on the condition of the skin around the wound; whether the wound is acute or chronic; the amount of its exudate; the presence or absence of necrosis; the wound's response to the dressing ordered; whether it is noninfected or infected; the degree of cleaning and packing required; the nature of the dressings needed; and how drainage is to be managed.

ACUTE WOUNDS
Care of traumatic or surgical wounds usually requires limited, local care to the site. If an optimal wound environment is provided, these wounds heal with minimal scarring after 4 to 14 days. Infection,

hemorrhage, dehiscence, evisceration, and fistula formation may delay healing. Acute wounds are typically approximated with the use of sutures, staples, or skin adhesives.

CHRONIC WOUNDS
Pressure ulcers and leg ulcers take longer to heal because of such underlying conditions as diabetes mellitus, poor circulation, poor nutritional status, immunodeficiencies, and infection. In many instances, chronic wounds require a multidisciplinary approach and involve several treatment modalities. (See *Adjunctive therapies in wound care,* pages 14 and 15.) Chronic wounds require a multidisciplinary approach to healing.

WOUND CARE GOALS
The goal of the health care professional in wound management is to keep the wound moist, clean, and free from physical trauma and to maintain the patient's skin integrity. Choosing the most effective dressings and implementing appropriate care procedures or techniques help achieve this goal.

Choosing a dressing
With more than 2,000 wound-care products on the market, choosing the correct dressing may be difficult and overwhelming. (See *Choosing the ideal dressing,* page 16.) Developing a management pathway and planning wound care require consideration of:

- wound and skin-related factors, such as cause, severity, environment, condition of periwound skin, wound size and depth, anatomic location, volume of exudate, and the risk or presence of infection
- patient-related factors, such as vascular, nutritional, and medical status; odor-control requirements; comfort and preferences; and cost-benefit ratio
- dressing-related factors, such as availability, durability, adaptability, and uses.

Wound and skin characteristics and patient status
In most instances, topical management choices are guided by the patient's skin and wound characteristics and the patient's health status, including any complicating physical condition. For example, a hydrated, yellow pressure ulcer in an otherwise healthy pa-

Adjunctive therapies in wound care

THERAPY	DESCRIPTION	EFFECTS
Hyperbaric oxygen	In a chamber at >1 atmosphere of pressure (14.7 psi), the patient breathes 100% oxygen	■ Increases tissue oxygenation and fosters wound healing by: – supporting white blood cell bacterial destruction – allowing fibroblasts to proliferate and build collagen – developing new epithelial tissue
Electrical stimulation	Electrical current applied to stimulate tissue regeneration	■ Increases oxygen and nutrient transport to tissues ■ Reduces edema ■ Reduces pain ■ Increases fibroblastosis and collagen development ■ Improves scar tissue elasticity
Hydrotherapy	Partial- or full-body immersion in which injected air produces water turbulence and agitation	■ Promotes debridement (thermal or nonthermal) ■ Cleans the wound ■ Induces circulatory and neurologic effects
Ultrasound	High-frequency sound waves transmitted through water or sonic gel to the wound	■ Increases collagen elasticity ■ Decreases muscle and joint stiffness ■ Diminishes pain ■ Decreases muscle spasms ■ Increases oxygen transport ■ Decreases hyperemia ■ Accelerates wound recovery ■ Decreases edema

Adjunctive therapies in wound care *(continued)*

THERAPY	DESCRIPTION	EFFECTS
Nutritional support	High-calorie, high-protein, moderate-fat diet that contains enough non-nitrogen calories to prevent the body from using amino acids for energy; vitamin or mineral deficiencies must be corrected; 2 qt (2 L)/day fluid intake is recommended	■ Decreases susceptibility of soft tissue to break down
Compression	Elastic stockings or bandages applied to the lower extremities	■ Promotes venous blood return ■ Prevents blood pooling ■ Decreases edema
Topical growth factors	Biologically developed product applied directly to the wound; effects depend on target cell of the specific product	■ Increases wound healing by: – increasing wound strength – controlling collagen deposition – increasing cellular content
Support surface	Available as cushions, (for chairs or wheelchairs), mattress overlays, and beds (air-fluidized or air-suspension); requires turning or repositioning schedule	■ Provides stability for the skeleton ■ Distributes body weight over a larger area and reduces tissue pressure ■ Controls shear forces on the skin surface

Choosing the ideal dressing

To confirm that you've chosen the proper dressing, answer the following questions.
- Does the dressing protect the wound from secondary infection?
- Does it provide a moist wound-healing environment?
- Does the dressing provide thermal insulation?
- Can it be removed without causing trauma to the wound?
- Does the dressing remove drainage and debris?
- Is it free from particulates and toxic products?

tient might require a debriding agent, a moist dressing, or a dressing that supports autolysis. The same wound in an immunocompromised patient might necessitate immediate surgical debridement to reduce the risk of infection.

Product selection guidelines

Familiarity with the major categories of skin and wound care products and their actions, indications, contraindications, advantages, and disadvantages will aid in the selection of the most appropriate dressing. (See Part II.) Also to be considered are a product's available forms and its application and removal procedures. In many cases, one product can help meet more than one therapeutic goal. For example, moist dressings can support wound healing and debride.

Clinical guidelines

Topical wound management algorithms and other guidelines can make choosing a dressing easier. (See Chapter 3, Pressure ulcers, for treatment guidelines for pressure ulcers, and the appendices for treatment guidelines for arterial, diabetic, and venous ulcers.)

Treatment order

The prescribing health care professional's order for wound and skin management should include:
- specific site
- cleansing solution and method
- primary dressing or drug
- secondary dressing, if applicable

- securement device, if applicable
- frequency of dressing changes
- time frame for evaluating treatment effectiveness.

Before applying or changing a dressing, the caregiver should verify these elements.

A typical wound and skin management order for a wound on the right hip might read as follows:

Clean right hip with normal saline solution. Fluff and loosely pack tunneling areas and base of wound with hydrogel-impregnated gauze. Cover with a dry dressing. Secure with a retention tape. Change daily and reevaluate in 14 days.

A change in local or supportive measures is indicated if a wound has not decreased in size after 2 to 4 weeks of management. An immediate change in management is indicated if a negative outcome occurs at any time during the course of management.

PROCEDURES

Proper wound management includes correctly implementing and performing various procedures. For example, large, deep, or obviously dirty wounds may require debridement and irrigation, and draining wounds may require dressing and application of a pouch. Wounds with minimal purulent drainage usually can be managed with a wound dressing for packing. Some procedures meet more than one therapeutic goal. For example, irrigation can clean and debride a wound.

Culturing a wound

All wounds are contaminated with various organisms. Infection— as evidenced by purulent exudate, induration, erythema, edema, fever, or leukocytosis—may delay healing. Culturing the wound allows identification of infecting organisms. Culture methods include surface swab culturing, fluid culturing (through needle aspiration), curettage of the wound base (after cleaning the surface of the wound), and deep-tissue biopsy. (See *Swab-culturing technique,* page 18.) It's important to remember that swab cultures identify contamination only on the surface of the wound. The Centers for Disease Control and Prevention recommend either ob-

Swab-culturing technique

Collect a wound culture when purulent or suspicious-looking drainage or signs of infection — induration, fever, erythema, or edema — are present. When collecting, don't use purulent matter to culture, and don't swab over hard eschar. Use a sterile calcium alginate or rayon swab, not a cotton-tipped swab. To obtain a wound culture with a swab, follow these steps:

- Thoroughly rinse the wound with sterile saline solution before culturing.
- Gently rotate the swab.
- Swab wound edges using 10-point coverage as shown in the illustration.
- Place the swab in the culture medium and take it to the laboratory as soon as possible.

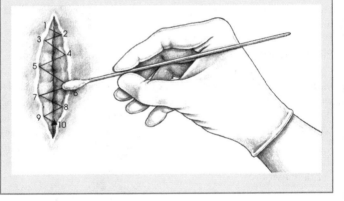

taining fluid from the wound through needle aspiration or obtaining tissue through a wound biopsy.

A wound that contains necrotic tissue or sinus tracts requires both an aerobic and an anaerobic culture. A wound that's open and viable needs only an aerobic culture. Bacteria levels greater than 105 or colony counts above 100,000 organisms/ml indicate that wound healing may be delayed. Notify the prescribing health care professional of culture results so that appropriate interventions can be ordered. If the wound doesn't respond to the prescribed antibiotic therapy after 2 to 4 weeks of optimal care, it should be reassessed, generally by means of a tissue biopsy. If the wound is full thickness, evaluate for the presence of osteomyelitis.

Removing a dressing

When removing a dressing, follow these guidelines:

- Use standard precautions.
- Remove the old dressing with the same care and attention you used to apply it.
- Carefully lift the adhesive barrier off the surrounding skin. If you meet resistance, you may need to use acetone-free adhesive remover or baby oil to ease removal (especially from hairy skin).
- Slowly remove the dressing, noting the amount, type, color, and odor of the drainage.
- Discard the dressing and gloves according to facility policy.

Irrigating a wound

Irrigation flushes cellular debris and drainage from an open wound. Irrigation with an antiseptic or antibiotic solution has been documented to be cytotoxic to exposed wound-healing cells. (See *Common antiseptic solutions,* page 20.) Wound irrigation requires sterile technique. After irrigation, open wounds usually are packed to absorb additional drainage.

Noninfected wound

For a clean, noninfected wound, gently cleanse with normal saline solution or other noncytotoxic solution to minimize disruption of healthy tissue. Use a bulb syringe, a gravity drip through I.V. tubing or surgical drains, or a piston syringe (without a needle) and a rubber catheter for low-pressure irrigation. Some health care professionals recommend cleaning only the surface around a clean wound because wound exudate contains growth factors, nutrients, and proliferating cells that aid healing.

Infected wound

For an infected wound, use flow pressures of less than 30 psi. This selectively debrides necrotic tissue while minimizing harm to healthier granulation tissue. Effective irrigation force (8 psi) can usually be obtained with a 35-ml syringe and a 19G needle.

Debridement

Debridement involves removing necrotic tissue to allow underlying healthy tissue to regenerate. (See *Debriding a wound,* pages 21 and 22.) Depending on the type of injury, a combination of debridement techniques may be used.

Common antiseptic solutions

SOLUTION	ACTIONS	SPECIAL CONSIDERATIONS
Acetic acid	■ Effective against *Pseudomonas aeruginosa* in superficial wounds	■ Toxic to fibroblasts in standard dilutions ■ Changes color of exudate, which may provide false assurance for elimination of infection
Hydrogen peroxide	■ Provides mechanical cleansing and some debridement by effervescent action	■ Can cause ulceration of newly formed tissue ■ Toxic to fibroblasts ■ Do not use to pack sinus tracts (can cause air embolism) ■ Do not use for forceful irrigation (can cause subcutaneous emphysema)
Povidone-iodine preparations	■ Broad-spectrum effectiveness when used on intact skin or small, clean wounds	■ Toxic to fibroblasts in normal dilutions ■ Not always effective in infected wounds ■ Long-term use in wounds may cause iodine toxicity
Sodium hypochlorite solution	■ Effective against *Staphylococcus* and *Streptococcus* species ■ Dissolves necrotic tissue ■ Controls odors	■ Toxic to fibroblasts in normal dilutions ■ Protects intact surrounding skin to prevent breakdown

Debriding a wound

Debridement is the removal of dead or devitalized tissue. Wounds can be debrided enzymatically, mechanically, autolytically, and by combination.

Enzymatic debridement
Enzymatic debridement breaks down necrotic tissue without affecting viable tissue. Agents used are prescription drugs that are ordered by the doctor. All enzymes are not equally effective, so follow the manufacturer's instructions carefully.

Mechanical debridement
The three techniques of mechanical debridement include applying a wet-to-dry dressing, using a whirlpool bath, or removing the necrotic tissue by surgery. Therapy may range from conservative to aggressive. To apply a wet-to-dry dressing, follow these steps:
- Moisten the gauze with a solution such as normal saline, and wring it out until it is slightly moist.
- Fluff the gauze completely and place it over the wound bed.
- Remove the dressing when it is almost dry. Tissue debris and drainage will adhere to the gauze.

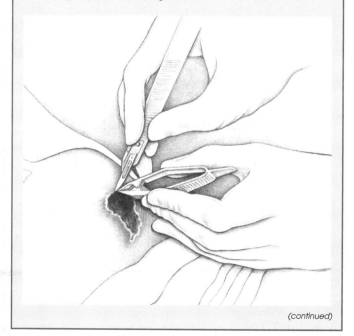

(continued)

Debriding a wound *(continued)*

Mechanical debridement *(continued)*

Surgical debridement involves a doctor removing dead or devitalized tissue with a sharp instrument or laser, either at the bedside or in the operating room. Surgical excision and skin grafting are usually re-served for deep burns or ulcers. Typically, the patient receives a local or general anesthetic. The term laser is an acronym for light amplifica-tion by stimulated emission of radiation. It is an electro-optical instru-ment that produces an intense beam of light in uniform wavelengths. This beam of light can deliver high energy levels to a small surface area, providing instant hemostasis and sterilization of the wound. Laser is generated from different media (for example, carbon dioxide) and is used in surgical excision and the debridement of pressure ulcers.

Autolytic debridement

Autolytic debridement allows the body to lyse or break down necrotic tissue by using the body's enzymes and defense mechanisms. Many dressings are designed to promote autolysis.

Combination debridement

Depending on the type of injury, debridement techniques may be combined. For example, mechanical methods may be used with en-zymatic methods such as wound-cleansing beads or topical agents that absorb exudate and debris.

Cleansing

The goal of wound cleansing is to remove bacteria and debris with as little chemical and mechanical force as possible and, at the same time, to protect healthy granulation tissue. Always cleanse a wound initially and before applying a new dressing. When cleansing a wound, observe the following:

- Use standard precautions.
- Carefully consider the choice of cleaner. Normal saline solution provides a moist environment, promotes granulation tissue for-mation, and causes minimal fluid shifts in healthy cells. Antiseptic solutions, such as acetic acid, hydrogen peroxide, sodium hypo-chlorite (Dakins solution), and povidone-iodine, may damage tissue and delay healing. Base your selection on the indications, contraindications, and benefits to healthy tissue.
- Use an appropriate technique. (See *Wound-cleansing technique.*)

Wound-cleansing technique

Using a sterile gauze pad moistened with the prescribed cleansing agent, wipe wound areas as shown: Clean a linear wound from top to bottom, and work outward from the incision in lines running parallel to it. Always wipe from the clean area toward the less clean area. Use a new swab or pad for each downward stroke.

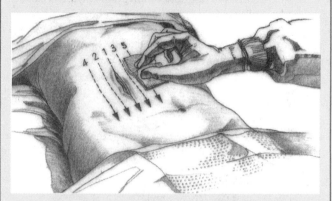

For an open wound, moisten a gauze pad with the cleaning agent and squeeze out excess solution. Clean the wound in full or half circles beginning in the center and working toward the outside. Clean to at least 1″ (2.5 cm) beyond the end of the new dressing or 2″ (5 cm) beyond the wound margins if you aren't applying a dressing. Use a new pad for each circle.

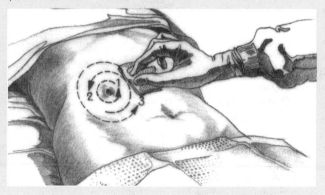

Packing

When packing a wound, use the following guidelines:

■ Carefully assess the size, depth, exudate or drainage, and configuration of the wound. These findings dictate the size and type of dressing to use.

■ Choose a dressing that is flexible enough to touch all the wound's surfaces.

■ Use solutions that provide a moist environment, are nontoxic to the body's cells, and do not interfere with healing.

■ Use synthetic or nonwoven gauze as the secondary dressing or to secure the primary dressing.

■ Don't pack the wound too tightly because it could inhibit the wound margins from contracting.

When packing is used for mechanical debridement, cotton mesh gauze has long been the common choice because it has large interstices that readily retain moisture and conform to the wound. Fluff the gauze before packing it into the wound. This exposes the maximum surface area of the gauze to the wound. (See *Packing a wound.*) However, many other topical wound management products have been indicated for wound packing and debriding based on wound size and exudate amount.

Applying a dressing

Before applying a dressing, take the following steps:

■ Check the wound care order.

■ Gather the supplies needed.

■ Check the patient's identification bracelet.

■ Explain the procedure to the patient.

■ Provide privacy for the patient.

■ Wash your hands and put on gloves.

To apply a new dressing, follow these guidelines:

■ Gently place the dressing at the wound center, extending it at least 1″ (2.5 cm) beyond the wound in each direction if the dressing is a pad. If the wound tunnels, loosely pack the tunneling area first, then fill the base of the wound.

■ The products chosen for topical wound management depend upon such wound characteristics as exudate or drainage amount. Select moisture-retentive dressings for wounds with light to moderate drainage. Choose absorbent dressings for wounds with moderate or heavier drainage.

Packing a wound

Loosely pack the wound cavity carefully with fluffed, moist sterile gauze pads. Make sure that all wound surfaces are covered and kept moist so that complete debridement can take place and granulation tissue can maintain hydration.

Loosely pack the wound only until wound surfaces and edges are covered. Packing that overlaps the edge can cause maceration of surrounding tissues.

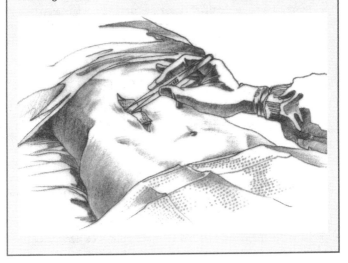

- When the dressing is in place, remove and discard your gloves to prevent the tape from sticking to them.
- Secure the edges of the dressing to the patient's skin with strips of tape. Or secure the dressing with a tie, such as Montgomery straps; a bandage, such as an elastic bandage or stockinette; a binder such as a T-binder; or a sling.
- Make sure the patient is comfortable.
- Clean or dispose of soiled equipment according to facility policy.

Drainage management
If a wound drains less than 1½ oz (50 ml) a day, use gauze dressings that are manufactured specifically to absorb drainage

and exudate. To protect the skin around a draining wound from maceration and breakdown, use skin sealants, petroleum-based products, or other water-resistant products. Estimate drainage (if unmeasurable) by counting the number of dressings saturated during each shift. Note the color, consistency, and odor of the exudate. Be sensitive to the patient's comfort level and provide emotional support, if needed.

Pouching

If a wound drains more than 1½ oz per day, apply a pouch to collect the excess drainage. Wound pouching provides accurate measurement of drainage, eliminates the need for frequent dressing changes, limits the spread of contamination, and improves the patient's comfort. If fitted and applied correctly, the pouch also protects the skin around the wound against breakdown. (See *Wound-pouching procedure.*)

Support surface therapy

Support surfaces (or tissue load management surfaces) are a major therapeutic means to manage pressure, friction, and shear on tissues. In addition, many support surfaces control moisture and inhibit bacterial growth. They're available in various sizes and shapes for use on beds, chairs, examination tables, and operating room tables. Used with proper topical wound care, turning, and repositioning, the correct support surface enhances healing of pressure ulcers and helps prevent new ones.

Types of support surfaces

Support surfaces can be divided into two categories: pressure-reducing devices and pressure-relieving devices. A pressure-reducing device for the trochanter or hip lowers pressure below that exerted by a standard hospital mattress or chair surface. A pressure-relieving device relieves pressure at the trochanter or hip below capillary closing pressure (26 to 32 mm Hg). Supportive devices for the heel or special positioning may be needed to eliminate pressure directly on the heel.

Wound-pouching procedure

To pouch a wound, follow the steps listed below.
- Always choose a pouch with an opening that is ⅛″ (0.3 cm) larger than the wound size.
- Note the condition of the skin around the wound. Apply a skin protectant as needed. Certain pouches have skin protectants incorporated in their barrier matrix.
- Check the drainage port at the bottom of the pouch to ensure closure.
- Put on gloves and gently apply the contoured pouch opening around the wound site. Begin at the lower edge of the pouch for adherence so that any drainage expressed can be contained.
- To empty the pouch, put on gloves and empty the contents into an appropriate container; note color, consistency, odor, and amount of fluid. Remember to follow isolation precautions when handling infectious drainage.

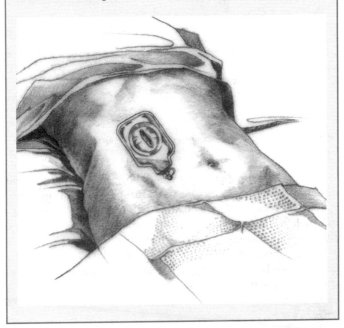

Selected characteristics for classes of support surfaces

PERFORMANCE CHARACTERISTICS	SUPPORT DEVICES	
	Air-fluidized bed	Low-air-loss bed
Increased support area	Yes	Yes
Low moisture retention	Yes	Yes
Reduced heat accumulation	Yes	Yes
Shear reduction	Yes	Unknown
Pressure reduction	Yes	Yes
Dynamic mattress or overlay	Yes	Yes
Cost per day	High	High

Support surfaces can be dynamic, with alternating inflation and deflation, or static, with the pressure load spread over a large area.

Static devices maintain constant inflation by use of materials that mold to the body surface, such as foam, gel, and water. (See *Selected characteristics for classes of support surfaces*.)

Each support surface must be carefully chosen, based on the patient's needs. (See *Managing tissue loads,* page 30.) The most common support surfaces are:

| | SUPPORT DEVICES | | |
Alternating air mattress	Static flotation (air or water) mattress	Foam overlay	Standard mattress
Yes	Yes	Yes	No
No	No	No	No
No	No	No	No
Yes	Yes	No	No
Yes	Yes	Yes	No
Yes	No	No	No
Moderate	Low	Low	Low

Source: Bergstrom, N., et al. Pressure Ulcer Treatment, Clinical Practice Guideline No. 15, AHCPR Publication No. 95-0652. Rockville, Md.: U.S. Department of Health and Human Services, Public Health Service, Agency for Health Care Policy and Research, December 1994.

- seating devices
- static air-filled overlays
- alternating air-filled mattress overlays
- gel- or water-filled mattress overlays
- replacement mattresses
- low-air-loss replacement mattresses
- low-air-loss specialty beds
- air-fluidized specialty beds. (See *Tissue load management surfaces*, pages 31 to 36.)

Managing tissue loads

A patient with one or more pressure ulcers may need one of several types of support surfaces and interventions to promote healing. This flow-chart shows which ones to choose, based on his condition.

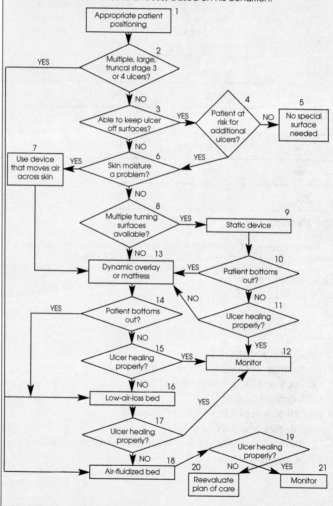

Source: Bergstrom, N., et al. *Pressure Ulcer Treatment*, Clinical Practice Guideline No. 15, AHCPR Publication No. 95-0652. Rockville, MD.: U.S. Department of Health and Human Services, Public Health Service, Agency for Health Care Policy and Research, December 1994.

Tissue load management surfaces

DESCRIPTION	**CONSIDERATIONS**

Beds

Air-fluidized bed

- Integrated system of support surface and frame
- Circulates air through silicone-like spheres to create a fluidlike state
- Also known as bead bed, sand bed, and high-air-loss bed
- Also helps control incontinence and large amounts of wound drainage and body fluids

- Not recommended for mobile patients, patients with pulmonary disease, or patients with unstable spine
- Continuous circulation of warm, dry air may dehydrate patient or desiccate wound bed
- Head of bed cannot be raised
- Weight of product needs to be taken into consideration when placed at a site of service
- Sharp objects may damage product
- Proper inflation necessary for optimal effectiveness

Low-air-loss bed

- Integrated support surface and bed frame
- Distributes the patient's body weight evenly over a sequence of pillows inflated with air by a motor
- Interconnected air cells have a minimum depth of 5" (12.5 cm)
- Low-air-loss therapy provides a generous amount of dry air flow between the patient and the surface, which controls moisture and heat buildup and prevents maceration and friction
- System has a dedicated power supply unit

- Slippery surface; patient may slide down or out of bed during transfers
- Motor may be noisy
- Sharp objects may damage product
- Proper inflation necessary for optimal effectiveness

Low-air-loss bed with adjuvant features

- Combines other therapies, such as pulsation, percussion, and kinetic therapy, with low-air-loss bed
- Distributes patient's body weight evenly over a sequence of pillows inflated with air by a motor

- Not recommended for patients who have cervical or skeletal traction
- Slippery surface; patient may slide down or out of bed during transfers

(continued)

Tissue load management surfaces *(continued)*

DESCRIPTION

CONSIDERATIONS

Low-air-loss bed with adjuvant features *(continued)*

- Integrated support surface and bed frame
- Interconnected air cells have a minimum depth of 5″
- Low-air-loss therapy provides a generous amount of dry air flow between the patient and the surface, which controls moisture and heat buildup and prevents maceration and friction
- System has a dedicated power supply unit

- Motor may be noisy
- Sharp objects may damage product
- Proper inflation necessary for optimal effectiveness

Mattress overlays

Air

- Dynamic overlays use alternating inflation and deflation to prevent constant pressure against skin and enhance blood flow
- Interconnected cells inflated with a pump
- Recommended cell depth not less than 3″ (7.5 cm)
- Cells with larger diameter and depth produce greater pressure relief over the body

- Assembly required
- Sensation of inflation and deflation may bother patient
- Electricity required
- Sharp objects may damage product
- Slippery surface; patient may slide down or out of bed during transfers
- Proper inflation necessary for optimal effectiveness

Foam

- For contoured foam, base height and height from bottom of foam to start of contour shouldn't be less than 2″ (5 cm) overall height shouldn't be less than 3½″ (8.8 cm)
- Foam density should range from 1.35 to 1.8 lb/ft³
- 25% indentation load deflection should be about 30 lb

- Types of foam vary considerably
- Effectiveness of foam needs monitoring
- Plastic protective sheet is usually necessary for incontinent patients
- Foam may trap perspiration and be hot
- Cleaning may remove flame-retardant coating

Tissue load management surfaces *(continued)*

DESCRIPTION	**CONSIDERATIONS**

Gel

- Provides flotation with pressure reduction
- May be manufactured in combination with foam
- Recommended depth not less than 2"

- Product is heavy and relatively expensive
- Research to prove effectiveness limited
- Sharp objects may damage product
- Some surfaces may be slippery; patient may slide down or out of bed during transfers
- Proper inflation necessary for optimal effectiveness

Water

- Provides lower interface pressures than standard hospital mattresses
- Recommended depth not less than 3"

- Water heater required to maintain comfortable temperature
- Fluid motions can make procedures and patient transfers difficult
- Precautions needed to prevent microorganism growth
- Product is heavy
- Sharp objects may damage product

Mattress replacements

Air

- Reduces interface pressures and replaces the standard hospital mattress
- May be manufactured in combination with other materials, such as foam
- May have removable shapes within the mattress
- Recommended height not less than 5"
- Waterproof cover should be applied to reduce shear and friction
- 2-year warranty recommended

- Moisture not always controlled
- Need for overlays reduced
- No therapeutic benefit when used with overlays
- Initial cost is high
- Low-maintenance product that's easy to clean
- Sharp objects may damage product
- Slippery surface; patient may slide down or out of bed during transfers
- Proper inflation necessary for optimal effectiveness

(continued)

Tissue load management surfaces *(continued)*

DESCRIPTION	CONSIDERATIONS

Foam

- Reduces interface pressures and replaces the standard hospital mattress
- May be manufactured in combination with other materials, such as gel
- May have removable shapes within the mattress
- For contoured foam, base height and height from bottom of foam to start of contour shouldn't be less than 2"; overall height shouldn't be less than $3\frac{1}{2}$"
- Foam density should range from 1.35 to 1.8 lb/ft^3
- 25% indentation load deflection should be about 30 lb
- Waterproof cover that reduces friction and shear is recommended.

- Moisture not always controlled
- Need for overlays reduced
- No therapeutic benefit when used with overlays
- Initial cost is high
- Low-maintenance product that's easy to clean

Gel

- Reduces interface pressures and replaces the standard hospital mattress
- May be manufactured in combination with other materials, such as foam
- May have removable shapes within the mattress
- Recommended height not less than 5"
- Waterproof cover should be applied to reduce shear and friction
- 2-year warranty is recommended

- Product is heavy
- Moisture not always controlled
- Need for overlays reduced
- No therapeutic benefit when used with overlays
- Initial cost is high
- Low-maintenance product that's easy to clean
- Sharp objects may damage product
- Some surfaces may be slippery; patient may slide down or out of bed during transfers

Water

- Reduces interface pressures and replaces the standard hospital mattress
- May be manufactured in combination with other materials, such as gel

- Moisture is not always controlled
- Reduces the need for overlays
- No therapeutic benefit when used with overlays
- Initial cost is high

Tissue load management surfaces *(continued)*

DESCRIPTION	CONSIDERATIONS

Water *(continued)*

- May have removable shapes within the mattress
- Recommended height not less than 5″
- Waterproof cover should be applied to reduce shear and friction
- 2-year warranty recommended

- Low maintenance and easy to clean
- Sharp objects may damage product

Enhanced overlays and mattresses

Alternating-pressure mattress

- Recommended depth not less than 5″
- Configuration of the system's chambers allows for cyclical changes in pressures in different chambers, creating a low- and high-pressure area
- Fabric covering generally air-permeable, bacteria-impermeable, and waterproof; cover should also reduce friction and shear

- Sensation of inflation and deflation may bother patient
- Motor may be noisy
- Moisture buildup may occur
- Sharp objects may damage product
- Slippery surface; patient may slide down or out of bed during transfers
- Proper inflation necessary for optimal effectiveness

Low-air-loss overlay

- Overlay connected to system of air cells with a minimum cell depth of 3″
- System allows for air to escape from the surface
- Fabric covering generally air-permeable, bacteria-impermeable, and waterproof; cover should also reduce friction and shear

- Motor may be noisy
- Sharp objects may damage product
- Some surfaces may be slippery; patient may slide down or out of bed during transfers
- Moisture buildup controlled
- Proper inflation necessary for optimal effectiveness

Nonpowered adjustable zone overlay

- Must have at least three independent adjustable zones
- Manifold system should provide constant force equalization within each section
- Cover material should have a low coefficient of friction

- Motor may be noisy
- Sharp objects may damage product
- Some surfaces may be slippery; patient may slide down or out of bed during transfers
- Proper inflation necessary for optimal effectiveness

(continued)

Tissue load management surfaces *(continued)*

DESCRIPTION	CONSIDERATIONS
Low-air-loss mattress ■ Interconnected air cells with a minimum depth of at least 5" ■ System allows air to escape from the surface ■ Dedicated power supply unit integrated into the system	■ Motor may be noisy ■ Sharp objects may damage product ■ Some surfaces may be slippery; patient may slide down or out of bed during transfers ■ Not recommended for patients who have cervical or skeletal traction ■ Proper inflation necessary for optimal effectiveness
Low-air-loss mattress with adjuvant therapies ■ Interconnected air cells with a minimum depth of at least 5" ■ System allows for air to escape from the surface ■ System has a dedicated power supply unit ■ System may provide other therapies, such as pulsation, percussion, and kinetic therapy	■ Not recommended for patients who have cervical or skeletal traction ■ Slippery surface: patient may slide down or out of bed during transfers ■ Motor may be noisy ■ Sharp objects may damage product ■ Proper inflation needed for optimal effectiveness
Seating devices ■ Cushions or other seating surfaces used for patients at risk for skin breakdown ■ Generally used in conjunction with a pressure-reducing or pressure-relieving device for the bed ■ May be static or dynamic and constructed of air, fluid, foam, or gel ■ May be powered or nonpowered	■ Each patient must be evaluated for correct product based on his needs ■ Products should be reevaluated routinely for effectiveness

2

Nutrition assessment and therapy

Nutrition has long been identified as one of the critical factors in wound healing. Providing nutrition therapy for wound healing includes a complete nutrition assessment, design of an individualized treatment plan, and periodic monitoring to evaluate the effectiveness of the treatment plan.

Assessment

A complete nutritional assessment includes body measurements, evaluation of laboratory test results, physical examination, and dietary interview. Based on the information collected in these four areas, the clinician can then determine a patient's nutrient needs, evaluate the adequacy and appropriateness of the current diet, and recommend changes.

BODY MEASUREMENTS

Anthropometric data collection is the measurement of a patient's body over time with comparisons to standards. In a wound-care clinic, hospital, or skilled nursing setting, anthropometric data collection typically is limited to the measurement of height and weight. To ensure accuracy, stature must be measured rather than self-reported by the patient.

If standing height can't be measured, knee height calipers may be used. These calipers measure the length of the lower leg from the bottom of the foot to the top of the patella. A mathematical formula converts the knee height to stature.

Current weight must be obtained using a scale that is calibrated often and treated gently to assure reliable readings.

Additional anthropometric measurements — triceps skin-fold measurement, midarm circumference, and midarm muscle circumference — have limited usefulness in most wound-care settings.

LABORATORY TEST RESULTS

Laboratory tests help evaluate the patient's nutrition and hydration status. A complete nutritional assessment includes an evaluation of both a standard multiple analysis and a complete blood count as well as protein stores, electrolyte and fluid balance, renal function, liver function, glucose levels, anemias, and immune status. It may also include other specific nutritional laboratory values, such as prealbumin, folic acid, B-12, ferritin, transferrin, and lymphocyte count. The accompanying table indicates the levels of mild, moderate, and severe depletion for common protein status lab values. (See *Markers of malnutrition*.) Many laboratory assays, such as albumin, are affected by hydration status. Repeating laboratory tests after a patient has been rehydrated is important.

Careful interpretation of laboratory data is imperative, as is evaluating current data, to provide the best information on the patient's condition. If lab data are several months old, they won't accurately reflect the situation today. If possible, new labs should be drawn to base the treatment on the most up-to-date condition of the patient.

PHYSICAL EXAMINATION

The physical examination provides evidence of deficiencies and signs of malnutrition. It also provides insight into the patient's functional status, including the ability to self-feed. The areas to examine and the clinical signs to look for include:

- *hair* — dry, sparse, brittle, or easily plucked
- *skin* — turgor, bruises, tears, pressure ulcers, or other skin integrity problems or xerosis
- *lips* — cheilosis or angular fissures
- *gums* — swelling or bleeding
- *teeth* — condition of natural teeth or denture fit and acceptance
- *tongue* — glossitis, pallor, atrophy, or sores
- *nails* — brittle or spoon nails
- *mucous membranes* — dry

Markers of malnutrition

Marker	Normal value	Mild depletion	Moderate depletion	Severe depletion
Percent of usual body weight	100%	85 to 95	75 to 84	<75
Albumin, g/dL	≥3.5	2.8 to 3.4	2.1 to 2.7	<2.1
Prealbumin, mg/dL	16 to 30	10 to 15	5 to 9	<5
Transferrin, mg/dL	>200	150 to 200	100 to 149	<100
Total lymphocyte count, mm³	2500	<1500	<1200	<800

Adapted with permission from Whitney, E.N.; Cataldo, C.B.; and Rolfes, S.R. Understanding Normal and Clinical Nutrition, 5th ed. Belmont, CA: West/Wadsworth, 1998.

- *hands*—arthritis and inability to open food containers
- *vision*—inability to see food on plate
- *mental status*—inability to communicate food preferences and understand diet instruction
- *height* and *weight*—visual confirmation of anthropometric data obtained
- *motor skills*—extent of hand-to-mouth coordination and any inability to hold utensils and self-feed.

DIETARY INTERVIEW

A thorough dietary history can provide important details that the clinician must take into account when writing the plan of care, and the patient interview is crucial to obtaining a dietary history. The extent of this history depends on the type of clinical setting.

A basic history may include a food frequency list or a three-day diet recall. Understanding the patient's usual eating pattern and the typical food consumed on a daily basis is important. The clinician should ask the patient about favorite foods, disliked foods, cultural preferences, food allergies, lactose intolerance, and other similar questions. They should also discuss digestive process concerns, such as problems with nausea, constipation, diarrhea, vomiting, chewing problems, swallowing trouble, and any flavor or taste changes.

In outpatient and clinical settings, obtaining additional details about grocery shopping and food preparation is important. Isolation and lack of socialization often result in poor intake and may lead to nutritional deficiencies. Any changes in the patient's weight, as well as a history of the weight change, should be examined to provide information about the patient's normal and usual weight. Interview family members if the patient is unable to provide a history due to illness or mental deficiency.

Evaluation

After completing the data collection, the clinician can make an evaluation of the patient's nutritional status and needs. The four components of the nutrition assessment (body measurements, laboratory test results, physical examination, and dietary interview) provide sufficient information on which to base clinical judgments.

WEIGHT TRENDS
The anthropometric height and weight data should be used for additional calculations to determine if malnutrition or a nutritional deficiency exists. Body mass index (BMI) is a helpful indicator of underweight and obesity, both of which may impede wound healing. BMI, an index of a patient's weight in relation to height, is calculated by the following formula: weight in kilograms divided by the square of the height in meters. BMI results less than 19 and greater than 25 require further investigation. (See *Body mass index*, Appendix A.)

Another calculation, the patient's "percent of usual body weight," indicates whether patients have deviated from their customary weight. To make this calculation, use the following formula: current weight divided by usual weight × 100. Patients who weigh less than 90% of their usual body weight require nutritional intervention to halt any further involuntary weight loss.

CALCULATING NUTRIENT NEEDS
Calculating the patient's nutrient needs for calories, protein, and fluids helps determine whether daily intake is meeting those needs. To calculate caloric needs, use the Harris-Benedict equation to predict basal energy expenditure (BEE):

$$\text{Females: } 655 + 9.56 \text{ W} + 1.85 \text{ H} - 4.68 \text{ A}$$
$$\text{Males: } 66.5 + 13.75 \text{ W} + 5.0 \text{ H} - 6.78 \text{ A}$$

(W = weight in kilograms; H = height in centimeters; A = age in years)

After calculating the BEE, you'll need to modify it for level of activity and extent of illness and injury. Activity factors add 20% to 30% to the BEE for most patients. Injury factors can add an additional 50% or more. Clinical judgment must be used to best estimate the patient's daily total energy expenditure (TEE); many different systems exist for arriving at this estimate. For example, a 75-year-old woman weighing 108 lb and standing 5′ tall has a BEE of 1,055 calories per day (655 + 469 + 282 − 351). If she is confined to bed, an activity factor of 1.2 is added. If she has a stage 3 wound, an additional injury factor of 1.3 is added. The resulting TEE is 1055 × 1.2 × 1.3 = 1,646 calories per day. If this patient has a history of losing weight or shows signs of malnutrition, an additional injury factor is added. Some health care professionals simply add 250 calories per day to the TEE for weight gain of about one-half pound per week.

An alternate system to the Harris-Benedict formula is calculating needs based on calories per kilogram of body weight. The accompanying table outlines guidelines for calculating calories, protein, and fluid needs based on this system. (See *Nutrient needs based on body weight*, page 42.)

Treatment plan

After completing the data collection and evaluation, the clinician can begin to formulate the treatment plan, starting with the least invasive and least costly interventions and progressing to more invasive and higher-cost interventions as needed. The accompanying treatment algorithm demonstrates how interventions should advance in a logical fashion. (See *Nutrition screening and assessment*, page 43.)

DIET

Typically in most health care settings, the patient will have a prescribed diet. The clinician must ensure that the diet meets the patient's estimated caloric, protein, and fluid needs. For example, if a patient doesn't drink milk, the diet plan must meet calcium and vitamin D needs through other means, such as yogurt, cheese, or

Nutrient needs based on body weight	
Nutrient	**Requirements**
Calories	
Normal	25 to 30 kcal/kg/d
Protein-calorie malnutrition (PCM)*	30 to 35 kcal/kg/d
Critically ill or injured*	35 to 40 kcal/kg/d
Protein	
Recommended daily allowance (RDA)	0.8 g/kg/day
PCM	1.5 g/kg/day
Critically ill or injured*	1.5 to 2.0 g/kg/day
Fat	< 30% kcal
Water	30 cc/kg body weight or 1 L/1000 kcal

*Nutrient supplementation required

supplements. The diet must also be appropriate for the patient. Appropriateness includes the proper texture in relation to the patient's dental status, the accurate therapeutic diet for disease states such as diabetes, and whether the diet is acceptable to the patient.

The chief dietary treatment goal for wound healing is to provide adequate calories and protein to promote anabolism and the building of new tissue. The very best local and nursing care will not heal wounds without the existence of sufficient nutritional substrate from which to build new tissue. However, after the food has been served, the patient must consume it to receive any benefit. Proper environment, socialization, verbal cues, praise for good intake, proper positioning, culturally appropriate meals, therapeutic silverware, and patient and family education are some of the steps that can help assure adequate mealtime intake.

SUPPLEMENTAL NUTRITION
Often, elderly and infirm patients dislike eating large meals and prefer smaller meals and snacks spaced throughout the day. Many high-calorie and high-protein beverages, cookies, bars, yogurts, and ice creams are available to supplement meals. The key to us-

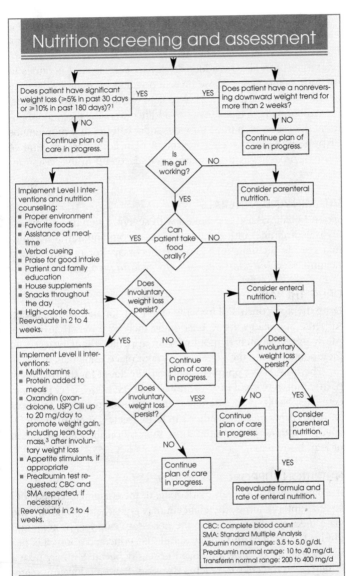

Nutrition screening and assessment

Does patient have significant weight loss (≥5% in past 30 days or ≥10% in past 180 days)?[1] — YES — YES — Does patient have a nonreversing downward weight trend for more than 2 weeks?

NO → Continue plan of care in progress.

NO → Continue plan of care in progress.

Is the gut working? — NO → Consider parenteral nutrition.

YES ↓

Implement Level I interventions and nutrition counseling:
- Proper environment
- Favorite foods
- Assistance at mealtime
- Verbal cueing
- Praise for good intake
- Patient and family education
- House supplements
- Snacks throughout the day
- High-calorie foods.

Reevaluate in 2 to 4 weeks.

Can patient take food orally? — YES / NO → Consider enteral nutrition.

Does involuntary weight loss persist? — YES / NO → Continue plan of care in progress.

Does involuntary weight loss persist? — NO → Continue plan of care in progress. / YES → Consider parenteral nutrition.

Implement Level II interventions:
- Multivitamins
- Protein added to meals
- Oxandrin (oxandrolone, USP) CIII up to 20 mg/day to promote weight gain, including lean body mass,[3] after involuntary weight loss
- Appetite stimulants, if appropriate
- Prealbumin test requested; CBC and SMA repeated, if necessary.

Reevaluate in 2 to 4 weeks.

Does involuntary weight loss persist? — YES[2] / NO → Continue plan of care in progress.

YES → Reevaluate formula and rate of enteral nutrition.

CBC: Complete blood count
SMA: Standard Multiple Analysis
Albumin normal range: 3.5 to 5.0 g/dL
Prealbumin normal range: 10 to 40 mg/dL
Transferrin normal range: 200 to 400 mg/d

1. American Health Care Association, Resident Assessment Instrument for Long Term Care Facilities. Version 2.0.
2. Strawford, A, et al. "Resistance exercise and supraphysiologic androgen therapy in eugonadal men with HIV-related weight loss: A randomized controlled trial." JAMA, 281:1282-90, 1999.
3. If, at any time, patient can't receive adequate nutrient intake, reevaluate gut function and consider nutritional support.

Adapted with permission from BTG Pharmaceuticals, Iselin, N.J. (2001).

ing these supplemental products is to avoid texture and flavor fatigue by offering a variety. Very few patients will readily accept the same product week after week.

Protein can also be added to drinks, cereals, and potatoes in the form of a powder. These protein powders do not vary the taste or texture of foods and are a convenient way to meet protein needs.

Additionally, recipes may be modified to make them more nutrient dense, so each meal provides more calories and more grams of protein. A multifaceted treatment plan combining several of these approaches is usually the most successful in increasing intake.

VITAMIN AND MINERALS

Wound healing has been linked with several vitamins and minerals plus arginine and glutamine. The accompanying table summarizes the vitamins and minerals necessary for proper wound healing. (See *Nutrients necessary for wound healing*.)

DRUG THERAPY

Drug therapy consists of appetite stimulants or an anabolic agent. Appetite stimulants act to encourage increased mealtime intake. Allow approximately 1 month for an appetite stimulant to reach therapeutic levels; the effects don't take place immediately.

The only FDA-approved oral anabolic agent for the treatment of involuntary weight loss, oxandrolone (Oxandrin; BTG Pharmaceuticals, Iselin, N.J.), attenuates the catabolic response to stress and stimulates protein synthesis in body tissues. Such an agent facilitates optimal protein utilization, thereby promoting restoration of lean body mass.

NUTRITION SUPPORT

If a patient's oral intake is inadequate to meet estimated needs despite all interventions, the clinician may consider enteral nutrition via a feeding tube to provide the necessary calories, protein, and fluids. The patient and family should be educated about this option before it becomes a medical necessity because it may take a family several weeks to reach a decision. Patient education materials explaining how tube feeding is performed may be useful, and all education and discussion sessions should be documented in the medical record.

Nutrients necessary for wound healing

NUTRIENT	FUNCTION	RESULTS OF DEFICIENCY
Proteins	■ Wound repair ■ Clotting factor production ■ White blood cell (WBC) production and migration ■ Cell-mediated phagocytosis ■ Fibroblast proliferation ■ Neovascularization ■ Collagen synthesis ■ Epithelial cell proliferation ■ Wound remodeling	■ Poor wound healing ■ Hypoalbuminemia and generalized edema, which slows oxygen diffusion and metabolic transport mechanisms from the capillaries and cell membranes ■ Lymphopenia ■ Impaired cellular immunity
Carbohydrates	■ Supply cellular energy ■ Spare protein	■ Body uses visceral and muscle proteins for energy
Fats	■ Supply cellular energy ■ Supply essential fatty acids ■ Cell membrane structure ■ Prostaglandin production	■ Inhibited tissue repair ■ Use of visceral and muscle proteins for energy
Vitamin A	■ Collagen synthesis ■ Epithelialization	■ Poor wound healing ■ Impaired immunity
Vitamin C	■ Membrane integrity ■ Antioxidant	■ Impaired immunity ■ Poor wound healing ■ Capillary fragility
Vitamin K	■ Normal blood clotting	■ Increased risk of hemorrhage and hematoma formation

(continued)

Nutrients necessary for wound healing (continued)

NUTRIENT	FUNCTION	RESULTS OF DEFICIENCY
Iron	• Collagen synthesis • Enhances leukocytic bacterial activity • Hemoglobin synthesis	• Anemia, leading to increased risk of local tissue ischemia • Impaired tensile strength
Zinc	• Cell proliferation • Cofactor for enzymes • Vitamin A utilization	• Impaired collagen cross-linkage • Slow healing • Alteration in taste • Anorexia • Impaired immunity
Copper	• Collagen cross-linkage • RBC synthesis	• Decreased collagen synthesis • Anemia
Pyridoxine, riboflavin, and thiamine	• Energy production • Cellular immunity • Red blood cell (RBC) synthesis	• Decreased resistance to infection • Impaired wound healing
Arginine	• Increases local wound immune system • Nitrogen-rich (32% nitrogen, whereas the average amino acid is 16% nitrogen) • Precursor to proline, which is converted to hydroxyproline and then to collagen	• Decreased local wound immune system
Glutamine	• Primary fuel for fibroblasts • Preservation of lean body mass	• Less fuel for fibroblasts

3

Pressure ulcers

Localized sites of cell death, pressure ulcers occur most commonly in areas of compromised circulation secondary to pressure. They may be superficial, caused by local skin irritation with subsequent surface maceration, or deep, originating in underlying tissue. Deep ulcers may go undetected until they penetrate the skin.

Cause

Most pressure ulcers develop when soft tissue is compressed between a bony prominence (such as the sacrum) and an external surface (such as a mattress or the seat of a chair) for a prolonged period. (See *Common pressure ulcer sites*, pages 48 and 49.) Pressure — applied with great force for a short period or with less force over a longer period — disrupts blood supply to the capillary network, impeding blood flow to the surrounding tissues and depriving tissues of oxygen and nutrients. This leads to local ischemia, hypoxia, edema, inflammation and, ultimately, cell death. The result is a pressure ulcer, also known as a bedsore, decubitus ulcer, or pressure sore.

Shear, which separates the skin from underlying tissues, and friction, which abrades the top layer of skin, also contribute to pressure ulcer development. Contributing systemic factors include infection, malnutrition, edema, obesity, emaciation, multisystem trauma, and certain circulatory and endocrine disorders.

Common pressure ulcer sites

These figures show the anatomic locations that are susceptible to pressure ulcer formation.

Lateral position

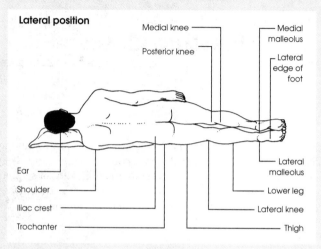

Prone position

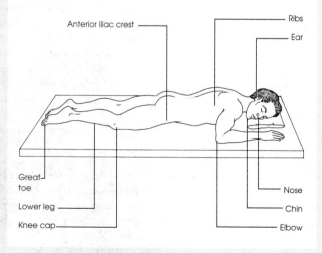

Common pressure ulcer sites *(continued)*

Posterior position

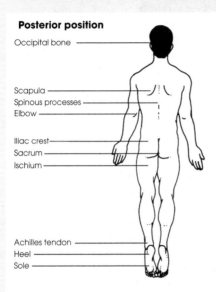

- Occipital bone
- Scapula
- Spinous processes
- Elbow
- Iliac crest
- Sacrum
- Ischium
- Achilles tendon
- Heel
- Sole

Sitting position

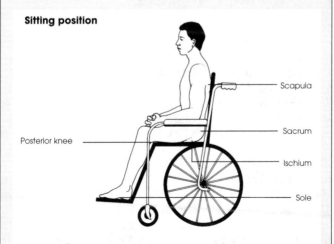

- Scapula
- Sacrum
- Ischium
- Sole
- Posterior knee

Assessment

An early sign that an ulcer may be forming over a bony prominence is blanching erythema, verified by finger compression. The condition may resolve without tissue loss if pressure is reduced or eliminated. Nonblanchable erythema, a more serious sign, suggests that tissue destruction is imminent or has occurred. The skin may appear bright red to dark red or purple. If deep tissue damage is also present, the area may be indurated or boggy when palpated. Wound management effectiveness and duration depend on wound severity.

Prevention

Pressure ulcers are most likely to develop in patients who have sustained pressure over bony prominences. Patients who spend most or all of their time in a bed or alternative seating device (such as a wheelchair) without shifting their body weight properly are at great risk. Risks increase with various cofactors, such as partial or total paralysis and malnutrition. (See *Patients at risk for pressure ulcers.*) To prevent pressure ulcers and achieve positive outcomes, a multidisciplinary team must design and implement a comprehensive program. Members of this team may include the following specialists:
- primary care provider, such as a physician
- wound care specialist, such as a wound, ostomy, or continence nurse
- physical therapist, occupational therapist, speech therapist
- registered dietitian.

A pressure ulcer prevention program provides guidelines to identify patients at risk and minimize risk factors. From these guidelines, standards of care can be established.

IDENTIFYING PATIENTS AT RISK

Rating scales are the most common risk assessment tools used by clinicians to identify potential pressure ulcer risk for each patient. These risk assessment tools include the Norton, Braden, Gosnell, and Waterlow scales, with the Braden scale being the most widely used. (See *Norton scale,* page 52. See also *Braden scale,* Appendix B.) Each scale has different number and patient parameters, which clinicians use to identify the factors most closely associated with

Patients at risk for pressure ulcers

At greatest risk for pressure ulcers are patients compromised by the following conditions:
- chronic illness that requires bed rest
- dehydration
- diabetes mellitus
- diminished pain awareness
- fractures
- history of corticosteroid therapy
- immunosuppression
- incontinence
- malnutrition
- mental impairment, possibly related to coma, altered level of consciousness, sedation, or confusion
- multisystem trauma
- paralysis
- poor circulation
- previous pressure ulcers
- significant obesity or thinness.

pressure ulcer formation. Some of the common parameters for these scales are:
- general physical condition
- mental status
- activity
- mobility
- incontinence
- nutritional status.

The numerical "cutscore," which signals the onset of risk for pressure ulcer formation, is unique to each scale.

CLINICAL GUIDELINES

As an aid to risk assessment and management, the Agency for Health Care Research and Quality (formerly the Agency for Health Care Policy and Research), a branch of the U.S. Department of Health and Human Services, published two booklets for health care professionals: *Pressure Ulcers in Adults: Prediction and Prevention* and *Treatment of Pressure Ulcers*. The agency also publishes handbooks in English and Spanish for patients titled *Preventing Pressure Ulcers: A Patient's Guide* and *Treating Pressure Sores*.

Norton scale

Assess the following five conditions and assign appropriate scores. A total score of 14 or less indicates risk of pressure ulcer. A score under 12 indicates high risk.

Name _____ Date _____

PHYSICAL CONDITION		MENTAL CONDITION		ACTIVITY		MOBILITY		CONTINENCE	
Good	4	Alert	4	Walks	4	Full	4	Good	4
Fair	3	Apathetic	3	Walks		Slightly		Occasional	
Poor	2	Confused	2	with help	3	limited	3	incontinence	3
Very poor	1	Stuporous	1	Sits in		Very		Frequent	
				chair	2	limited	2	incontinence	2
				Remains in		Immobile	1	Urine and	
				bed	1			fecal	
								incontinence	1
TOTAL		**TOTAL**		**TOTAL**		**TOTAL**		**TOTAL**	

TOTAL SCORE _____

Treatment

Successful pressure ulcer management requires a comprehensive approach that includes prevention, relieving pressure, restoring circulation, managing the wound, and minimizing related disorders. To help clarify the ongoing assessment and care, follow an algorithm that clearly maps out a course of action. (See *Topical management algorithm for wound care,* pages 54 and 55.)

Ensuring adequate skin care, nourishment, and mobility (to relieve pressure and promote circulation) may help prevent pressure ulcers from occurring, possibly reverses a stage 1 pressure ulcer, and aids in the management of deeper pressure ulcers.

PREVENTION AND EARLY INTERVENTION

Customizing a prevention and early intervention program for an at-risk patient is a necessary component to the patient's plan of care. The components that comprise these steps as outlined by the Agency for Health Care Research and Quality include:

- identification of at-risk individuals who need preventive interventions and of the specific factors that place them at risk
- maintenance and improvement of tissue tolerance
- protection against the adverse effects of external mechanical forces, including pressure, shear and friction
- reduction of the incidence of pressure ulcers through educational programs.

SKIN CARE

Proper care is crucial to preventing further skin breakdown. To maintain and improve tissue tolerance to pressure, perform the following interventions:

- Systematically inspect the skin at least once a day, paying particular attention to the skin over bony prominences.
- Clean the skin at frequent intervals with warm water and a mild cleansing agent; then apply moisturizers and a barrier cream. During skin care, minimize the force applied to the skin. Avoid massaging bony prominences because this may damage capillaries.
- Minimize skin exposure to moisture caused by incontinence, perspiration, or wound drainage. If the patient is incontinent, clean the skin at the time of soiling. When sources of moisture cannot be controlled, use linen-saver pads or briefs made of materials that absorb moisture and present a quick-drying surface to the skin.
- Minimize environmental factors, such as low humidity (less than 40%) and exposure to cold, which may lead to dry skin.
- Use proper positioning, transferring, and turning techniques to minimize skin injury caused by friction and shear forces. To reduce friction injuries, use lubricants (such as cornstarch and creams), protective films (such as transparent films and skin sealants), protective dressings (such as hydrocolloids), and protective padding.

NUTRITION

A balanced diet that includes adequate protein and calories is essential to wound healing. Patients with pressure ulcers may need greater amounts of protein to help ensure a positive nitrogen balance and to replace protein lost through their ulcers. They may

Topical management algorithm for wound care

Use this chart to help you effectively assess, plan, intervene, and evaluate wounds. You'll need to exclude patients with diabetic or neurotrophic ulcers and those with stages 3 and 4 osteomyelitis, systemic infection, or venous stasis ulcers.

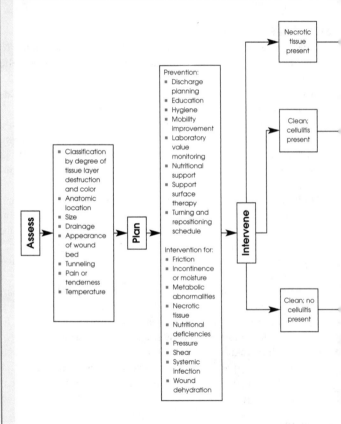

*Debridement performed according to practitioner's state practice, professional regulation standards, and competency validation

Hess, C.T., Clinical Wound Manager Manual Series for the Wound Care Department. © Wound Care Strategies, Inc., 2001.

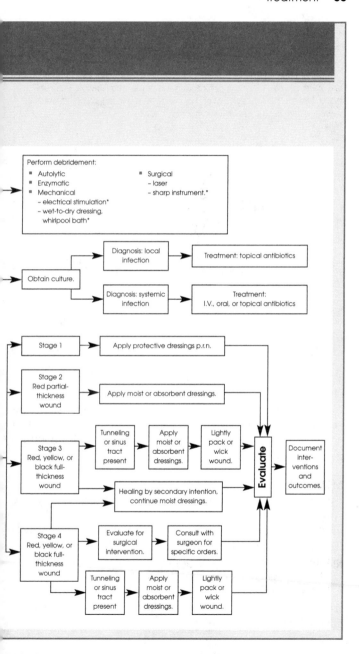

Turning and repositioning schedule

Turn and reposition the patient at least every 2 hours or as the plan of care dictates. Adjust the schedule to coincide comfortable positioning with the patient's activities. For instance, position him on his back when he eats. These two clocks show a sample schedule.

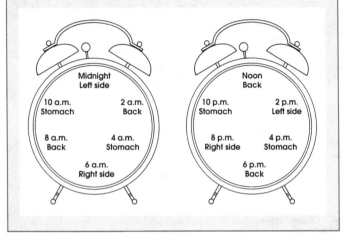

also need vitamin and trace element supplementation, especially of vitamin C and zinc. When a patient is unable or unwilling to eat, he may require enteral or parenteral feeding. Expect to individualize the nutritional support plan for each patient, consistent with the overall goals of therapy. (See Chapter 2, Nutrition assessment and therapy.)

MOBILITY

For most patients, maintaining current activity level, mobility, and range of motion is usually sufficient to prevent pressure ulcers or for their early treatment. If a patient has a mobility or an activity deficit, implement the interventions listed below to help protect him from the adverse effects of pressure, friction, and shear.

For the patient confined to bed:
- Systematically turn and reposition the patient at least every 2 hours, following a customized, written schedule. (See *Turning and repositioning schedule.*)

- Use pillows or foam wedges to keep bony prominences (such as knees and ankles) from direct contact with the mattress or skin-to-skin contact.
- For a completely immobile patient, use devices that relieve pressure on the heels.
- When using the side-lying position, avoid positioning the patient directly on the trochanter.
- Maintain the head of the bed at the lowest degree of elevation appropriate for the patient, and limit the amount of time it is elevated.
- During transfers and position changes, use lifting devices.
- Place the at-risk patient on a pressure-reducing device, such as a foam overlay.

   For the patient confined to a chair:

- Reposition the patient, shifting the points under pressure at least every hour.
- Have the patient shift body weight every 15 minutes, either independently or with assistance, following a customized, written schedule.
- Use a pressure-reducing device, such as a foam overlay, on the seating surface.
- When positioning the patient, consider pressure relief, postural alignment, and distribution of weight and balance.

CLASSIFICATION BY STAGES

Several classification systems identify pressure ulcers by stages. These staging systems identify wounds by the tissue layers involved. They don't describe a wound completely and are only an anatomic description of the wound's depth. The National Pressure Ulcer Advisory Panel (NPUAP) system for describing pressure ulcers is a combination of the most commonly used staging systems. It's also used to classify other wound types. (See *Staging pressure ulcers,* pages 58 and 59.)

STAGING AND DOCUMENTING PRESSURE ULCERS

When documenting the stages of pressure ulcers, the health care professional should be familiar with the vocabulary necessary for accurate description and measurement.

Staging pressure ulcers

The following staging system is consistent with the recommendations of the National Pressure Ulcer Advisory Panel (Consensus Conference, 1991).

Stage 1

A stage 1 pressure ulcer is an observable pressure-related alteration of intact skin whose indicators as compared to the adjacent or opposite area on the body may include changes in one or more of the following: skin temperature (warmth or coolness), tissue consistency (firm or boggy feel), and/or sensation (pain, itching). The ulcer presents as a defined area of persistent redness in lightly pigmented skin, whereas in darker tones, the ulcer may appear with persistent red, blue, or purple hues.

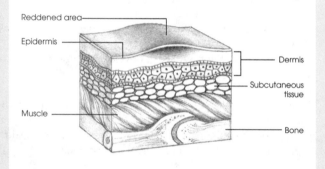

Stage 2

Partial-thickness skin loss involving the epidermis or dermis. The ulcer is superficial and presents clinically as an abrasion, blister, or shallow crater.

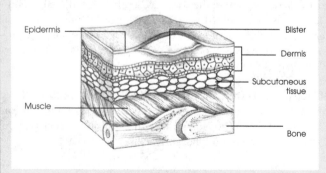

Staging pressure ulcers *(continued)*

Stage 3
Full-thickness skin loss involving damage or necrosis of subcutaneous tissue, which may extend down to, but not through, underlying fascia. The ulcer presents clinically as a deep crater with or without undermining of adjacent tissue.

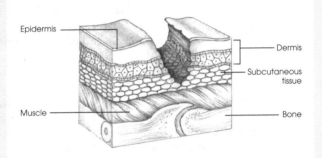

Stage 4
Full-thickness skin loss with extensive destruction, tissue necrosis, or damage to muscle, bone, or support structures (for example, tendon or joint capsule). Tunneling and sinus tracts may also be associated with stage 4 pressure ulcers.

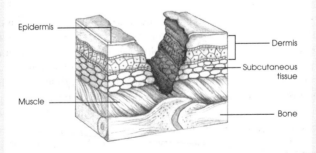

Stage 1

- Document and describe length and width only. No measurable depth exists because the epidermis is intact, although underlying tissue may be damaged. Assessment of stage 1 pressure ulcers may be difficult in patients with darker skin.

Stage 2

- Document and describe length, width, and depth. All stage 2 pressure ulcers have depth because the wound has penetrated through the epidermis. For superficial pressure ulcers, the depth may be documented as less than 0.1 cm. Any depth equal to or greater than 0.1 cm can be accurately measured with a measuring device.

Stage 3

- Document and describe length, width, and depth as well as tunneling, if present. When necrotic tissue is present, accurate staging of the pressure ulcer isn't possible until the slough or eschar has been debrided and the wound base is visible.

Stage 3

- Document and describe length, width, and depth as well as tunneling (if present) and underlying support structures (fascia, muscle, and bone). When necrotic tissue is present, accurate staging of the pressure ulcer isn't possible until the slough or eschar has been debrided and the wound base is visible.

Reverse staging

Staging is intended to describe the amount of tissue destroyed rather than the amount of tissue healed. Reverse staging rests on the misconception that a stage 4 ulcer becomes a stage 3 ulcer and then a stage 2 ulcer as it heals. However, original tissue that was destroyed by the wound (such as subcutaneous tissue, muscle, and bone) is instead replaced with granulation tissue and new epithelium. You can review the NPUAP position statements about reverse staging by visiting their Web site (www.npuap.org).

Because tools to measure pressure ulcer healing didn't exist until after 1900, and because it's essentially required for reimbursement (particularly in long-term care settings), some clinicians do reverse staging. A better way to describe wound healing includes use of tools such as the Pressure Sore Status Tool (PSST),

Pressure Ulcer Scale for Healing (PUSH), Sessing scale, or Sussman tool or documentation of the following:

■ dimensions of size (length and width)
■ dimensions of depth
■ dimensions of tunneling or undermining
■ tissue amount and type (eschar, slough, or granulation)
■ amount and qualitative description (color, thickness, and odor) of exudate.

Comparison with the depth of the wound and the depth at worst point, as documented on admission, allows an accurate evaluation of wound healing. Health care professionals should develop specific wound care policies and procedures based on standard guidelines, such as those of the Agency for Health Care Research and Quality; the Wound, Ostomy, Continence Nurses Society; or the NPUAP.

ADDITIONAL MANAGEMENT

All stages of pressure ulcers require topical wound care, and surgical intervention may be required for stages 3 and 4.

Topical wound care

Care varies with the management modalities used and the ulcer's stage. (See *Interventions in topical wound care*, page 62.)

Support surfaces

The interventions used to reduce pressure over bony prominences are vital to the success of the plan of care. (See Chapter 1, Fundamentals of wound healing.)

Surgical interventions

If infection develops or the patient is immunocompromised, immediate surgical debridement may be necessary. In stage 3 pressure ulcers, spontaneous closure may take months and may cause scar tissue that can predispose the patient to recurrent pressure ulcers. For these reasons, surgical excision and closure may be used to manage these ulcers. Stage 4 ulcers are handled similarly, but debridement may be more radical when a bony prominence is involved.

Tissue flaps are the most common procedure used for surgical management of pressure ulcers. They involve the transfer of skin and underlying structures to fill a defect. Tissue flaps are clas-

Interventions in topical wound care

The following interventions will help you to effectively manage a pressure ulcer.

- Determine the stage of the ulcer to ensure consistency of care and to help plan therapy.
- Withhold corticosteroids, if possible, for 4 to 5 days after the appearance of an ulcer because they can inhibit healing.
- Clean the wound with normal saline solution, an antiseptic solution, or another agent, as ordered.
- Apply topical antibiotics to areas of local infection, if prescribed.
- Debride necrotic tissue from the pressure ulcer using enzymatic, mechanical, autolytic, or sharp debridement methods.
- Cover the ulcer with dressings, such as gauzes, absorbent sponges, nonocclusive dressings, or transparent films, as indicated.
  - Apply a transparent film to maintain a moist environment in stages 1 and 2 pressure ulcers and to enhance autolysis of necrotic tissues in stages 3 and 4.
  - Use a hydrocolloid dressing to maintain a moist environment in stages 2, 3, and 4 and to enhance the autolytic process in the presence of necrosis.
  - Apply an absorptive dressing such as a wound filler to maintain a moist environment, fill dead space, and absorb exudate in stages 3 and 4 pressure ulcers.
- Maintain skin integrity and circulation.
- Protect the ulcer from pressure or trauma by using effective pressure-relieving devices and following repositioning and turning schedules for patients with limited mobility.
- Assess nutrition. Encourage adequate calorie, protein, and fluid intake.

sified according to the tissue layers included and the surgical methods used to transfer the tissue. All flaps require partial detachment of the tissue from its original site (with the base remaining attached).

Venous and arterial ulcers

Health care professionals commonly encounter lower extremity ulcers caused by venous and arterial disease. Managing these frequently problematic wounds can be difficult, exacting a costly toll on the patient's well-being. In addition, health care expenditures in the United States related to the evaluation and management of these vascular wounds are estimated in the billions of dollars.

Statistics about vascular ulcers in the United States show the magnitude of the problem:

- Approximately 1% of the general population and 3.5% of people over age 65 have venous ulcers. The number is rising as the population ages.
- The recurrence rate of venous ulcers approaches 70%.
- The estimated per-episode cost of care for venous ulcers can exceed $40,000.
- If an estimated 2.5 million people have venous ulcers, the total cost of treatment is believed to be approximately $2.5 to $3.5 billion.
- An estimated two million workdays per calendar year are lost due to chronic venous ulcers.

Management of vascular ulcers has improved over the past decade as health care professionals have come to realize the importance of proactive measures and a multidisciplinary team approach. Additionally, the introduction of newer treatment modalities, such as the use of growth factors and biologic skin replacements, hold the promise of treating difficult wounds, accelerating the wound-healing process, and preventing new wound formation.

Venous ulcers

Venous ulcers are believed to account for approximately 70% to 90% of chronic leg ulcers. The incidence of venous ulceration increases with age.

Venous ulcers can be difficult to heal. In some studies, 50% of patients had venous ulcers that persisted for more than 9 months, and 20% had ulcers that did not heal for more than 2 years. After healing, depending on compliance with use of compression stockings, more than 60% of patients experienced recurrence of venous ulcers.

PATHOGENESIS

The proper diagnosis and management of venous ulcers begins with a basic understanding of the venous system of the lower extremities. The components of the venous system include:

- deep veins, including the femoral, popliteal, and tibial veins
- superficial veins, including the greater and lesser saphenous veins
- communicating veins (perforators) that connect the superficial and deep venous systems
- calf muscles that force blood to move toward the heart when they contract
- valves that prevent reflux of blood away from the heart and toward the distal and more superficial veins.

The veins and muscles of the lower leg form a physiological unit called the calf-muscle pump. Activation of the calf-muscle pump during activity, such as walking or running, forces blood in the deep veins toward the heart, resulting in a drop in pressure within the deep venous system. This drop in pressure facilitates the movement of blood from the superficial system to the deep system via a series of communicating (perforator) veins.

Damage to any component of the calf-muscle pump can lead to reflux, typically referred to as venous insufficiency. An impaired calf-muscle pump is unable to appropriately lower pressure (often due to reflux) in the deep venous system, resulting in venous hypertension. Ultimately, venous hypertension is considered the root cause of the various manifestations of venous disease, including varicose veins, acute and chronic lipodermatosclerosis (LDS), and venous leg ulcers. Other medical problems can adversely affect the function of the calf-muscle pump, including heart failure, muscle weakness secondary to paralysis, obesity, pregnancy, deep vein thrombosis, and valvular damage or dysfunction.

ASSESSMENT

Diagnosis of venous ulceration depends on a thorough patient history and physical examination. In obtaining the history, the clinician should focus on risk factors such as prior venous disease, trauma, deep vein thrombosis, pregnancies, congestive heart failure, family history of venous disease, obesity, and advanced age. Women are three times more likely than men to develop venous leg ulcers.

Characteristic clinical findings include the presence of varicosities, hyperpigmentation, LDS, and dermatitis. (See *Signs and symptoms of venous leg ulcers*, page 66.) The shape of the leg may also provide a clue, because the "inverted bottle shape" is a sign of LDS. Venous ulcers tend to be superficial and thus to have flat wound edges without undermining.

Several findings that tend to go against the diagnosis of venous ulceration include the presence of eschar in the wound bed, exposed tendons in the base of the ulcer, *livedo reticularis* (net-like vascular pattern that extends from the wound edges) in the surrounding skin, and a round shape or "punched-out" ulcer.

A number of conditions are associated with the formation of ulcers that can look like venous leg ulcers. (See *Conditions that mimic venous leg ulcers*, page 67.)

Complications associated with venous ulceration include the development of dermatitis, wound infection (bacterial and fungal), osteomyelitis, squamous cell carcinoma, and basal cell carcinoma. Venous ulceration can be further complicated by the presence of acute or chronic LDS or arterial insufficiency.

While most leg ulcers are caused by venous insufficiency, the clinician must also carefully assess for the presence of arterial insufficiency because concomitant arterial disease can delay or prevent healing. Additionally compression therapy, the cornerstone of treatment for venous insufficiency, can cause tissue necrosis and ulceration in patients with underlying arterial disease.

DIAGNOSTIC TESTS

Performing the appropriate diagnostic tests is paramount when evaluating the patient with a suspected venous ulcer. The results of the tests will provide the basis for proper interventions and pa-

Signs and symptoms of venous leg ulcers

FACTOR	SIGNS AND SYMPTOMS
Wound location	Typically on the medical lower leg, superior to the medial malleolus (near the saphenous vein)
Appearance of wound bed	Referred to as "ruddy" or "beefy red"; granular in appearance
Wound shape and margins	Flat, irregular wound margins without undermining
Drainage and exudate	May be moderate to heavy
Surrounding skin	Venous dilatation, including submalleolar venous flare (typical of mild venous insufficiency), telangiectasias, reticular veins, varicose veins, edema (typical of more advanced venous disease), atrophie blanche (white plaques with dotlike capillaries) maceration, hyperpigmentation (from hemosiderin staining), and lipodermatosclerosis. Scarring from prior healed ulcers may be noted.
Pain	Controversial. Many believe that pain is usually not present. However, several studies have reported severe pain occurring in as many as 76% of patients with venous ulcers. Deep ulcers, particularly around the malleoli, or small venous ulcers surrounded by atrophie blanche are the most painful

tient management. Tests that can be performed include the following:

- *Ankle-brachial index (ABI)* — a simple, noninvasive test that determines the difference in blood pressure between the upper and lower extremities. The ABI assesses for the presence of arterial insufficiency, which is present in approximately 25% of

Conditions that mimic venous leg ulcers

- Antiphospholipid syndrome
- Arterial insufficiency
- Cryofibrinogenemia
- Cryoglobulinemia
- Factitial ulcers
- Homocysteinemia
- Infection
- Pyoderma gangrenosum
- Sickle cell disease
- Trauma
- Vasculitis

patients with venous disease. An ABI less than 0.6 is abnormal; as the valve diminishes, a declining ABI correlates with worsening of arterial insufficiency. An exceedingly low ABI contraindicates the use of compression therapy until further evaluation for the presence of arterial disease is performed.

- *Contrast venogram* — provides a radiographic picture of the venous system through use of radiopaque dye injected into a dorsal pedal vein. Its invasive nature makes it a less desirable test. This test carries a risk for inducing local thrombophlebitis and deep vein thrombosis. Nonionic dye should be used in patients with renal insufficiency.
- *Doppler ultrasonography* — a noninvasive test to establish the absence or presence of venous reflux and obstruction. Accuracy of this test is subject to the quality of operator interpretation.
- *Duplex scan* — locates venous reflux in the superficial, deep, and perforator systems.
- *Impedance plethysmograph* — assesses venous outflow in the lower extremities by measuring variations in electrical impedance that may occur with blood volume changes.
- *Photoplethysmography* — measures vascular volume and vascular competence via a transducer with infrared light.
- *Radionuclide venography* — assesses the venous system utilizing the radiopharmaceutical technetium 99.

MANAGEMENT

Management of the patient with a venous ulcer frequently requires a multi-disciplinary approach. The main goal is to heal the wound by promoting the wound-healing process. Important secondary goals include alleviating pain, reducing edema, improving LDS, and preventing ulcer recurrence. To achieve these goals, the effects of venous hypertension must be diminished and the underlying risk factors that promote venous insufficiency must be addressed. Medical conditions that accompany venous ulcers, such as arterial insufficiency, also need to be addressed.

While compression therapy remains the favored treatment, improvements have been made in the areas of biosynthetic dressings, growth factors, chemical debriding agents, antiseptics, elastic compression therapy, and bioengineered skin equivalents.

Dressings

Topical management of venous ulcers depends on the wound's characteristics, including amount of exudate, size of the wound, presence or absence of infection, and characteristics of the surrounding skin. Moisture-retentive dressings should be selected for wounds with light to moderate drainage. Examples of these product categories include hydrocolloids, transparent films, and certain foams. Absorbent dressings should be selected for wounds with moderate to heavy exudate. Examples of these product categories include foams, alginates, and specialty absorptive dressings.

Debridement

Debridement of the wound bed has classically been considered the first step in the treatment of venous ulcers. Debridement can be accomplished using autolytic, chemical, mechanical, and biological methods. Evidence supporting the efficacy of many of these methods is sparse.

- *Autolytic debridement*— is accomplished by using occlusive dressings, which can help maintain a moist wound environment, thereby promoting reepithelialization. They also have been shown to reduce pain and provide a barrier to infection.
- *Chemical debridement*— involves the use of enzyme debriding agents, including Accuzyme, collagenase, deoxyribonuclease, fibrinolysin, papain, and trypsin.
- *Mechanical debridement*— can be accomplished by several methods, including application of wet-to-dry dressings, hydrotherapy, irrigation, surgery, and dextranomers. The major disadvantage of mechanical debridement is that it is nondiscriminatory, frequently removing viable tissue along with necrotic tissue. Sharp surgical debridement of venous ulcers is often not

needed because venous ulcers are typically free of frank necrotic tissue or eschar.

Leg elevation

Edema is clearly an impediment to the healing process. The simplest method to reduce edema is bed rest with leg elevation. However, this is usually impractical and difficult to enforce except in the inpatient setting. Leg elevation of 18 cm above the heart for 2 to 4 hours each day produces the best results. Prolonged elevation of the legs above heart level allows edema to subside and improves microcirculation in patients with chronic venous insufficiency.

Compression

Leg elevation alone is usually not enough for most patients with venous disease. Compression remains the cornerstone of therapy for patients with venous ulcers, improves the rate of ulcer healing, reduces the incidence of recurrence, and prolongs the time to first recurrence. Fifty to sixty percent of patients heal with compression therapy alone over a 6-month period. Some of the physiologic changes reported to occur with compression therapy include improvement of lymphatic drainage, reduction of superficial venous pressure, improvement of blood flow velocity through unoccluded deep and superficial veins, and reduction of reflux in the deep veins. Studies have shown that venous ulcers that demonstrate healing after 4 weeks of compression therapy are likely to be completely healed by 24 weeks. In contrast, venous ulcers that don't show healing after 4 weeks of compression therapy tend to remain problematic.

Relative contraindications for compression include arterial insufficiency and uncompensated congestive heart failure. A low ABI warrants referral to a vascular surgeon for further testing and evaluation.

A number of modalities are available for the application of compression therapy. Products can be categorized into two main types: rigid compression and elastic compression. Elastic compression bandages can be further categorized into three classes: class 1— conforming stretch bandage, class 2— light support bandage, and class 3— compression bandage.

Rigid compression

Unna's boot has been the most popular option for controlling edema in the lower extremities. The boot is made of a gauze bandage impregnated with a gelatinous substance and zinc oxide paste. Initially applied wet to the affected lower extremity, the device becomes a rigid compression bandage as it dries. When the calf muscles press against this inelastic bandage, they pump more effectively, facilitating removal of fluid from the leg.

Several disadvantages are associated with Unna's boot. The rigid bandage is unable to conform to the leg's reduced circumference as edema decreases, making this product less effective over time. Additionally, Unna's boot can't absorb large amounts of drainage; it usually becomes soiled. Subsequently, the peri-wound skin may become macerated, and an unpleasant odor may be noticeable. Finally, it doesn't provide compression during periods of inactivity.

Elastic compression

Compression stockings, elastic wraps, and compression pumps aid venous return when used in conjunction with leg elevation. Compression stockings, which are available in different pressure grades, can be applied often. However, they may be difficult to use and may need to be replaced every 6 months.

Inexpensive, elastic wraps maintain pressure at about 20 mm Hg, if the wraps are new. However, after being washed, these wraps lose some of their compression capability.

Compression pumps assist in venous return, decreasing edema and enhancing fibrolytic activity. Inflation and deflation of select chambers on a given cycle provide the "pumping" action needed to assist in resolving venous hypertension. Although this process may prove to be effective for some patients, it may be too time-consuming for the patient or caregiver.

Sustained, graduated compression with an elastic, multilayered bandage system decreases edema throughout the day regardless of the lower extremity volume. This compression system, comprised of several different components, has been clinically proven to achieve pressures of 30 mm Hg to 40 mm Hg at the ankle, graduating to 12 mm Hg to 17 mm Hg below the knee. Padding is applied as the initial layer. This padding assists in redistributing the pressure around bony prominences and absorbing wound exudate. The remaining layers are elastic and cohesive bandages that achieve sustained graduated compression. The multilayer system is appropriate for both ambulatory and nonambulatory patients. It is flexible and comfortable and can control heavy drainage. Therapeutic pressures are sustained for at least seven days, opposed to other bandage systems in which the pressure decreases rapidly after application.

Other treatments

New technologies, such as skin substitutes and biologics, growth factors, and gene therapy, provide greater choices for the treatment of chronic venous ulcers.

Antiseptics

The use of topical antiseptics is controversial. In the past, studies revealed that cytotoxicity of these agents exceeded their bactericidal activity. Antiseptics are also associated with side effects such as dermatitis. More recent clinical trials have shown that products containing cadexomer iodine have significant antimicrobial activity, stimulate formation of granulation tissue, and promote wound healing with minimal side effects.

Bioengineered skin equivalents

Apligraf, a bioengineered human skin equivalent, is effective in the treatment of venous ulcers. The Food and Drug Administration (FDA) has approved Apligraf for the treatment of venous ulcers that fail to heal after 4 weeks of therapy.

Growth factors

Several studies suggest that growth factors, such as human recombinant epidermal growth factor, can improve healing rates in venous ulcers. Preliminary results have been variable, and further clinical trials are needed before growth factors can be considered a viable adjunct to proven therapies.

Surgery

There are no specific indications for autologous skin grafting for the treatment of venous ulcers. Split-thickness skin grafts, pinch grafts, and meshed grafts have variable efficacy in treating these ulcers. Superficial vein surgery, such as ligation or sclerosis of the long and short saphenous veins, has not been shown to improve the rates of venous ulcer healing or recurrence.

Systemic therapy

Some systemic pharmacotherapy, including systemic antibiotics and fibrinolytic agents, may be useful as adjuvant therapy for the treatment of venous ulcers.

Use of systemic antibiotics should be limited to ulcers with clinically proven infection. They haven't been shown to increase the rate of healing of uncomplicated venous ulcers.

Fibrinolytics, such as stanozolol and pentoxifylline, have been studied in several clinical trials. Stanozolol, an anabolic steroid, appears to be effective at reducing pain and induration associated with LDS, but it doesn't appear to increase the rate of ulcer healing. Pentoxifylline may accelerate the healing rate of venous ulcers but needs to be further studied.

Some clinicians have suggested that the use of oral zinc may help accelerate healing rates. However, a review of six randomized controlled clinical trials studying the use of zinc sulfate administered orally revealed no benefit.

Arterial ulcers

An estimated 5% to 20% of leg ulcers result from ischemia due to arterial insufficiency, which most commonly results from progression of atherosclerosis. The incidence of atherosclerosis increases in the elderly, and patients with arterial ulcers are typically older than age 50. The reported incidence of arterial insufficiency ranges from 2.2% in patients ages 50 to 59 to 7.7% in patients ages 70 to 74. Since arterial disease tends to be progressive, management of these ulcers typically requires revascularization. Accompanying medical conditions frequently include diabetes mellitus and venous stasis.

PATHOGENESIS

Arterial insufficiency refers to impairment of arterial blood flow leading to tissue ischemia and, potentially, necrosis. Such impairment can occur acutely, for example, due to trauma or thrombosis, or chronically, due to diseases such as atherosclerosis. Both acute and chronic arterial insufficiency can lead to the formation of leg ulcers. Arterial insufficiency can occur at any level, from large arteries, to arterioles and capillaries. Tissue ischemia that leads to leg ulcers occurs more in large vessels or in mixed disease.

Diseases associated with arterial insufficiency and ulcer formation

Large vessel disease
- Acute thrombosis (any cause)
- Arteriosclerosis obliterans
- Arteriovenous malformation
- Thromboangiitis obliterans

Small vessel disease
- Raynaud's phenomenon

Microthrombotic disease
- Antiphospholipid syndrome
- Cholesterol emboli
- Cryofibrinogenemia

Vasculitis
- Hypersensitivity vasculitis
- Polyarteritis nodosa group
- Rheumatoid arthritis
- Systemic lupus erythematosus
- Takayasu arteritis

Other
- Acute trauma
- Polycythemia vera
- Sickle cell anemia

Obstruction of arterial flow can be classified as *anatomic* or *functional*. Anatomic causes of obstruction include thrombosis, embolism, and atherosclerosis. Functional impairment occurs in the context of conditions such as Raynaud's disease, where abnormal vasomotor function leads to reversible obstruction. Reversible ischemia tends to cause pain and infrequently results in ulceration. Aside from obstruction, other potential causes of impaired arterial blood flow include disruption such as from trauma, fistulas, or aneurysms.

The most common cause of arterial ulcers is atherosclerosis. Risk factors for the development of atherosclerosis include age, smoking, diabetes mellitus, hypertension, dyslipidemia, family history, obesity, and sedentary lifestyle. Arterial insufficiency might occur at the same time as other pathologic mechanisms leading to tissue necrosis and ulceration. Diabetic foot ulcers, for example, may result from the combination of neuropathy, trauma, and arterial insufficiency. Certain diseases are associated with arterial insufficiency. (See *Diseases associated with arterial insufficiency and ulcer formation.*)

Some conditions are also associated with the formation of ulcers that can mimic arterial leg ulcers. (See *Conditions that mimic arterial leg ulcers,* page 74.)

Conditions that mimic arterial leg ulcers

- Eosinophilic vasculitis
- Hypertensive ulcers
- Pressure
- Pyoderma gangrenosum
- Scleroderma
- Spider bite
- Trauma
- Venous insufficiency

ASSESSMENT

Initial assessment of any ulcer begins with a thorough patient history and physical examination.

While taking the history, the clinician should screen for risk factors for atherosclerosis, especially smoking, diabetes, hyperlipidemia, and hypertension. A history of coronary artery disease (angina pectoris or myocardial infarction) or carotid disease (transient ischemic attacks or ischemic stroke) increases the likelihood that peripheral arterial disease is present. Claudication, a burning sensation of the calf muscles during ambulation that's relieved by rest, is the physical manifestation of arterial insufficiency of the large arteries of the legs.

Ischemic ulcers tend to have a "punched-out" appearance, being small, round, and with smooth, well-demarcated borders. The wound base is typically pale and lacks granulation tissue. Wet or dry gangrene may be present. Arterial ulcers tend to occur over the distal part of the leg, especially the lateral malleoli, dorsum of the feet, and the toes. They can be shallow or deep and are frequently painful.

In addition to these common features, the physical examination may reveal decreased peripheral pulses; lack of hair over the distal leg; and cyanosis, pallor, or atrophy of the surrounding skin. Lifting the leg more than 30 degrees can induce pallor in the ischemic limb. When dropped to a dependent position, the leg may become very red.

Vasculitic ulcers tend to have some characteristics similar to ischemic ulcers, including their location, size, and shallow depth. However, there are several typical differences. Vasculitic ulcers frequently have irregular shapes and borders. Additionally, the base of the wound tends to be necrotic with significant vascularity. The surrounding skin is usually hyperemic rather than pale. Vasculitis may also feature other cutaneous manifestations including palpable purpura, petechiae, and persistent urticaria.

DIAGNOSTIC TESTS

Tests to assess the patient with a suspected arterial ulcer include the following:

- *ABI.* This simple calculation can be performed in the clinic to assess for the presence of arterial insufficiency. Systolic blood pressure is measured over the brachial artery and the posterior tibial artery. The ankle pressure, measured using a hand-held Doppler, should be the same as or slightly higher than the brachial pressure. Claudication typically occurs when the ABI is less than 0.8. An ABI of 0.5 to 0.75 represents severe arterial disease, while an ABI less than 0.5 is limb threatening. The ABI has the advantages of being inexpensive, noninvasive, and has a reported high sensitivity and specificity.

- *Segmental pressure.* Arterial insufficiency can be confirmed through noninvasive studies to measure segmental pressures. Supine systolic pressures are recorded at the thigh, below the knee, and above the ankle. These segmental pressures should be approximately the same and similar to the brachial systolic pressure. A fall-off in the segmental pressure of more than 30 mm Hg indicates the presence of arterial occlusion.

- *Arterial waveform analysis.* Arterial waveforms can be obtained using pulse volume recording or Doppler waveform analysis. The normal arterial waveform is triphasic. A monophasic waveform points to moderate arterial occlusive disease, whereas a severely blunted waveform indicates severe disease.

- *Transcutaneous oxygen measurement.* The transcutaneous oxygen measurement ($TcPO_2$) can assess for the presence of microvascular insufficiency. A measurement greater than 30 mm Hg indicates adequate perfusion, while a value less than 20 mm Hg indicates disease. If the tissue surrounding an ulcer has a $TcPO_2$ less than 20 mm Hg, the wound typically won't heal.

- *Lower extremity angiography.* The "gold standard" for diagnosing arterial vascular disease, this procedure is indicated for those patients who are candidates for revascularization procedures. The test has associated risks, including cholesterol plaque embolization, acute vascular occlusion, arterial damage, and contrast-induced nephropathy.

- *Magnetic resonance angiography (MRA).* A noninvasive means of determining the presence and severity of arterial obstruction, MRA has become an increasingly important tool in the diagnosis of peripheral arterial disease and may ultimately supplant contrast arteriography as the premier test. Due to MRA's strong magnetic field, patients with metallic foreign bodies (such as cardiac pacemakers or vascular clips) can't undergo MRA. Additionally, patients who suffer from severe claustrophobia are frequently unable to tolerate the small confines of the MRI machine.

Other testing that may assist in the diagnosis or management of patients with arterial ulcers includes complete blood count; hemoglobin electrophoresis; serologies such as antinuclear antibody, anti-deoxyribonucleic acid, and rheumatoid factor; erythrocyte sedimentation rate; and biopsy.

MANAGEMENT

Managing arterial ischemic ulcers classically involves conservative debridement, pain control, use of occlusive dressings, and improvement of circulation. Treatment is also directed at the causes of arterial disease. For example, the management of arteriosclerosis includes exercise therapy, reduction of cholesterol, smoking cessation, and control of blood pressure and blood sugar. Antiplatelet agents (aspirin, ticlopidine, and clopidogrel) and xanthine derivatives (pentoxifylline) are commonly used to treat the symptoms associated with peripheral arterial disease. However, medical treatment alone typically has been of limited effectiveness for arterial ulcers. Newer modalities, including human growth factors and bioengineered skin substitutes, hold significant promise in the treatment of these frequently difficult-to-heal wounds.

Occlusive dressings

Occlusive dressings provide several beneficial effects. By providing immediate coverage, they reduce pain and protect the wound from infection. The dressings also help control exudate, enhance autolytic debridement, and maintain a moist wound environment, which accelerates the healing process.

Revascularization

Surgical intervention to improve circulation is the mainstay of treatment for severely ischemic extremities. Procedures include percutaneous balloon angioplasty with or without stent placement, percutaneous laser angioplasty, and arterial bypass surgery.

Vascular endothelial growth factor

Also known as vascular permeability factor, vascular endothelial growth factor (VEGF) is a secreted endothelial cell mitogen that plays an important role in angiogenesis following injury. It has been demonstrated that, in normal skin, tissue hypoxia increases levels of VEGF as well as the number of VEGF receptors in microvascular endothelial cells. Several studies have shown VEGF administration can induce angiogenesis, stimulating formation of collateral circulation in severely ischemic limbs. In one study, VEGF was also shown to heal or improve ischemic ulcers in four of seven patients. This treatment has not yet received FDA approval, and further testing needs to be done to assess its safety and efficacy.

Vacuum compression therapy

Some studies have suggested that vacuum compression therapy (VCT) favorably alters blood flow to the extremity and is useful for treating ischemic ulcers. VCT has two phases: the negative-pressure phase, during which blood vessels are enlarged and blood is pulled into the leg, and the positive-pressure phase, during which blood is pushed out of the leg. Further studies need to be completed to examine VCT's efficacy and safety for the treatment of arterial ulcers.

Bioengineered skin equivalents

Several studies report the efficacy of bioengineered skin in the treatment of arterial ulcers. Bioengineered skin offers the advantage of immediate wound coverage, reduction of pain, and protection against wound infection. Some of the substitutes also contain growth factors that stimulate wound healing.

Hyperbaric oxygen therapy

Several studies report the benefits of hyperbaric oxygen therapy in the treatment of problematic ischemic wounds. This therapy uses a special chamber to deliver 100% oxygen under increased atmospheric pressure, significantly increasing tissue oxygenation. The greatest benefit is seen in tissues with compromised blood flow.

Symptomatic therapy
Certain drugs are used to provide symptomatic relief.

Antiplatelet agents
In general, antiplatelet agents, such as ticlopidine and clopidogrel, reduce the symptoms associated with arterial insufficiency but don't accelerate wound healing. A newer agent, cilostazol, is a type III phosphodiesterase inhibitor that decreases platelet aggregation and increases vasodilation. The FDA has approved cilostazol for the treatment of intermittent claudication but not for the treatment of arterial ulcers. This drug also reduces pain and increases exercise tolerance in patients with arterial insufficiency.

Pentoxifylline
Also known as Trental, pentoxifylline is a xanthine derivative that is effective in decreasing claudication but hasn't been shown to assist in healing arterial ulcers. The optimal response to this agent typically isn't seen until 6 to 8 weeks after initiation of therapy.

Diabetic foot ulcers

Approximately 16 million people in the United States have diabetes, with 798,000 new cases reported annually. Fifteen percent of those with diagnosed and as-yet-undiagnosed diabetes will develop at least one foot ulcer during the chronic state of the disease, and the leading risk factor for ulceration is previous ulceration. Diabetes is responsible for 56% to 83% of the estimated 125,000 lower extremity amputations performed annually.

The financial and emotional costs and the potential complications associated with the effect of this disease on the foot are overwhelming. Preventing the loss of limb and function is the goal of the multidisciplinary team members caring for the patient with a diabetic foot ulcer. To achieve this end, clinicians must understand the scope and severity of diabetes and its physiological results.

Contributing factors

As the diabetic patient's disease progresses, underlying clinical conditions, such as neuropathy, vascular disease, foot deformity, and infection, become more prevalent. These conditions may occur alone or in combination with other factors. An estimated 60% to 70% of diabetic patients have peripheral neuropathy; 15% to 20% have peripheral vascular disease; and 15% to 20% of patients have both.

DIABETIC NEUROPATHY
A common accompaniment to long-term diabetes, diabetic neuropathy is often overlooked and undiagnosed until an ulcer or

pain in the extremity develops. However, early diagnosis and an aggressive ulcer prevention plan can be very successful. Both are imperative to decreasing the number of amputations in this population.

Diabetic neuropathy involves components of the sensory and autonomic nervous systems and the motor system. Sensory damage leads to an abnormal sensation in which the patient loses the sensation of pain or loses all sensation, which results in partial or total numbness of the foot. Due to this loss of sensation, also known as a loss of protective sensation, the patient may be unaware of a damaging event or process in the foot region. The patient would discover even significant blisters, wounds, or infections only by doing a visual foot check or experiencing systemic signs of infection.

Motor neuropathy, another facet of diabetic neuropathy, can cause changes in the biomechanics of the weightbearing foot. Imbalances of the foot occur when some muscles atrophy and opposing muscles are unchecked in their action. This can lead to changes in which particular surfaces bear weight in phases of the gait cycle. Deformities such as claw toes, which are not accommodated in normal shoes, can result and may produce pressure or friction areas.

Diabetic neuropathy may also affect the autonomic nervous system, which controls the functions of smooth muscle, glands, and visceral organs. Possible effects include changes in the vascular tone, which result in abnormal blood flow, and anhidrosis, which leads to fragile, dry skin that is easily damaged and very difficult to heal.

Damage associated with diabetic neuropathy cannot be reversed. However, controlling glucose can prevent or delay further damage. Pain that may accompany diabetic neuropathy can be treated in various ways. Some of the risk factors for developing diabetic neuropathy are modifiable, such as hyperglycemia, hypertension, smoking, cholesterol levels, and heavy alcohol use. Patient education about these risk factors and the benefits of controlling these areas is imperative.

PERIPHERAL VASCULAR DISEASE

Peripheral vascular disease is a serious medical problem in both the nondiabetic and diabetic populations. In diabetes mellitus, the process of atherosclerosis is accelerated and involves vessels of the entire body. Treatment for narrowing of the arteries and thrombosis includes antiplatelet therapy, surgery for the damaged and blocked vessels, and noninvasive techniques for better evaluation of the vascular status. Presently, new research with very interesting possibilities is under way.

DIABETIC FOOT STRUCTURE AND BIOMECHANICS

When all of these physiological processes occur in the lower extremity, they lead to structural and functional changes in the foot. The majority of diabetic foot ulcers result from mechanical forces that exceed what the tissue is able to bear and repair. As previously described, diabetic neuropathy leads to the loss of protective sensation, which otherwise would allow the patient to feel the overloaded tissue. Diminished blood flow and the skin's weakened state mean that the tissue may have difficulty bearing normal stresses, much less the stresses that are increased in particular areas due to muscle imbalance, poor footwear, and gait changes.

Several structural changes can occur in the diabetic foot. The most severe cases are seen in diabetic patients who develop Charcot foot (neuroarthropathy). Charcot foot usually first presents with erythema, increased local skin temperature, swelling, bounding pulses and, sometimes, moderate pain. Distinguishing Charcot foot from cellulitis can be difficult. However, the patient with Charcot foot doesn't have a fever or an elevated white blood cell count, which would be present with infection.

In patients with long-term Charcot foot, actual osseous destruction can be viewed on X-ray. This bony destruction occurs at the distal ends of the metatarsals and the anklebones. Since the patient usually has neuropathy and decreased sensation, chronic cases generate little pain. Continued ambulation results in further bony destruction and stress fractures. Resulting bony fracture changes cause the arch structure to collapse. The foot then takes on a new weightbearing rocker-bottom shape. The major pressure area of the gait cycle now becomes the arch, an area of ulceration for many patients with Charcot foot.

Many ulcerations occur in diabetic patients without Charcot factors. The heads of the metatarsals are major areas of ulceration. Although pressure is known to increase on the tissue in the area of eventual ulceration, the cause of this increased pressure is under investigation. One theory holds that weakness of the intrinsic muscles results in the claw toe deformity and the displacement of the fatty pads that normally cushion the metatarsal heads. This loss of cushioning results in easier ulceration. However, some new studies examine the integrity of the plantar fascia as the source of the claw toe deformities.

Weakness of the musculature responsible for dorsiflexion and plantarflexion of the foot and ankle complex is another effect of long-term diabetes and may play a role in load patterns on the plantar surface. Changes also occur in the joint mobility of foot structures. The first ray (the first metatarsal and phalange) may lose mobility, thus increasing pressure on the first metatarsal head. Other areas of limited joint mobility are associated with possible increased ulcerations. These include the subtalar joint with increased plantar pressure and the fourth and fifth metatarsals and phalanges.

Plantar callus formation in diabetic feet is commonly the focus of treatment. Callous formations occur in weightbearing and nonweightbearing areas of the diabetic foot. Many presume that the callous is a response to increased pressure on the specific point. However, it may also stem from the autonomic effects of neuropathy and the resulting skin changes. Once present, the callous does cause increased pressure and should be trimmed off regularly.

Diabetic foot management

The goal of the wound care team, which should always include the patient and the family, is to prevent as much damage as possible and to ensure maximum function and quality of life. This means reduction of and the possible elimination of amputations and loss of life related to the diabetic foot.

Interventions to achieve this goal are currently available. Patient education, prevention, and management programs are common denominators when attacking this problem. The first line of defense begins with a thorough understanding of the assessment parameters of the diabetic foot patient.

ASSESSMENT

Wound care team members need to be proactive when assessing and managing the diabetic foot patient. For clinical management to be effective, the team must have a keen understanding of the disease state and the patient's current overall health, not just the

Assessment questions

- When was the patient diagnosed with diabetes?
- What is the medication regimen for this patient?
- Does the patient have a clear understanding of the disease process and potential complications?
- How often does the patient self-monitor his blood glucose level?
- Has the patient had a blood test to check the glycosylated hemoglobin levels (a measure of glycemic control) in the past 3 months?
- Has a licensed professional, that is a Certified Diabetic Educator, Dietician, counseled the patient?
- Does the patient complain of lower limb or foot pain — indicative of claudication?
- Has the patient ever experienced foot ulcers?
- Has the patient suffered any known heart disease?

Adapted from Hess, C.T. *Clinical Wound Manager Manual Series for the Wound Care Department.* ©Wound Care Strategies, Inc., 2001

status of the foot. In-depth understanding of the patient's medical condition in combination with his actual and potential risk factors helps determine the best plan of care for a successful outcome.

Patient history

A thorough patient history is paramount to the treatment plan. Clinical team members must ask specific questions to determine the status of the patient's diabetes. (See *Assessment questions.*)

The clinician can't take for granted the patient's ability to care for himself. Rather, the patient should be asked to provide both verbal descriptions of self-care techniques — including foot care, foot checks, and insulin administration — and physical demonstrations of self-care, for example, demonstrating the ability to assess the feet and between the toes. The clinician's responsibility is to accurately document the goals thus far achieved by the patient.

Physical examination

Obtaining a verbal patient history provides the clinician with only half of the clinical picture. Next comes a thorough evaluation of the patient's lower legs, feet, and toes for muscular tone, skin and

---

Physical assessment checklist

- Has the team member performed a general physical examination that assesses the patient for signs of neuropathy and muscle wasting?
- Has the team member evaluated the patient's popliteal and pedal pulses?
- Has the team member described the condition of the patient's foot or feet? Is there evidence of Charcot foot, healed or existing areas of breakdown, or poor nail condition?
- Has the team member noted the overall status of the skin and presence of any scars from previous ulcers or surgery?
- Has the team member noted any other lower extremity conditions such as venous insufficiency, which may complicate treatment?

Adapted from Hess, C.T. *Clinical Wound Manual Series for the Wound Care Department.* ©Wound Care Strategies, Inc., 2001

---

tissue integrity, and vascular status. (See *Physical assessment checklist.*)

Assessment strategies to evaluate the diabetic foot should also include:

- performing the Semmes-Weinstein test.
- obtaining the patient's ankle-brachial index (ABI) to assess blood flow, or referring the patient for more advanced arterial vascular studies. ABI results should be interpreted with caution in patients with diabetes secondary to a high degree of calcified or stenotic vessels, which give falsely elevated values.
- examining the patient's feet for ulcers, especially the plantar aspect of the toes, laterally to the foot, between the toes, and the tips of the toes
- evaluating the footwear the patient commonly wears. Does it protect the feet, or does it promote rubbing?

Semmes-Weinstein test

The most widely used test for identifying loss of protective sensation in the diabetic patient's foot is the Semmes-Weinstein test. It involves applying a 10-gram nylon monofilament to certain strategic areas of the foot. The patient who can't feel the monofilament is at risk for ulcerations and needs a customized pathway and prevention plan. Annual screening with the Semmes-Weinstein test is recommended for all patients with diabetes. (See *Monofilament test to assess protective sensation.*)

Monofilament test to assess protective sensation

A Semmes-Weinstein monofilament is commonly used to assess protective sensation in the feet of patients with diabetes. A 10-gram (5.07 log) monofilament wire is applied to each foot at 10 sites — the plantar aspect of the first, third, and fifth digits; the plantar aspect of the first, third, and fifth metatarsal heads; the planter midfoot medially and lat-

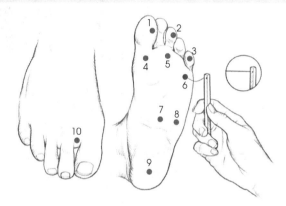

erally; the plantar heel; and the dorsal aspect of the midfoot. Loss of protective sensation generally is indicated by a patient's inability to feel the monofilament at 4 or more of the 10 sites. The following pointers should assist in ensuring that the procedure is done correctly:

- Place the patient in a supine or sitting position with legs supported and shoes and socks removed. Touch the Semmes-Weinstein monofilament to the patient's arm or hand to demonstrate what it feels like. During the test, the patient should respond "yes" each time he feels the pressure of the monofilament on his foot.
- Make sure the patient's feet are in a neutral position, with toes pointing straight up. Have the patient close his eyes. Hold the Semmes-Weinstein monofilament perpendicular to the patient's foot, then press it against the first site, increasing the pressure until the monofilament wire bends into a C shape. Make sure it does not slide over the skin. The device should be held in place for about 1 second. After the patient responds, record the response on a foot screening form. Use a "+" for a positive response and a "−" for a negative response. Then move to the next site.
- Remember to test sites in random order and to vary the time between applications. That way, the patient won't be able to guess the cor-

(continued)

Monofilament test to assess protective sensation *(continued)*

rect response. If the patient has an ulcer, scar, callus, or necrotic tissue at the test site, apply the Semmes-Weinstein monofilament along the perimeter of the abnormality, not directly on it.

- Refer the patient for an intensive education and follow-up program to learn how to inspect and protect the feet if the test indicates that he's experiencing loss of protective sensation. The patient can be taught self-assessment with the Semmes-Weinstein monofilament, but it doesn't replace a professional evaluation.

Adapted with permission from Sloan, H.L., and Abel, R.J. "Getting in touch with impaired foot sensitivity," Nursing98 1998;28(11):50-51.

After completing a thorough patient history and physical assessment, the clinician should document the findings in detail. The next step is to educate the patient about the disease process and the importance of the patient's role in the care plan. This also involves assessing the patient's preferred learning style and accommodating that style in the teaching plan.

Providing the patient with the proper skills and products needed to prevent foot ulceration is a team approach.

Risk factor evaluation

Assessment also involves evaluating the patient's risk for foot ulcers. Risk factors in the diabetic population include the following:

- absent protective sensation
- vascular insufficiency
- foot deformity causing high-pressure focal points
- autonomic neuropathy causing fissure and integument and osseous hyperemia
- limited joint mobility
- obesity
- impaired vision
- poor glucose control causing advanced glycosylation and impaired wound healing
- poorly designed or poorly fitting footwear, causing or inadequately protecting from tissue breakdown
- history of lower extremity amputation
- history of foot ulceration.

University of Texas diabetic foot classification system

Stage	Grade 0	Grade I	Grade II	Grade III
A	Pre- or postulcerative foot at risk for further ulceration	Superficial ulcer without tendon, capsule, or bone involvement	Ulcer penetrating to tendon or joint capsule	Ulcer penetrating to bone
B	Infection present	Infection present	Infection present	Infection present
C	Ischemia present	Ischemia present	Ischemia present	Ischemia present
D	Infection and ischemia present	Infection and ischemia present	Infection and ischemia present	Infection and ischemia present

Reprinted with permission from "Best Practices for the Prevention, Diagnosis, and Treatment of Diabetic Foot Ulcers, *Ostomy/Wound Management* 46(11):55-68, November 2000.

Classifying diabetic foot ulcers

Diabetic ulcers are described according to their depth and classified using a grading system. Many tools exist for classifying diabetic ulcers; the most commonly used system has been the Wagner Ulcer Grade Classification developed by Wagner and Meggitt. (See *Wagner ulcer grade classification,* Appendix C.) According to the Wagner scale, the ulcer classified with a lower grade tends to be less complex and may respond to medical intervention. Higher grades may dictate surgical management or amputation.

However, some difficulties in using the Wagner scale have led to the development of different assessment scales. One example is the Brodsky scale, which combines depth and ischemia. A second classification system in use is the University of Texas Treatment Base Diabetic Foot Classification System. (See *University of Texas diabetic foot classification system.*)

Infection in the diabetic foot

Diabetic foot infections are always serious and should be considered limb threatening. The diabetic patient doesn't provide the typical response to infections in many cases, and the result is a delay in diagnosis and management.

Diabetes itself, diabetic neuropathy, vasculopathy, and faulty wound healing mechanisms all contribute to the problem of infection in patients with diabetes. The disease compromises the immune system, which results in decreased function of defense mechanisms. Diabetic patients also have increased problems with nail fungi and skin infections, which can damage the skin and allow access for bacteria.

Infection spreads easily in the foot because of its very compartmentalized structure. Edema associated with infections can cause elevated compartmental pressures, which lead to ischemia and further foot damage. This problem of compartmental spread can be seen frequently in ulcerative infections that move rapidly through the plantar fascial plane and compartment.

A diagnosis of infection depends on the presence of two or more signs of infection, including purulent drainage, crepitus, fluctuance, loss of glycemic control, and any systemic signs. Many times the patient doesn't provide the normal response to an infection, so white blood cell count and erythrocyte sedimentation rate may not be elevated.

Bone infection results in destructive bone changes that may mimic those of neuropathy or Charcot disease. Bone infections are difficult to diagnose with radiographs, bone scans, or other procedures. Destructive changes may not be visible on a radiograph for 3 to 4 weeks. Hence, the clinician should strongly consider the presence of osteomyelitis when bone can be palpated through a chronic open wound. Correlation with localized wound status, drainage, systemic signs, and location supports a diagnosis of bone infection. Identifying the organism that has invaded the bone requires a bone culture, and the organism may not be the same one that is swab-cultured from the surrounding wound itself.

Treatment of the ulcer infection centers around debridement of the necrotic tissue in the wound, glycemic control, administration of systemic antibiotics, and good local wound care. If the patient has peripheral vascular disease, achieving adequate antibiotic levels in the area of tissue damage may be very difficult due to poor tissue perfusion. If the patient has osteomyelitis, the treatment regimen is usually prolonged (6 weeks or more) to allow for the poor penetration of antibiotic into the bone in most cases. In some cases, removing the bone is the only way to eliminate the infection.

Nonsurgical management

Nonsurgical management of the diabetic foot includes maximizing good wound care by maintaining an appropriately moist wound environment, debriding necrotic tissue, eliminating pressure areas on the foot, and improving the muscular strength and length of the lower extremity.

Achieving the goal of relieving pressure areas on the foot may sound easier than it is. Off-loading, or pressure relief of the diabetic foot, relies on patient compliance, clinician understanding of biomechanics, and availability of the appropriate products or materials.

Total contact casting is considered by many to be the best method of off-loading diabetic foot wounds. The pressure is redistributed across the rest of the plantar surface and away from the wound through careful cast application. Casting materials are widely available in most clinics, and patient compliance is relatively high because the cast is applied and removed by the clinical team.

Other methods of off-loading appropriate for many patients include custom-molded ankle-foot orthoses, posterior splints, orthotic dynamic splints (which are bivalved and similar to a total contact cast), and custom-molded healing sandals. Prefabricated products, such as cast walkers, are also available. These walkers may be more appropriate for patients with vascular compromise or wounds that require frequent care. Other options include customizable postoperative shoes and shoe materials provided through trained professionals.

Whatever the options for off-loading available in a facility, they all require a complete education plan for the patient, a level of commitment on the patient's part, and close monitoring, with any necessary modifications made promptly. Compliance is key to successful wound healing.

Physical therapy can also assist in diabetic wound healing with programs that address muscular imbalances in the lower extremity and foot, gait changes, off-loading, and exercise programs to assist in glycemic control. Electric stimulation, another modality widely available through physical therapy, is highly effective in assisting the wound-healing process. Additionally, physical therapists in many states are able to perform sharp debridement and are active members of the wound care team in both inpatient and outpatient settings.

Surgical options

Many patients require surgical intervention to aid in healing the diabetic foot ulcer. This may involve debridement procedures to remove necrotic tissue; to address nail issues; or to change the wound from a chronic, nonhealing state to an active, inflammatory (acute) state, which jump-starts the wound-healing process. When osteomyelitis is present, the infected section of the bone usually must be removed to allow the ulcer to heal. If the bone is structurally a source of pressure during weight bearing, partial bone removal may be necessary, a procedure known as an osteotomy. Some osteotomies as well as tendon releases to address structural changes are performed as preventative measures in foot areas that are highly prone to breakdown. However, this approach is still controversial.

Vascular issues in the diabetic foot also need assessment for possible surgical intervention. If the foot does not have adequate blood supply, healing will not occur despite the wound care team's best efforts. Vascular assessment and frequent reassessment are imperative throughout the patient's care.

6

Wound assessment, documentation, and outcome management

Designing a clinical pathway for wound healing begins with a comprehensive patient assessment, which details the patient's medical history inclusive of the wound's status. Appropriate interventions are predicated upon the assessment and documentation outlining the findings.

Developing documentation guidelines is a critical building block necessary to evaluate the clinical efficiency and cost-effectiveness of your contracted providers. Proper documentation provides guidance for appropriate treatment decisions, evaluation of the healing process, support for reimbursement claims, and a defense for litigation. Documentation may be provided in many forms, such as manual on paper, telephonic, photographic, or computer-generated. Once established, the documentation system should become the framework of clinical practice for all wound-care team members.

CLINICIAN'S CHECKLIST
The health care professional's thorough mastery of the assessment and documentation components is imperative. These skills become the link to ensure effective management and healing of wounds.

Evaluating the effectiveness of the plan of care and the status of the wound requires documenting assessments and interventions. Wound care documentation can combine a variety of information-gathering tools reflecting the wound's status across the healing continuum. When assessing a wound and documenting findings, include the following factors:

- *classification* by degree of tissue layer destruction or color
- *anatomic location,* including extremity and nearest bony prominence or other anatomic landmark
- *size,* specifying length, width, depth, and tunneling, and using consistent units of measure
- *appearance* of the wound bed and surrounding skin
- *drainage,* specifying amount, color, and consistency
- *pain or tenderness,* which may indicate infection, underlying tissue destruction, or vascular insufficiency
- *temperature,* which may indicate pressure ulcer formation, if the skin is intact, or an underlying infection.

Awareness of the cause of each wound for each patient is also important. (See *Understanding wound etiology.*)

Wound classification

Wound classification establishes a common language for wound assessment and wound healing. It helps to foster sound clinical judgments, provides a universal scheme for documentation, and allows better evaluation of treatments.

Accurate measurements of wound length, width, depth, and tunneling complement and complete the classification of a wound. Other essential documentation elements include a description of the skin around the wound, the wound's surface (intact, exuberant granulation tissue, or necrotic tissue), and the drainage or exudate found in the wound. Three main types of classification systems are used; two are based on the degree of tissue layer destruction, and one is based on the color of the wound bed.

Several classification systems identify certain types of wounds by grades (diabetic ulcers), stages (pressure ulcers), or other factors.

CLASSIFICATION BY STAGE OR GRADE

Staging systems identify certain types of wounds by stage (pressure ulcers) or grade (diabetic ulcers). See Chapter 3, Pressure ulcers, and Chapter 5, Diabetic foot ulcers.

CLASSIFICATION BY DEPTH

Partial-thickness and full-thickness are terms commonly used to classify wounds whose primary cause is something other than pressure. Partial-thickness wounds extend through the first layer of

Understanding wound etiology

The health care professional must evaluate each patient's wound by identifying:
- the wound's cause
- any underlying medical conditions
- the wound's history and treatment to date.

Establishing the cause will help identify the correct classification and management. For example, a wound caused primarily by pressure would be classified as a pressure ulcer and documented according to the pressure ulcer staging system. Other wounds such as vascular ulcers that result from arterial or venous insufficiencies may be classified by depth and documented as partial- or full-thickness wounds.

Underlying medical conditions, such as poor nutrition, diabetes mellitus, or neuropathy, may explain why the wound is healing slowly. These underlying conditions need to be treated concurrently.

Finally, treatment history is significant because the health care professional may learn which treatments have been tried and proved unsuccessful.

---

skin (the epidermis) and into, but not through, the second layer of skin (the dermis). Partial-thickness wounds heal by reepithelialization.

Full-thickness wounds extend through both the epidermis and the dermis and may involve subcutaneous tissue, muscle and, possibly, bone. Full-thickness wounds primarily heal by granulation, contraction, and reepithelialization. Examples of partial- and full-thickness wounds are skin tears, lacerations, surgical wounds, and vascular (venous and arterial) ulcers.

Describing a wound as partial or full thickness identifies the depth of the wound. However, it doesn't identify the condition of intact skin, the identifiable layers of tissue exposed (for example, bone), or the color of the exposed wound bed.

CLASSIFICATION BY COLOR

A three-color concept of wound classification was adapted by Marion Laboratories for use with traumatic, surgical, and other wounds that heal by secondary intention (open wound bed). It can be used as a component of wound assessment and as a tool to help direct treatment.

The three-color concept classifies wounds as red, yellow, or black.

- *Red* indicates clean, healthy granulation tissue. When a wound begins to heal, a layer of pale pink granulation tissue covers the wound bed, which later becomes beefy red.
- *Yellow* indicates the presence of exudate or slough and the need for wound cleaning. Exudate can be whitish yellow, creamy yellow, yellowish green, or beige.
- *Black* indicates the presence of eschar. Necrotic tissue slows healing and provides a site for microorganisms to proliferate.

If a wound displays two or even all three colors at once, base your intervention strategy on the least desirable color present. For example, if a wound is both yellow and black, base your intervention strategy on a black wound. Some facilities classify mixed wound colors by percentages, for example, 75% black and 25% yellow.

Wound location

The anatomic location of existing skin breakdown (for example, left hip, right lateral malleolus, or right ischial tuberosity) should be documented consistently. Generally, a documentation form with diagrams of different anatomic sites is a helpful tool. (See *Wound and skin assessment tool.*) One way to use this form is to circle the areas involved and assign a different letter for each location to ensure consistency of documentation.

Wound measurement

Accurate wound measurements are tools that assist the wound care team in designing an appropriate plan of care. Size is determined by measuring length, width, and depth, usually in centimeters, or by measuring volume. Several methods exist for measuring wounds, including linear measurement, wound tracings, and wound molds. The direction and depth of any tunneling should also be described. Consistent vocabulary and consistent units of measure are essential when documenting and describing wound measurements.

LENGTH AND WIDTH

The length and width of any wound are measured as linear distances from wound edge to wound edge. To ensure accurate and

Wound and skin assessment tool

Primary diagnosis _Left CVA_

Secondary diagnosis _Diabetes_

Pertinent medical history _Right-side weakness, depression, IDDM_

WOUND ANATOMICAL LOCATION:

Site _Right heel_   Date of outset _10/18/01_

(circle affected area)

DATE (M/D/Y)	TERM	TYPE #	LENGTH, WIDTH (cm)	DEPTH (cm)	TUNNELING (cm, o'clock)	COLOR (R/Y/B/M)	DRAINAGE (amount and type)	ODOR & TYPE (Y/N)
10/18/01	ST 2	2	4 x 3	< 0.1	Ø	10	Scant, serous	N

(continued)

Wound and skin assessment tool *(continued)*

CLASSIFICATION	TERMS	TYPE
Pressure ulcers	**ST1**—nonblanchable erythema of intact skin; heralding lesion of skin ulceration	**1.** Stage 1
	ST2—partial-thickness skin loss involving epidermis or dermis; ulcer is superficial; presents as an abrasion, blister, or shallow crater	**2.** Stage 2
	ST3—full-thickness skin loss involving damage or necrosis of subcutaneous tissue that may extend down to, but not through, underlying fascia; ulcer presents as a deep crater with or without tunneling of adjacent tissue	**3.** Stage 3
	ST4—full-thickness skin loss with extensive destruction, tissue necrosis, or damage to muscle, bone, or support structures	**4.** Stage 4
	ST3 or ST4(?)—wound completely covered with necrotic tissue; cannot be staged until wound base is visible	**5.** Stage 3 or 4 (?)
Wound	**PTW** (partial-thickness wound)—loss of epidermis and partial loss of dermis	**6.** Skin tear
	FTW (full-thickness wound)—tissue destruction, extending through the dermis and involving the subcutaneous layer; may involve muscle or bone	**7.** Surgical **8.** Vascular ulcer **9.** Other
Color	**R**—clean, healthy, granulating tissue	**10.** Red
	Y—presence of slough or fibrotic tissue	**11.** Yellow
	B—presence of eschar	**12.** Black
	M—two or more colors present in wound (specify color by letters)	**13.** Mixed
Skin condition	**SC** (skin condition)—an abnormal finding on the surface of the skin	**14.** Rash **15.** Incontinence-related **16.** Bruises **17.** Other

PAIN (Y*/N)	PHOTO (Y/N)	ADJUNCTIVE THERAPIES OR PRODUCTS AND ADDITIONAL COMMENTS	SIGNATURE, TITLE
		☒ Support Surface ☒ Nutritional Intervention ☐ New Orders Obtained	
N	Y	T & P 2 hours, heel protectors, heels elevated	B. Carey, RN

Patient's Name (Last, Middle, First)	Attending Physician	Room Number	ID Number
Brown, Ann	Dr. A. Dennis	123-2	01726

consistent measurements, establish landmarks for wound measurements. For example, look at the wound as if it were the face of a clock.

The top of the wound — 12 o'clock — is toward the patient's head. Conversely, the bottom of the wound — 6 o'clock — is in the direction of the patient's feet. Therefore, length can be measured from 12 to 6, using the patient's head and feet as guides. Width can be measured from side-to-side or hip-to-hip or from 3 o'clock to 9 o'clock.

Length and width can also be documented by making a tracing of the wound on transparent paper with a permanent marker. The tracing should be placed in a plastic bag (for infection control) and may be kept in the patient's chart for reference throughout treatment. If the wound is healing normally, subsequent tracings will show a progressive decrease in size.

DEPTH

The depth of a wound can be described as the distance from the visible surface to the deepest point in the wound base. If the depth varies, measure different areas of the wound bed to confirm the deepest site. Document your findings according to your facility's policy. (See *Measuring wound depth,* pages 98 and 99.)

When assessing a pressure ulcer, also document the depth of tissue loss by staging it on a scale of 1 to 4. Stages 3 and 4 are the most serious, sometimes requiring surgical closure or grafting.

VOLUME

An alternative method for measuring a wound cavity is to determine wound volume. This can be done by filling the wound cavity with an amorphous material (such as dental alginate paste), allowing the material to solidify, removing the resulting mold of the wound, and submerging the mold in a calibrated container that contains a set amount of water. The amount of water displaced is the wound volume. This technique is used mainly in research and laboratory studies, rather than daily clinical practice.

TUNNELING

Tunneling, also referred to as rimming or undermining, is tissue destruction underlying intact skin. Both the direction and the depth of tunneling should be documented. (See *Measuring wound tunneling,* page 100.)

Measuring wound depth

To properly evaluate healing, the health care professional must measure the wound initially and regularly during treatment. One method is to use a sterile, flexible applicator and follow the procedure below.

- Put on gloves. Gently insert the applicator into the deepest portion of the wound that you can see.

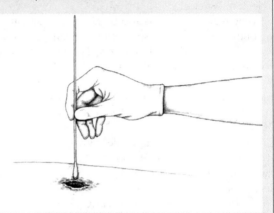

- Grasp the applicator with the thumb and forefinger at the point corresponding to the wound's margin.

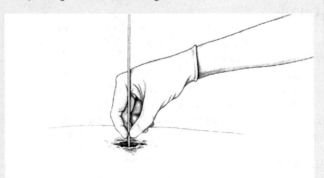

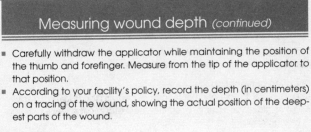

Measuring wound depth *(continued)*

- Carefully withdraw the applicator while maintaining the position of the thumb and forefinger. Measure from the tip of the applicator to that position.
- According to your facility's policy, record the depth (in centimeters) on a tracing of the wound, showing the actual position of the deepest parts of the wound.

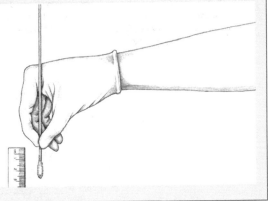

MEASURING PARTIAL- AND FULL-THICKNESS WOUNDS

When documenting partial- and full-thickness wounds, include length, width, depth, and tunneling (if present) in full-thickness wounds. All partial-thickness wounds have depth because the wound has penetrated through the epidermis. Because measuring superficial wounds is difficult, some health care professionals choose to document the depth as less than 0.1 cm. Any depth equal to or greater than 0.1 cm can be measured with a measuring device. Other parameters to use when describing partial- and full-thickness wounds are the color of the wound bed, appearance of the skin around the wound (periwound skin), and the presence of tunneling, drainage, and odor.

MEASURING PRESSURE ULCERS

When documenting the stages of a pressure ulcer, be familiar with the vocabulary necessary for accurate description and measurement. (See Chapter 3, Pressure ulcers.)

Measuring wound tunneling

The health care professional should document both the direction and depth of tunneling, as outlined below.

Direction of tunneling

To determine the direction of tunneling, perform the following steps:

- Put on gloves and gently insert the applicator into the sites where tunneling occurs.
- View the direction of the applicator as if it were a hand of a clock (12 o'clock points in the direction of the patient's head).
- Progressing in a clockwise direction, document the deepest sites where the wound tunnels (for example, 3 o'clock).

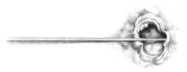
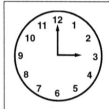

Depth of tunneling

To measure the depth of tunneling, perform the following steps:

- Insert the applicator into the tunneling areas.
- Grasp the applicator where it meets the wound's edge.
- Pull the applicator out, place it next to a measuring guide, and document the measurement (in centimeters).

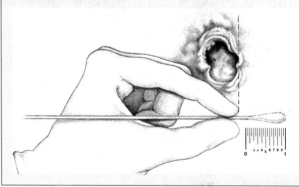

Wound appearance

Examination of a wound includes determining wound bed color, characterizing the skin around the wound, and observing for the presence of foreign objects.

COLOR

The color of a wound bed should always be documented. It's one universal tool used to distinguish viable tissue from nonviable tissue and may also guide wound management. For example, if a wound bed begins to change from red to yellow or black, this may indicate that the wound is becoming dehydrated and may need an alternative plan of care.

However, using colors such as red, yellow, and black to describe a wound bed may not always characterize what is seen within the wound. Other colors, such as pink, gray, and white, may be better descriptors when assessing the wound and documenting color.

SURROUNDING SKIN

Also assess the skin around the wound (periwound skin) and document your findings. Observe for color and feel for temperature. Note if the skin is intact or open, moist or weepy. A ring of redness, or halo of erythema, may indicate an underlying infection. Notify the primary care provider if signs of infection appear, such as redness, swelling, warmth, pain, exudate, or strong odor, and expect to take appropriate interventions such as starting antibiotic therapy as prescribed.

Finally, evaluate the epithelial edge for continuity. Local trauma may cause new epithelial tissue to erode. Epithelialization may be delayed if granulation tissue is covered with exudate or if it is dry or too moist.

PRESENCE OF FOREIGN OBJECTS

Assess the wound for foreign material, such as sutures, staples, or environmental debris, which can increase the risk of infection and may delay healing. If foreign material is present, document your findings and notify the primary care provider.

Wound drainage

Document drainage amount, color, consistency, and odor. Amount is documented as light, moderate, or heavy or as scant, moderate, large, or copious. Drainage color and consistency can be described as follows:

- *serous* — clear, watery plasma
- *sanguineous* — bloody (fresh bleeding)
- *serosanguineous* — plasma and red blood cells
- *purulent* — thick drainage, white blood cells and living or dead organisms, possibly with a yellow, green, or brown color that can suggest the type of infecting organism.

A pungent, strong, foul, fecal, or musty odor suggests infection.

Pain or neuropathy

Document the presence of severe pain or tenderness within or around the wound, and report it to the primary care provider. Pain may indicate infection, underlying tissue destruction that isn't visible, or vascular insufficiency. Also document the absence of pain, which may indicate nerve destruction or neuropathy. Work with the patient who can't communicate verbally but can understand commands to locate the site of any pain. If the patient is unable to respond verbally or with simple commands, observe for signs of pain, such as facial grimaces, retraction of a body part, or tenseness during the procedure. Document the patient's nonverbal as well as verbal responses because both are important descriptors to include in the comprehensive assessment. Specific information related to pain, tolerance of the dressing change procedure, patient's ability to provide self-care, and response to adjunctive therapies and treatments (such as rehabilitation) assist in developing a proactive plan of care.

The Joint Commission on Accreditation of Healthcare Organizations (JCAHO) has developed evidenced-based pain management standards that have been incorporated into the requirements for JCAHO accreditation. To comply with these standards, facilities need to implement policies and procedures to inform patients of their right to pain relief and demonstrate that pain is being routinely addressed, reassessed, treated, and managed effectively. Assessment data collected to determine the patient's pain level include:

- *pain intensity*—Use a pain intensity rating scale appropriate for the patient population. Document pain intensity at present, worst, and least levels. If possible, use the same pain rating scale consistently in the organization and among disciplines.
- *location*—Ask the patient to mark the site on a diagram, or point to the site of pain.
- *quality; patterns of radiation, if any; and character*—Elicit and record the patient's own words whenever possible.
- *onset, duration, variations, and patterns*
- *alleviating and aggravating factors*
- *present pain management regimen and effectiveness*
- *pain management history*—Include a medication history, presence of common barriers to reporting pain and using analgesics, past interventions and response, and patient's manner of expressing pain.
- *effects of pain*—Ask about pain's impact on daily activities, such as function, sleep, appetite, relationships with others, emotions, and concentration.
- *patient's pain goal*—Include goals for managing pain intensity and goals related to function, activities, and quality of life.
- *physical examination and observation of the pain site.*

Skin temperature

When assessing for potential skin breakdown or assessing the skin around an existing pressure ulcer or other wound, begin with temperature. Warmth may indicate pressure ulcer formation, if the skin is intact, or the presence of an underlying infection.

Additional assessment factors

Check for local factors (such as infection and necrosis) and systemic factors (such as chronic disease and vascular insufficiency) that may impede wound healing. (See Chapter 1, Fundamentals of wound healing.) If you identify such factors, you may need to extend your assessment.

Differentiating arterial, diabetic, and venous ulcers

ARTERIAL ULCERS	DIABETIC ULCERS	VENOUS ULCERS
Predisposing factors		
■ Peripheral vascular disease (PVD) ■ Diabetes mellitus ■ Advanced age	■ Diabetic patient with peripheral neuropathy ■ Long-term uncontrolled or poorly controlled diabetes	■ Valve incompetence in perforating veins ■ History of deep vein thrombophlebitis and thrombosis ■ Previous history of ulcers ■ Obesity ■ Advanced age
Anatomic location		
■ Between toes or tips of toes ■ Over phalangeal heads ■ Around lateral malleolus ■ At sites subjected to trauma or rubbing of footwear	■ On plantar aspect of foot ■ Over metatarsal heads ■ Under heel	■ On medial lower leg and ankle ■ On malleolar area
Patient assessment		
■ Thin, shiny, dry skin ■ Hair loss on ankle and foot ■ Thickened toenails ■ Pallor on elevation and dependent rubor ■ Cyanosis ■ Decreased temperature ■ Absent or diminished pulses	■ Diminished or absent sensation in foot ■ Foot deformities ■ Palpable pulses ■ Warm foot ■ Subcutaneous fat atrophy ■ Arterial assessment findings if patient also has PVD	■ Firm edema ■ Dilated superficial veins ■ Dry, thin, scaly skin ■ Evidence of healed ulcers ■ Periwound and leg hyperpigmentation ■ Possible dermatitis

Differentiating arterial, diabetic, and venous ulcers *(continued)*		
ARTERIAL ULCERS	**DIABETIC ULCERS**	**VENOUS ULCERS**
Wound characteristics		
■ Even wound margins	■ Even wound margins	■ Irregular wound margins
■ Gangrene or necrosis	■ Deep wound bed	■ Superficial wound
■ Deep, pale wound bed	■ Cellulitis or underlying osteomyelitis	■ Ruddy, granular tissue
■ Blanched or purpuric periwound tissue	■ Granular tissue present unless PVD is present	■ Usually minimal to moderate pain
■ Severe pain	■ Low to moderate drainage	■ Frequently moderate to heavy exudate
■ Cellulitis		
■ Minimal exudate		

LOWER-EXTREMITY ULCERS

Ulcerations, particularly on the lower legs or feet, commonly occur from arterial insufficiency, venous hypertension, neuropathy, or a combination of these conditions. A common cause is a decrease in blood supply to the area. Predisposing factors, such as the anatomic location of the ulcer and distinctive wound characteristics, help to distinguish among ulcers of the lower extremities. (See *Differentiating arterial, diabetic, and venous ulcers*. See also Chapter 4, Venous and arterial ulcers, and Chapter 5, Diabetic foot ulcers.)

Monitoring wound status

After the patient has been assessed, a plan of care implemented, and appropriate management modalities initiated, monitor the wound's progress (or lack of progress). In some facilities, monitoring wound status is accomplished by skin care teams. Such teams perform the following functions:

■ *monitoring* patients with select wounds, pressure ulcers, and skin conditions

- *assessing* selected wounds weekly and evaluating their progress or lack of progress
- *making collaborative decisions* regarding wound management effectiveness, so that dressings may be reordered or alternative modalities selected.

Photographic documentation

Wound documentation is usually supplemented with a photograph of the wound when needed for legal or medical purposes. Photographic documentation helps the practitioner assess the wound and measure changes over time. Typically, the wound is photographed in color on initial assessment and then at select intervals according to facility policy. Photographic documentation for legal purposes is discussed in Chapter 7, Legal and payment issues.

Patient outcomes

The *art and science* of wound care management directly impacts the patient's clinical and financial outcomes. An outcome is the overall condition of a patient that results from all health care processes performed on or for that patient. It refers not only to the patient's medical condition but also to the resulting quality of life the patient experiences. To achieve the best possible wound care outcomes while controlling costs, a comprehensive wound management system, based on validated protocols, should be established. (See *Establishing a wound management system*.)

An effective tool for managing outcomes is the clinical pathway. Such a pathway can serve as a guideline for the health care team to follow for a specific diagnosis. A wound-healing pathway designed for a specific diagnosis should include accurate assessment, documentation, and intervention processes and the expected outcome.

- *Assessment*, both initial and ongoing, describes the overall condition of the patient, including wound status.
- *Documentation*, both written and photographic, lays the foundation for management decisions, evaluation of the wound-healing process, and reimbursement decisions. It also serves as a defense in litigation.

Establishing a wound management system

The following steps can guide you through the process of establishing a wound management system for your institution. Once in place, such a system can help achieve positive outcomes and control costs.

Define the tools and build the team
The tools essential to building a wound management system include patient and practitioner education, information systems, and utilization review and outcomes management tracking systems to assess the program's effectiveness and measure clinical, functional, and financial outcomes. To maximize the wound-healing process, you will also need to develop a multidisciplinary team of wound care practitioners who are dedicated to continuous quality improvement practices for each patient.

Define your clinical practice guidelines
Develop and use protocols in a systematic wound care system. To ensure consistent care and achieve the best possible outcomes, institute validated protocols, such as the clinical practice guidelines for preventing and treating pressure ulcers published by the Agency for Health Care Policy and Research.

Select your wound care products
Choose from topical wound care products, tissue load management products, support surfaces, nutritional interventions, and adjunctive therapies and products. When choosing products and developing the plan of care for a particular patient, the practitioner should consider the type of wound, the patient's individual needs, and the specific product.

Develop an educational pathway
With the other members of the wound care team, define the common terminology for documenting wound care. Also, define the terminology for wound classification and cause to establish a baseline for assessment and intervention. Measurements and descriptions of wounds should include length, width, depth, tunneling, odor, drainage, color of the wound bed, and other pertinent characteristics. Such standardization of documentation is crucial for quality care, outcomes research, and reimbursement.

Develop a wound management information system
Develop an information system that allows for the assessment of each patient's wound and overall medical condition. Such a system should provide clinically effective and cost-efficient pathways to achieve successful outcomes. The system should assess outcomes through utilization review to ensure that existing wounds heal, to prevent the deterioration of existing wounds, and to reduce the incidence of new or recurring wounds.

- *Interventions*, guided by the multidisciplinary wound care team, include topical treatments, use of support surfaces, use of adjunctive therapies and products, and nutritional supplements.
- *Expected outcome* describes the overall condition of the patient that should result from all the processes performed on or for that patient.

Monitoring the competency of staff members and patients, evaluating the clinical research for each product used, and assessing outcomes through utilization management tools can help ensure positive outcomes, despite the many variables that can affect wound care outcomes.

Competency is the common thread found in both the *art* and *science* of wound care that directly impacts the overall care of the patient. JCAHO defines competency as a determination of an individual's capability to perform per expectations. Competency affects all health care professionals across the continuum. Providers need to be competent in delivering care, and payers need to be competent in understanding the clinical practices for which they are paying on behalf of the patient.

Wound care competency is mandatory for all professionals delivering care in this disease management approach. These programs need to be monitored, evaluated, and modified as the facility deems appropriate.

One way to improve wound care competency is to structure ongoing education and training that will maintain and improve the clinician's knowledge level. Then, the facility has the responsibility to perform ongoing competency assessment through a defined, continuous process. This ongoing monitoring will identify those professionals who are experts in both the *art* and *science* of wound care. The benefit of competency testing in all facilities is great. It increases patient satisfaction and clinician satisfaction and retention as well as improves the facility's public relations.

7

Legal and payment issues

To the typical jury member or judge, a patient who has a wound that looks terrible and smells awful means that the patient has suffered something terrible — and someone is to blame. The most obvious place to lay the blame is on the wound-care practitioners who treated the patient. Because of this need to assign blame for the patient's suffering, wound-care practitioners are at high risk for becoming involved in legal action. At the same time, they must deal with new payment and reimbursement practices that stem from recent changes in Medicare payment rules. This chapter examines the legal and reimbursement issues that wound-care practitioners face.

Legal risks

Because legal actions that involve wound care are among the hottest areas of litigation, wound-care practitioners are increasingly concerned about the legal risks of providing care. Certain factors increase these risks.

■ As our understanding of why patients develop wounds and what works best to heal wounds evolves, standards for appropriate wound care change and many practitioners fail to keep up with the changes.

■ Some patients and their families incorrectly believe that appropriate standards of care now dictate that patients only develop wounds because providers have been negligent.

- The "folk medicine" component of wound care — including such practices as applying sugar water, shortening, honey, and other inappropriate substances to wounds — interferes with proper wound healing.

  In particular, wound-care practitioners may face liability for:
- negligence
- violations of Medicare and Medicaid fraud and abuse prohibitions
- abandonment for terminating services to patients.

LIABILITY FOR NEGLIGENCE

A provider may incur liability for negligence for failing to provide necessary and appropriate wound care for a patient. To prove negligence, a patient must show that:

- the provider owed the patient a duty
- the provider breached the duty owed to the patient
- the breach of duty resulted in injury or damage to the patient.

  If the patient fails to meet even one of these requirements, he will lose his lawsuit. To take the necessary steps to avoid liability, the provider must understand what each requirement means.

Owing a duty

The provider owes the patient a duty of reasonable care as defined by national standards of care. Sources of these standards include licensure statutes, guidelines set forth by such accrediting organizations as the Joint Commission on Accreditation of Healthcare Organizations, court decisions, requirements of third-party payers, and standards of professional associations related to wound care.

Breaching a duty

The provider may breach his duty to the patient by doing something he shouldn't have done (an act) or by failing to do something that he should have done (an omission). In most court cases that involve provider negligence, more than one act or omission occurred. However, the patient only has to prove that a single act or omission occurred to meet the requirement.

Causing injury

The patient must demonstrate that the provider caused the patient's injuries. The best way to define causation is with the phrase

Potential for negligence claims

A negligence lawsuit can arise from several types of failures on the part of the wound care provider. Common examples include failure to:
- follow the legally authorized prescriber's orders
- refuse to provide care when a legally authorized prescriber orders inappropriate wound care
- monitor and observe a patient properly
- report changes in a patient's condition to the appropriate practitioners
- document properly all care provided
- provide proper care.

"but for": But for the provider's act or omission, the patient would not have been injured.

The most important aspect of proving negligence is injury or damage. If no injury occurred, the provider has no legal liability. The patient is almost always required to show physical injury or damage to prove liability; a patient whose claim rests on emotional damage alone will probably lose his lawsuit.

Premature discharge or failure to provide care
Wound-care patients may use this legal theory of negligence to attempt to show that practitioners are legally liable when a patient is injured as a result of the practitioner's failure to provide care because he would not be paid. For example, the patient may claim that he was prematurely discharged from the practitioner's care. Or he may claim that care was not rendered in the first place because the payer would not authorize it.

Other types of situations can give rise to claims of negligence. (See *Potential for negligence claims*.) What steps can a wound-care practitioner take to protect against liability in these situations?

Protecting against negligence claims
To protect against claims of negligence, the practitioner should:
- protest decisions to deny payment and document that protest
- obtain valid informed consent from the patient, especially for relatively invasive types of wound care
- document all wound care.

Protesting adverse payment decisions

Providers should attempt to use payers' grievance procedures, which vary from payer to payer. If grievance procedures are inappropriate or ineffective, practitioners should protest via telephone and confirm the conversation in writing.

Obtaining valid informed consent

Following all the steps necessary to obtain valid informed consent provides significant protection against legal liability. For informed consent to be valid, an adult patient must meet two prerequisites. First, he must have the *capacity* to understand information the practitioner gives him about proposed treatments. Second, he must consent *voluntarily*; any fraud or duress used to obtain the consent invalidates it.

If the patient meets these two prerequisites, the practitioner must then:
- specifically describe the proposed treatments
- describe the possible benefits of the proposed treatments
- provide information about significant risks associated with the proposed treatments
- describe alternative treatments
- affirm the right of the patient to refuse treatment.

Documenting care

A practitioner can also protect against negligence claims by documenting all wound care completely, accurately, and in a timely manner. Such documentation should routinely include:
- photographs of the wounds (with the patient's written permission for such photos)
- measurements of the wounds, including depth and circumference
- amount, color, and odor of any discharge.

LIABILITY FOR FRAUD AND ABUSE

A practitioner can face liability for fraud and abuse violations when submitting claims for reimbursement from Medicare or Medicaid. Specifically, the federal False Claims Statute affirms that a practitioner who documents anything that is untrue and sends that documentation to the government as part of a reimbursement claim to Medicare or Medicaid is submitting a false or fraudulent claim. For example, a practitioner who submits a claim for payment for wound-care treatment that was not provided has submitted a false claim and, as a result, may face both criminal and civil liability.

The federal government also takes the position that, when a provider submits a claim for payment, the provider promises that the care given was both necessary and appropriate. If the care given is later determined to be substandard, reimbursement claims for that care are also false or fraudulent. For example, when a practitioner applies povidone-iodine to a wound based on the primary care provider's orders and submits a claim for that care, the practitioner has engaged in fraud because povidone-iodine is no longer considered an acceptable wound-care treatment.

Protection against false claims violations

How can a provider avoid allegations of making false claims? As with negligence, the best protection is careful and complete documentation, including photographs of the wounds. The adage "A picture is worth a thousand words" holds true in wound care; many auditors and investigators who have doubted the appropriateness of services provided have been convinced otherwise after examining photographs of the wounds. The practitioner's facility should also have a fraud and abuse compliance plan in place to help all providers avoid fraud and abuse of all types, including false claims.

LIABILITY FOR ABANDONMENT

Wound-care providers are likely to encounter situations in which discontinuing services to a patient is advisable. For example, when a patient or his primary caregiver or both are noncompliant with the plan of care, the wound-care provider may wish to terminate services. Termination may be justified because the provider's risk of liability for negligence is greatly enhanced due to the difficulty of distinguishing patient noncompliance from substandard provider care.

Prior to discontinuing services for noncompliance, however, the provider should carefully document instances of noncompliance as follows:

- The provider should document specific instances of noncompliance by the patient or primary caregiver in plain English. General statements such as "Patient and primary caregiver noncompliant" are insufficient.

- After each documented instance of noncompliance, the provider should counsel the patient and primary caregiver regarding these instances and document such counseling.
- If the noncompliance resulted from a need for additional patient education, the provider must reeducate the patient and document the instruction, including the patient's successful return demonstration.

When the above actions don't result in compliance, the provider must consider whether to terminate services.

Wound-care providers who must terminate services to a patient — a situation that is becoming more common in wound care — may be justifiably concerned about liability for abandonment. To prove abandonment, the patient must demonstrate that the provider unilaterally terminated the provider-patient relationship without reasonable notice when the patient needed further attention. If any element is missing — if the patient and provider both agreed to termination, if the patient received reasonable notice, or if the patient didn't need further attention — the patient can't prove abandonment.

Such a definition seems to give practitioners a way to protect themselves from such liability by giving reasonable notice of termination. But what is reasonable notice? A practitioner needs to determine reasonable notice for each patient by holding team meetings or case conferences to consider all the circumstances of that case. Once team members have decided what constitutes reasonable notice for that situation, the practitioner should carefully document the results of the meeting and give the patient both verbal and written notice of termination. In most instances, 3 to 5 days' notice is appropriate for a noninstitutionalized patient.

Payment systems

Most payers have implemented some form of prospective payment system that requires providers in all sites of service to manage skin and wound care, achieve cost-effective outcomes, maintain excellent quality assurance reviews, and achieve high levels of patient satisfaction. Providers must understand the major payment systems' rules for wound-care services, procedures, dressings, drugs, and devices. To successfully coordinate care, providers must also understand the major payment systems of their referral sources and of the providers and sites of service to whom they will refer patients. Providers should review contracts they have with payers and contact other major payers to determine their coverage criteria, coding, and payment rates for the services, procedures, and products they provide for patients as well as for orders they write to other providers for follow-up services, procedures, and products. (See *Medicare payment systems for skin and wound care*, pages 116 and 117.)

Fortunately, many skin- and wound-management modalities are available in the marketplace. After conducting a complete patient history and physical, assessing the wound, evaluating the patient's ability to participate in his own care, and reviewing the payer's coverage criteria, providers can determine a plan of care that offers the best clinical and financial outcomes for patient, payer, and provider. At times, providers will be forced to design a less-than-optimum plan of care due to patient preference or payer coverage. Therefore, providers should capture assessment, documentation, clinical, and financial outcome data in an electronic database. This data can then be used to improve critical pathways, product formularies, contract fees with payers, and patient satisfaction. Over time, the providers with the best clinical and cost-effective skin and wound-care outcomes, the best quality assurance results, and the highest level of patient satisfaction will have the most referrals and the most profitable business.

Providers can achieve their clinical and financial goals by following these necessary steps:

- obtain the services of a wound-care consultant in the early stages of developing wound-management service
- write policies and procedures for skin- and wound-management service
- develop research-based wound-care pathways (care maps)
- design a skin- and wound-care modality formulary based on clinically proven efficacy and cost-effectiveness, availability, ease of use, function, and direct cost (the last consideration)
- use technology to reduce the length of stay, the number of dressing changes, the number of professional visits, the time to heal, and the total cost of care
- design a supply management system that controls product utilization internally or externally, to control costs and waste
- obtain cost reductions based on volume purchases, due to standardization of products

Medicare payment systems for skin and wound care

	FACILITY
Hospital	Diagnosis Related Group (DRG)[1]
Hospital outpatient department	Ambulatory Payment Classification (APC)[3] ■ Transitional Pass-Through and New Technology Payments[4] ■ Surgical Dressing Policy[5] (if the hospital has a National Supplier Clearinghouse Number)
Physician office	
Skilled nursing facility	■ Part A: Resource Utilization Group, revision III (RUG-III)[6] ■ Part B: Surgical Dressing Policy
Home health agency	Home Health Resource Group (HHRG)[7]
Durable medical equipment supplier	■ Surgical Dressing Policy ■ Negative-Pressure Wound Therapy Pump Policy[8]

1 DRG — Patients are classified into a DRG by diagnosis, procedures performed, age, and discharge status. A payment rate is assigned to each DRG, adjusted geographically, and is meant to cover all the costs of the hospital admission. The code used to determine the DRG is the ICD-9-CM code.

2 RBRVS — Services and procedures are assigned values based on the resources used: physician work, practice expenses (including cost of surgical dressings), and malpractice insurance. A conversion factor, updated annually, converts the relative values into a Physician Fee Schedule, which is geographically adjusted. The code used to determine the RBRVS/Physician Fee Schedule is the CPT code.

3 APC — Services and procedures performed are identified by CPT codes, which are grouped based on resource utilization and clinical comparability. A payment rate is assigned to each APC group and is geographically adjusted. The APC payment rate covers use of the procedure or treatment room, most drugs, most biologics, most medical supplies (including surgical dressings), and care provided by hospital employees who are included on the Medicare cost report.

4 Transitional Pass-Through and New Technology Payments — In addition to APC payments, hospital outpatient departments can receive payments for certain drugs, biologics, and innovative devices that haven't been included in the APC payment calculations.

5 Surgical Dressing Policy — Level II Healthcare Common Procedure Coding System (HCPCS) codes, utilization guidelines, and documentation guidelines are assigned to each Health Care Financing Administration (HCFA)-covered category of surgical dressing. A payment rate is listed for most categories on the Durable Medical Equipment Regional Carrier (DMERC) fee schedule.

PHYSICIAN	NURSE PRACTITIONER / CLINICAL NURSE SPECIALIST
Resource-Based Relative Value Scale (RBRVS)[2] — Physician Fee Schedule	RBRVS — 85% of Physician Fee Schedule, if professional isn't included in hospital cost report
RBRVS — Physician Fee Schedule	RBRVS — 85% of Physician Fee Schedule, if professional isn't included in hospital cost report
■ RBRVS — Physician Fee Schedule ■ Surgical Dressing Policy (if physician has a National Supplier Clearinghouse number)	■ RBRVS — 85% of Physician Fee ■ Schedule, if professional is isn't billed "incident to" the physician
RBRVS — Physician Fee Schedule	RBRVS — 85% of Physician Fee Schedule, if professional isn't included in the skilled nursing facility's cost report
RBRVS — Physician Fee Schedule	RBRVS — 85% of Physician Fee Schedule, if professional isn't included in the home health agency's cost report

6 RUG-III — Assessment of resources needed by the patient for a particular period of time is conducted through a standardized tool called the Minimum Data Set. This information assigns each patient to a RUG-III group, which translates into a Health Insurance Prospective Payment System (HIPPS) rate code. The HIPPS rate code is then used to determine a per-diem rate, which is geographically adjusted for each patient for a designated period of time. This rate must cover all skin and wound management modalities during the Part A-covered stay.

7 HHRG — The Outcome and Assessment Information Set (OASIS) is completed for every patient prior to each 60-day episode of care. It identifies the clinical, functional, and service resources needed by the patient. An OASIS score groups the patient to an HHRG based on the patient's level of severity. A national payment rate for each 60-day episode of care is assigned to each HHRG and is geographically wage-adjusted.

8 Negative-Pressure Wound Therapy Pump Policy — Level-II HCPC codes, utilization guidelines, and documentation guidelines are assigned to the negative-pressure pumps, to the accompanying dressing set, and to the accompanying canister set. A payment rate is listed for each code on the DMERC Fee Schedule.

Reprinted from Schaum, K.D. "Medicare Payment System for Skin and Wound Care," in Hess, C.T. Clinical Wound Manager Manual Series for the Wound Care Department. © Wound Care Strategies, Inc., 2001.

- implement a delivery system that prevents delays in management and oversupplying products
- plan for disposal of medical waste
- identify all ICD-9-CM, CPT, HCPCS, Pass-Through and New-Technology, and local codes that represent the diagnosis, evaluation and management service, procedures, and products that need to be included on payer claim forms
- implement a photodocumentation system
- install outcomes tracking program on computer
- educate and validate the competency of all staff members, including the physicians, on the ability to assess, aggressively manage, and appropriately document skin and wound care
- prevent skin breakdown
- develop a multidisciplinary plan of care, with clearly defined endpoints
- implement early, aggressive, state-of-the-art skin and wound management
- assess wound accurately and document findings completely
- accurately select the primary diagnosis that is the most appropriate
- order the wound-management modality based on the assessment, the outcome-oriented care plan, skill of the patient and caregiver, and payer guidelines
- assure physician orders include all required components and document the medical necessity for modalities ordered
- educate the patient and caregiver about the efficient use of appropriate dressings, drugs, and medical equipment
- reach achievable clinical and financial outcomes and patient satisfaction in the least amount of time, using the least amount of labor and material resources
- establish method of transferring documentation: origin of wound, surgery date (if applicable), type of debridement (if applicable), original stage of wound, wound assessment, diagnosis, and physician's orders
- initiate timely referral to the next level of care
- prepare a discharge summary that includes information required for the next provider to manage care and supplies in a cost-efficient manner
- obtain new referrals for well-managed wound care, which generates more revenue.

Part Two

WOUND CARE PRODUCTS

Dressings

Overview

For centuries, humans have been combining substances for use in topical wound care. Early Egyptians mixed concoctions of naturally occurring products such as honey, animal fat, and vegetable fibers. Shamans and witch doctors created poultices of plant extracts and animal products. As the culture progressed, mixtures became more complex, and the relative amounts of various ingredients became more important for a successful mixture, so the compounders began keeping records of specific compositions and preparation methods.

In the 19th and 20th centuries, synthetic ingredients such as polymers joined the list of naturally occurring ingredients in a variety of products. The complexity of products soared along with the explosion of new products. And with this explosion has come confusion over dressing selection.

Clinical Guide: Wound Care can help you, the practitioner, choose the proper skin and wound care products to facilitate healing based on the classification of the wound and skin condition. To utilize this tool properly, remember that the composition of a product is often key to its success and may be kept a trade secret. However, the U.S. Food and Drug Administration requires a basic level of disclosure regarding the ingredients in a product for fundamental safety reasons. Some products may contain ingredients that cause an allergic reaction in certain people or ingredients that shouldn't be mixed with certain other ingredients. For example, many people are allergic to latex and need to know if it's a component of a certain product. Labels of most food and household products contain information about their ingredients, which are listed in order of abundance in the mixture. In addition to the label, a Material Safety Data Sheet (or MSDS) is available upon request from any manufacturer for any of its products. An MSDS contains health and safety information on the product and its ingredients. Practitioners should be careful when mixing products, even unintentionally, and should always read the product label and package insert before use.

Practitioners must provide comprehensive product choices for wound care management, including topical wound care products, support surfaces, nutritional products, and adjunctive therapies that promote healing.

Part II provides quick-reference descriptions of wound care products grouped under generic categories. Included are alginates, collagens, composites, contact layers, drugs and biologics, foams, gauzes, hydrocolloids, hydrogels, miscellaneous surgical dressings, specialty absorptives, transparent films, and much more. (Part III provides a comprehensive listing of additional products: abdominal dressing holder/binders, tapes and closures, wound pouches, wound cleansers, gauzes, elastic bandages, and compression bandage systems). For each product, you'll find the size and configuration of the product, the action, indications, contraindications, and instructions for application and removal as well as the product's HCPCS code. (Note: Product names may be copyrighted or trademarked even when unaccompanied by copyright or trademark characters.) For specific packaging information, you may want to contact the manufacturer. (See Manufacturer resource guide, pages 470 to 473).

No single wound care product provides an optimum environment for healing all wounds. It remains your responsibility to understand the dressing's characteristics, function and appropriateness for each patient's wound.

HCPCS code overview

To ensure uniform Medicare claim coding by all suppliers of wound care dressings, the Statistical Analysis Durable Medical Equipment Regional Carrier (SADMERC) performs a Coding Verification Review. If manufacturers wish to have a Health Care Financing Administration Common Procedure Coding System (HCPCS) code assigned to their products, they must submit a formal application to SADMERC.

SADMERC and the four Durable Medical Equipment Regional Carriers (DMERCs) conduct reviews of products to determine the correct HCPCS codes for Medicare billing. These reviews result in a consensus coding decision. The assignment of a HCPCS code to a product should not be construed as an approval or endorsement of the product by SADMERC or Medicare and does not imply or guarantee reimbursement or coverage. Many other payers also require the assigned HCPCS codes on their claim forms.

If a manufacturer has provided proof of the SADMERC-assigned HCPCS code(s) for its product(s), the author has placed the five-digit alphanumeric code beside the size of each product. If a manufacturer has not requested a HCPCS Coding Verification Review, the author did not include any HCPCS information for that product. The provider and supplier are ultimately responsible for verifying the correct HCPCS codes before submitting claims to any payer.

Alginates

Action

Alginates are derived from brown seaweed. The products are composed of soft, nonwoven fibers shaped as ropes (twisted fibers) or pads (fibrous mats). Alginates are absorbent and conform to the shape of a wound. When packed, an alginate interacts with wound exudate to form a soft gel that maintains a moist healing environment. An alginate can absorb up to 20 times its weight.

Indications

An alginate may be used as a primary dressing on partial- and full-thickness, draining wounds; wounds with moderate to heavy exudate; tunneling wounds; infected and noninfected wounds; and "moist" red and yellow wounds.

Advantages

- Absorb up to 20 times their weight
- Form a gel within the wound to maintain a moist wound environment
- Facilitate autolytic debridement
- Fill in dead space
- Are easy to apply and remove.

Disadvantages

- Aren't recommended for wounds with light exudate or dry eschar
- Can dehydrate the wound bed
- Require a secondary dressing.

HCPCS code overview

The HCPCS codes normally assigned to alginate wound covers are:

A6196 — pad size ≤ 16 sq. in.

A6197 — pad size > 16 sq. in. but ≤ 48 sq. in.

A6198 — pad size > 48 sq. in.

The HCPCS code normally assigned to alginate wound fillers is:

A6199 — wound filler, per 6 in.

Alginates

NEW PRODUCT
AlgiCell Calcium Alginate
Dumex Medical

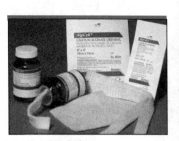

How supplied
Disc: 1″, 2″, 4″
Pad: 2″ × 2″, 4″ × 4″
      4″ × 8″
Rope: ¾″ × 12″, ¾″ × 36″

Action
Highly absorptive soft, white, sterile calcium alginate dressings, which form a soft gel in contact with wound fluids to maintain a moist environment.

Indications
For use as a primary dressing in the management of moderately to highly exudating partial- and full-thickness wounds. Rope may be used for deep wound packing to fill wound. Discs may be used for smaller wounds such as biopsy sites.

Contraindications
- Contraindicated for third-degree burns.
- Contraindicated for surgical implantation.

Application
- Cleanse wound with PrimaDerm Dermal Cleanser or saline solution according to facility policy.
- Apply AlgiCell to the wound bed.
- Loosely pack deeper wounds.
- Cover with an appropriate secondary dressing.

Removal
- Remove the secondary dressing.
- Gently rinse to remove remaining gel.
- Reapply daily or as indicated by amount of exudate and facility policy.

AlgiDERM Calcium Alginate Dressing or Packing

Bard Medical Division, C.R. Bard, Inc.

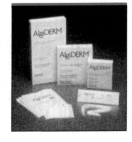

How supplied
Sheet: 5 × 5 cm, 9.5 × 9.5 cm; A6196
    10 × 20 cm; A6197
Rope: 2 g (30 cm); A6199

Action
AlgiDERM Calcium Alginate Dressing or Packing is a soft, sterile, nonwoven pad composed of fibers of pure calcium alginate. This highly absorbent alginate packing conforms to wound shape and interacts with exudate—wicking it away from the wound surface and into the packing—to form a soft gel that maintains a moist environment.

Indications
To manage pressure ulcers (stages 2, 3, and 4), partial- and full-thickness wounds, leg ulcers, abrasions, lacerations, donor sites, and superficial burns. Also used in the treatment of tunneling wounds, infected and noninfected wounds, red and yellow wound beds, and wounds with moderate to heavy drainage.

Contraindications
- Contraindicated for third-degree burns and nondraining wounds.
- Contraindicated in patients with known hypersensitivity to calcium alginate, although such sensitivity hasn't been reported to date.
- Should not be used with alkaline solutions.

Application
- Before applying AlgiDERM, debride necrotic tissue and eschar, then carefully cleanse the wound site with Biolex Wound Cleanser or normal saline solution. Don't dry the wound. Exudate must be present for dressing to gel.
- Before applying the dressing to a dry or lightly exudating wound, soak the dressing with saline solution.
- Apply AlgiDERM to the wound site and cover it with a secondary dressing, such as gauze, film dressing, or hydrocolloid.

Alginates

Removal

- Change the dressing when it becomes saturated with exudate or as follows. A heavily exudating wound may require frequent dressing changes; moderately to heavily exudating wounds require dressing changes every 2 to 4 days or as directed by the primary care provider.
- Don't leave the dressing in place for more than 7 days.
- Carefully remove the secondary dressing, according to the directions on the package insert for that product.
- Remove the dressing.
- Gently irrigate the wound with Biolex Wound Cleanser or normal saline solution to remove the residual gel without disrupting the delicate granulation tissue.
- Prepare and redress the moist wound site with new packing, then cover it with a secondary dressing.

AlgiSite M

Smith & Nephew, Inc.
Wound Management Division

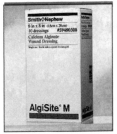

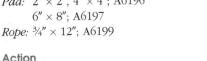

How supplied
Pad: 2" × 2", 4" × 4"; A6196
6" × 8"; A6197
Rope: ¾" × 12"; A6199

Action

AlgiSite M dressings create and maintain a moist wound environment, enabling epithelial cells to migrate freely across the wound surface. When gelled, AlgiSite M assists in promoting the passage of water vapor, oxygen, and carbon dioxide to maintain the hydrophilic environment.

Indications

To manage partial- and full-thickness wounds with moderate to heavy exudate, such as leg ulcers, pressure ulcers (stages 3 and 4), diabetic foot ulcers, and surgical wounds.

Contraindications

Contraindicated for third-degree burns and for wounds that don't produce enough exudate to cause the alginate to gel.

Application

- Cleanse the wound with normal saline solution or an appropriate wound cleanser.
- Choose a dressing that is slightly larger than the wound. Press the dressing into the wound so that it makes contact with the wound bed. The dressing should cover the entire wound surface, but it shouldn't extend beyond the edges. Cut off extra dressing or fold it over the wound.
- If the wound is deep and undermined, use the rope dressing. Loosely pack the rope into the wound, making sure the entire wound surface is covered.
- Cover the packing with an appropriate dressing. The dressing shouldn't block evaporation of wound exudate from the upper surface of the gel.

Removal

Change dressings daily if the wound is heavily draining or exudate begins to pool on the wound surface.

Alginates

CarboFlex Odor Control Dressing
ConvaTec

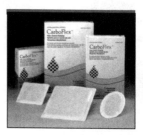

How supplied
Pad: 4″ × 4″; A6196
3″ × 6″ oval, 6″ × 8″; A6197

Action
CarboFlex is a sterile nonadhesive dressing with an absorbent wound contact layer (containing alginate and hydrocolloid), an activated charcoal central pad, and a smooth water-resistant top layer.

Indications
To manage acute and chronic wounds. May be used as a primary dressing for shallow wounds or as a secondary dressing over wound fillers for deeper wounds. May also be used on infected malodorous wounds under medical supervision together with appropriate therapy and frequent monitoring of the wound.

Contraindications
Contraindicated in patients with a known sensitivity to the dressing or its components.

Application
- If required, debride the wound and remove necrotic tissue. Cleanse the wound site, rinse well, and dry the surrounding skin.
- Don't cut the dressing.
- Choose a dressing that is larger than the wound area to ensure that the dressing overlaps the wound edge by at least 1¼″ (3.2 cm). For shallow wounds, the dressing may be placed directly onto the wound as a primary dressing; for cavity wounds, CarboFlex can be laid over a wound filler or gel as a secondary dressing.
- Place the fibrous (nonshiny) surface on the wound or cavity filler.
- Secure CarboFlex in place over the wound with tape or other appropriate material. The wound contact layer absorbs exudate and forms a soft gel.

Removal

- Change the dressing when clinically indicated, when exudate strike-through to the top layer occurs, or when the odor is no longer being absorbed. With noninfected malodorous wounds, CarboFlex may be left undisturbed for up to 3 days. If the wound is infected, CarboFlex should be changed more frequently.
- Carefully lift the dressing away from the wound by grasping it at one corner.

Alginates

CarraGinate High G Calcium Alginate Wound Dressing with Acemannan Hydrogel
Carrington Laboratories, Inc.

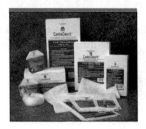

How supplied
Pad: 2″ × 2″, 4″ × 4″; A6196
4″ × 8″; A6197
Rope: 14″; A6199

Action
CarraGinate is a nonwoven, preservative-free, nontoxic absorptive dressing with Acemannan Hydrogel manufactured from seaweed.

Indications
To manage pressure ulcers, diabetic ulcers, venous ulcers, arterial ulcers, traumatic wounds, dermal lesions, donor sites, and partial- and full-thickness wounds with moderate to heavy wound exudate.

Contraindications
- Contraindicated for surgical implantation.
- Contraindicated for third-degree burns.

Application
- Flush the wound with a suitable wound cleanser, such as CarraKlenz, UltraKlenz, or MicroKlenz.
- Apply the dressing and cover it with a secondary dressing, such as CarraFilm or CarraSmart Film.

Removal
When changing, rinse away the remaining gel with a suitable wound cleanser, such as CarraKlenz, UltraKlenz, or MicroKlenz.

CarraSorb H Calcium Alginate Wound Dressing
Carrington Laboratories, Inc.

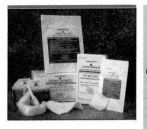

Alginates

How supplied
Pad: 2″ × 2″, 4″ × 4″; A6196
Rope: 12″ (30 cm); A6199

Action
CarraSorb H is a nonwoven, preservative-free, nontoxic absorptive dressing manufactured from seaweed. A soft gel forms as calcium in the alginate exchanges with sodium in the exudate. This sterile primary wound dressing insulates, absorbs, and fills in dead space.

Indications
To manage pressure ulcers (stages 3 and 4), arterial ulcers, venous ulcers, diabetic ulcers, donor sites, traumatic wounds, and dermal lesions. May also be used on tunneling wounds, wounds with undermining or sinus tracts, wounds with necrotic tissue and exudate, infected and noninfected wounds, wounds with moderate to heavy exudate, wounds with serosanguineous drainage, and red or yellow wounds.

Contraindications
- Contraindicated for surgical implantation.
- Contraindicated for third-degree burns.

Application
- Flush the wound with a suitable wound cleanser, such as UltraKlenz Wound Cleanser, CarraKlenz Wound Cleanser, or MicroKlenz Antiseptic Wound Cleanser.
- Apply the dressing to a moist wound bed; loosely pack it into deep wounds to allow room for expansion as it absorbs drainage. Use rope packing in undermined or tunneled areas.
- Cover the dressing with a secondary dressing, such as gauze, CarraFilm, or CarraSmart Film.

Removal
- Change the dressing according to the wound condition and amount of exudate or as directed by the primary care provider.

In general, a heavily draining wound may require one or two changes per day. As drainage decreases, gradually reduce the number of changes to once every 2 to 3 days.

- Remove the secondary dressing and nongelled CarraSorb H dressing.
- Rinse away any remaining gel residue with gentle irrigation.

Comfeel SeaSorb Alginate
Coloplast Corporation

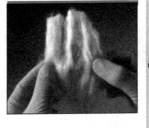

Alginates

How supplied
Dressing: 1½″ × 2½″, 4″ × 4″;
A6196
Rope: 16″; A6199

Action
Comfeel SeaSorb is a sterile, fiber-free, highly absorbent dressing composed of a xerogel of calcium-sodium alginate. On contact with wound exudate, the dressing forms a moist gel through a process of ion exchange. Comfeel SeaSorb dressing is easy to apply and remains intact after absorbing exudate, allowing one-piece removal.

Indications
To manage wounds with heavy exudate, such as leg ulcers and pressure ulcers. May also be used in clinically infected wounds, for which concurrent systemic antibiotic therapy may be given if indicated.

Contraindications
- Contraindicated for dry wounds and third-degree burns.
- Contraindicated for deep, undermined ulcers in which wound edges are at risk for collapsing.
- Contraindicated in patients allergic to one or more of the components.
- Consult the primary care provider before using this product on wounds with a high risk of infection or on lesions caused by syphilis, tuberculosis, leprosy, or cancer.
- Comfeel SeaSorb dressing must be removed before the start of long-term radiation treatment (with X-rays, ultrasound, diathermy, or microwaves).

Application
- Choose a dressing large enough to allow an overlap of ⅜″ (1 cm) onto the surrounding skin. The Comfeel SeaSorb dressing may be cut to size if necessary.

Alginates

- Apply the Comfeel SeaSorb dressing so that the printed side of the dressing is up and the nonprinted side is in contact with the skin surface.
- Use a secondary dressing, such as Biatain Foam Dressing or a semipermeable film dressing.

Removal

- Change when the dressing is saturated with exudate and has reached maximum absorption capacity.
- Change every 7 days, or more often if necessary. Dressing change may be required every day for the first few days. As granulation occurs, however, exudation decreases, and fewer changes are needed.

CURASORB
CURASORB Zinc
Kendall Healthcare Products
Company

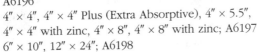

How supplied
Pad: 2″ × 2″, 4″ × 4″, 4″ × 4″ Plus
(Extra Absorptive), 2″ × 2″
with zinc, 4″ × 4″ with zinc;
A6196
4″ × 4″, 4″ × 4″ Plus (Extra Absorptive), 4″ × 5.5″,
4″ × 4″ with zinc, 4″ × 8″, 4″ × 8″ with zinc; A6197
6″ × 10″, 12″ × 24″; A6198
Rope: 12″, 24″, 36″, 12″ with zinc; A6199

Action
CURASORB and CURASORB Zinc absorb large volumes of exudate and maintain a moist wound surface.

Indications
To manage wounds with moderate to large amounts of exudate. May also be used on pressure ulcers (stages 2, 3, and 4), tunneling wounds, infected and noninfected wounds, full-thickness wounds, and red or yellow wounds.

Contraindications
- Contraindicated for wounds with dry eschar.
- Contraindicated for wounds with minimal exudate.

Application
- Apply the dressing dry.
- Cover the dressing with a secondary dressing.

Removal
Remove the dressing when strike-through to the secondary dressing occurs.

Alginates

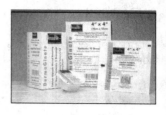

NEW PRODUCT
DermaGinate
DermaRite Industries

How supplied
Pad: 4″ × 4″
Rope: 12″

Action
DermaGinate is a sterile, nonwoven dressing of calcium-sodium alginate fiber designed to promote and maintain a moist wound environment. The fibers absorb wound exudates to form a firm, viscous gel-fiber material.

Indications
To manage infected and noninfected wounds, pressure ulcers, venous ulcers, and diabetic ulcers. May be used for partial- and full-thickness wounds, dermal lesions, tunneling wounds, and wounds with moderate to heavy drainage.

Contraindications
- Contraindicated for dry to lightly exudating wounds.
- Contraindicated for third-degree burns.
- Contraindicated in patients with known sensitivity to calcium alginate materials.

Application
- Cleanse the wound by irrigating with DermaKlenz solution.
- Pat dry surrounding areas.
- Apply dressing to the wound surface or wound bed; if wound is deep, pack DermaGinate rope gently at site.
- Cover the dressing with a secondary dressing and secure it.

Removal
- Remove the secondary dressing.
- For wounds with minimal exudate, dampen the dressing with normal saline solution to loosen, then lift.
- If necessary, gently rinse away the remaining gel or dressing fibers.

Hyperion Advanced Alginate Dressing
Hyperion Medical, Inc.

How supplied
Pad: 2″ × 2″, 4″ × 4″; A6196
   4″ × 8″; A6197
Rope: 12″; A6199

Action
Hyperion Advanced Alginate Dressings are used to manage exudate. The alginate dressing forms a gel when in contact with exudate to maintain a moist wound environment.

Indications
Indicated for partial- and full-thickness wounds, wounds with moderate to heavy exudate, wounds with tunneling or sinus tracts, wounds with necrotic tissue and exudate, and infected and noninfected wounds.

Contraindications
Not recommended for wounds with light exudate or dur eschar.

Application
- Cleanse the wound with normal saline solution or according to facility policy.
- Apply the dressing dry, avoiding periwound area, and cover with a secondary dressing.

Removal
- Carefully remove the dressing from the wound bed.
- Irrigate the wound with wound cleanser.

KALGINATE Calcium Alginate Wound Dressing
DeRoyal

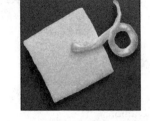

How supplied
Pad: 2″ × 2″, 4″ × 4″; A6196
4″ × 8″; A6197
Rope: 6″, 12″; A6199

Action
KALGINATE is a sterile, nonwoven, calcium alginate dressing of heavy fiber. Thick and substantial, it provides maximum absorption of exudate with minimal dressing changes. It allows for gaseous exchange, can be layered or packed for absorbency, and maintains its shape and integrity during removal.

Indications
To manage pressure ulcers (stages 3 and 4); full-thickness wounds; tunneling, infected, and draining wounds; and wounds with moderate to heavy exudate.

Contraindications
- Contraindicated for nondraining wounds.
- Contraindicated for third-degree burns.

Application
- Cleanse the wound area with normal saline solution.
- Place KALGINATE pad or rope into the wound, packing deep wounds loosely.
- Cover the dressing with an absorptive cover dressing, and secure in place.

Removal
- Change the dressing when the outer dressing is saturated with drainage.
- Remove the outer dressing.
- Irrigate the wound with normal saline solution, and lift the dressing from the wound bed.

KALTOSTAT Wound Dressing
ConvaTec

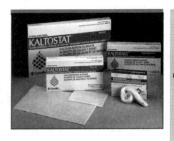

How supplied
Pad: 2″ × 2″, 3″ × 4¾″; A6196
4″ × 8″; A6197
6″ × 9½″, 12″ × 24″;
A6198
Rope: 2 g; A6199

Action
KALTOSTAT Wound Dressing is a soft, sterile, nonwoven dressing of calcium-sodium alginate fiber. The alginate fibers absorb wound exudate or normal saline solution and form a firm gel-fiber mat. The mat maintains a moist, warm environment at the wound-dressing interface and allows removal of the dressing with little or no damage to newly formed tissue.

Indications
To manage pressure ulcers, venous stasis ulcers, arterial ulcers, diabetic ulcers, donor sites, abrasions, lacerations, superficial burns, postoperative incisions, and other external wounds inflicted by trauma. May also be used for nosebleeds, dental extraction sites, and postoperative wound debridement.

Contraindications
- Contraindicated for third-degree burns.
- Not intended to control heavy bleeding.
- Not intended for use as a surgical sponge.

Application
- Debride the wound of excessive necrotic tissue and eschar, and irrigate with an appropriate cleansing solution.
- Trim the dressing to the exact size of the wound.
- For heavily exuding wounds, apply the dressing dry.
- For lightly exuding wounds or nonexuding wounds, place the dressing on the wound and moisten it with normal saline solution. Reapply normal saline solution as necessary to maintain the gel.
- Apply an appropriate secondary dressing to secure the dressing.

- To effect hemostasis on bleeding wounds, apply the dressing to the bleeding area. Remove the dressing after bleeding has stopped, then apply a new dressing.

Removal

- Change the dressing on heavily exuding wounds when strikethrough to the secondary dressing occurs or whenever clinical practice dictates. Depending on the wound, leave the dressing in place for up to 7 days.
- Removal is easy because the dressing forms a gel at the wound-dressing interface.
- To remove a dressing from a nonexuding or lightly exuding wound, saturate the dressing with normal saline solution. If the gel has dried, rehydrate it by saturating it with normal saline solution; softening may take several hours if severe drying has occurred.
- Cleanse the wound site before applying a new dressing; any alginate fibers and gels inadvertently left in the wound will be absorbed by the body.

Maxorb CMC/Alginate Dressing
Medline Industries, Inc.

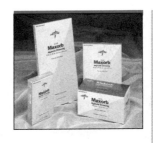

How supplied
Pad: 2″ × 2″, 4″ × 4″; A6196
    4″ × 8″; A6197
Rope: 12″ (2 gm); A6199
    Dressings are supplied in sterile form in single pouches or a lidded tray. The lidded tray package on the rope version is important because it keeps the fibers from compressing. As a result, fluid-handling capacity is increased.

Action
Maxorb CMC/Alginate Dressing's nonwoven alginate and carboxymethylcellulose fiber combination reacts with wound exudate to form a gel, providing a moist healing environment. The added presence of carboxymethylcellulose in Maxorb improves the wicking and fluid-handling ability of this dressing and increases wet strength. Because the product doesn't wick exudate laterally, it reduces the potential for damage to delicate periwound tissue.

Indications
To manage partial- and full-thickness wounds with moderate to heavy exudate, including venous stasis ulcers, pressure ulcers (stages 2, 3, and 4), arterial ulcers, diabetic ulcers, donor sites, lacerations, abrasions, postsurgical incisions, and second-degree burns. May also be used for infected and noninfected wounds, tunneling wounds, wounds with serosanguineous or purulent drainage, and red, yellow, or black wounds.

Contraindications
- Contraindicated for third-degree burns.
- Not intended for use as a surgical sponge.

Application
- Cleanse the wound with normal saline solution or an appropriate wound cleanser, such as Skintegrity Wound Cleanser.

Alginates

- Apply the dressing to a moist wound bed. The dressing doesn't need to be trimmed to fit the wound bed because it won't wick fluid laterally. Loosely pack deep or tunneling wounds.
- Cover with an appropriate secondary dressing such as Stratasorb Composite Dressing.

Removal

- Change dressing when strike-through to the secondary dressing occurs, every 2 to 5 days, or as directed by the primary care provider.
- The gelatinous pad may be easily lifted away in one piece from the wound bed, making dressing changes easier.
- Remove the secondary dressing as well as gelled and non-gelled Maxorb dressing.
- Irrigate with normal saline solution or another appropriate solution, such as Skintegrity Wound Cleanser, to remove any remaining gel.
- If the dressing is dry at time of removal, moisten it with saline or wound cleanser before removal. This may indicate the need to consider replacing this type dressing with a moistening, hydrogel product instead.

Melgisorb
Mölnlycke Health Care

How supplied
Pad: 2″ × 2″, 4″ × 4″; A6196
        4″ × 8″; A6197
Rope: 12½″; A6199

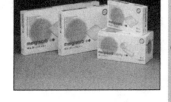

Action
Melgisorb is a hydrophilic alginate that absorbs wound exudate. As the alginate fibers absorb exudate, they form a moist gel.

Indications
To manage infected and noninfected wounds with moderate to heavy exudate, such as pressure ulcers, venous ulcers, arterial ulcers, diabetic ulcers, donor sites, postoperative wounds, and dermal lesions.

Contraindications
- Contraindicated for dry wounds.
- Contraindicated on third-degree burns.
- Not recommended for surgical implantation.

Application
- Cleanse and flush the wound with normal saline solution, then dry the healthy surrounding skin.
- Apply Melgisorb dry to a moist wound bed. For shallow wounds, choose the correct size of the flat dressing to cover the entire wound. For deep or tunneling wounds, choose and cut an appropriate length of rope and pack loosely.
- Cover with an appropriate secondary dressing.

Removal
Gently flush the wound with normal saline solution or another appropriate solution. Any nongelled Melgisorb can be moistened with saline and removed.

Alginates

Restore CalciCare Wound Care Dressing
Hollister Incorporated

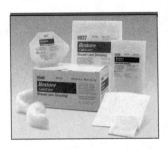

How supplied
Pad: 2" × 2", 4" × 4"
          4" × 8"
Rope: 12" (2 g)

Action
Restore CalciCare Wound Care Dressings are absorptive and made from calcium and sodium alginate. They conform to the wound and form a gel when in contact with exudate, creating a moist interface with the wound, which provides a moist healing environment.

Indications
To manage partial- and full-thickness wounds with moderate to heavy exudate, including pressure ulcers (stages 1, 2, 3, and 4), arterial and venous stasis ulcers, postsurgical incisions, donor sites, trauma wounds, diabetic ulcers, and dermal lesions.

Contraindications
- Contraindicated for dry to lightly exuding wounds.
- Contraindicated in patients with known sensitivity to calcium alginate or with other known allergic conditions.

Application
- Prepare the wound according to facility policy, or as directed. Make sure that the skin is clean and dry.
- Measure the wound with a wound-measuring guide.
- Apply the dressing to the wound surface. Loosely pack deep wounds with rope dressing.
- Cover the dressing with a secondary dressing and secure it.

Removal
- Remove the secondary dressing according to facility policy.
- Remove the Restore CalciCare dressing.
- If necessary, gently rinse away the remaining gel or dressing fibers, using Restore Wound Cleanser or normal saline solution.

Sorbsan Topical Wound Dressing
Bertek (Dow Hickam)
Pharmaceuticals

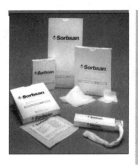

Alginates

How supplied
Pad: 2" × 2", 3" × 3", 4" × 4"; A6196
    4" × 8"; A6197
Rope: 12"; A6199

Action
When in contact with wound exudate, the surface of Sorbsan Topical Wound Dressing forms a soft, hydrocolloid gel. This gel maintains a moist environment at the wound surface that is conducive to granulation tissue formation, more rapid epithelialization, and healing. The gel provides a more adherent interface with the wound bed, allows for exchange of gases to and from the wound surface, is strongly hydrophilic, wicks exudate into the wound dressing, and provides a physical barrier.

Indications
To manage infected and noninfected wounds, pressure ulcers, venous ulcers, arterial ulcers, diabetic ulcers, donor sites, and other bleeding surface wounds. May also be used for partial- and full-thickness wounds, dermal lesions, traumatic injuries, incisions, tunneling wounds, wounds with moderate to heavy drainage, wounds with serosanguineous or purulent drainage, and red, yellow, or (moist) black wounds.

Contraindications
Contraindicated for third-degree burns.

Application
- Cleanse the wound by irrigating with normal saline solution.
- Blot dry the skin surrounding the wound.
- Remove the dressing from the package, and apply it to the moist wound surface.
- Cover the dressing with an appropriate secondary dressing.

Alginates

Removal

- Frequency of dressing changes depends on the volume of exudate. Change the dressing when the secondary dressing shows signs of strike-through or when Sorbsan has totally gelled. A heavily draining wound may require one or two dressing changes each day for the first few days. The average frequency of dressing change is daily to every other day.
- As the wound begins to heal and drainage decreases, change the dressing every 2 or 3 days or as directed by the primary care provider.
- Gently lift and remove the secondary dressing.
- For wounds with minimal exudate, dampen the dressing with normal saline solution before removal, if necessary.
- After removing the dressing, irrigate the wound with normal saline solution to wash away the remaining gel without disrupting granulation tissue.
- Redress the moist wound site as directed previously.

3M Tegagen HI Alginate Dressing

3M Tegagen HI Alginate Dressing
3M Health Care

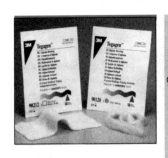

Alginates

How supplied
HI (High Integrity)
Pad: 2″ × 2″, 4″ × 4″; A6196
4″ × 8″; A6197
Rope: 12″; A6199
HG (High Gelling)
Pad: 2″ × 2″, 4″ × 4″; A6196
4″ × 8″; A6197
Rope: 12″; A6199

Action
3M Tegagen is a gel-forming, absorbent, versatile alginate, which provides for optimal wound healing. 3M Tegagen HI offers high integrity for quick dressing changes. 3M Tegagen HG offers high gelling properties, which may be preferable for gentle removal of the dressing from fragile tissue.

Indications
To manage wounds with moderate to heavy exudate, pressure ulcers, arterial ulcers, venous ulcers, diabetic ulcers, trauma wounds, and other dermal lesions.

Contraindications
- Contraindicated for surgical implantation.
- Contraindicated for third-degree burns.

Application
Pad:
- Moisten the wound site with normal saline solution or other sterile irrigation solution, according to facility policy. Dry the periwound skin.
- If the patient's skin is fragile or wound drainage may contact the periwound skin, apply 3M No Sting Barrier Film around the wound.

- Select the appropriate dressing size for the wound. Tegagen HG and HI alginate dressing may be trimmed to fit the wound site.
- Apply the dressing to the wound bed with minimal overlap to the periwound skin.
- Loosely pack deep wounds.
- Cover with an appropriate secondary dressing.

Rope:

- Fluff the rope dressing as needed for light packing.
- Ensure that the dressing lightly contacts all wound surfaces, including areas of undermining.
- Loosely pack deep wounds by fluffing and layering the dressing back and forth into the wound.
- Cover the rope dressing with an appropriate secondary dressing.
- Extend the cover dressing at least 1″ (2.5 cm) beyond the edge of the wound.

Removal

- Remove secondary dressing and nongelled alginate dressing. Rinse away remaining gel with gentle irrigation.
- If the dressing appears dry, saturate with sterile saline to aid in removal.
- Dressing may be removed using sterile forceps or gentle irrigation.

Collagens

Action
Collagen, the most abundant protein in the body, is fibrous and insoluble and is produced by fibroblasts. Its fibers are found in connective tissues, including skin, bones, ligaments, and cartilage. During wound healing, collagen encourages the deposition and organization of newly formed collagen fibers and granulation tissue in the wound bed. It also stimulates new tissue development and wound debridement, creating an environment conducive to healing. Collagen dressings are manufactured in sheets, pads, particles, and gels.

Indications
Collagen dressings may be used as primary dressings for partial- and full-thickness wounds, infected and noninfected wounds, tunneling wounds, wounds with minimal to heavy exudate (depending on the form of collagen dressing), skin grafts, donor sites, and red or yellow wounds.

Advantages
- Are absorbent
- Maintain a moist, wound-healing environment
- May be used in combination with topical agents
- Conform well to a wound surface
- Are nonadherent
- Are easy to apply and remove.

Disadvantages
- Aren't recommended for third-degree burns
- Aren't recommended for black wounds
- Require a secondary dressing.

HCPCS code overview
The HCPCS codes normally assigned to collagen dressings are:
A6021 — pad size ≤ 16 sq. in.
A6022 — pad size > 16 sq. in. but ≤ 48 sq. in.
A6023 — pad size > 48 sq. in.

The HCPCS code normally assigned to collagen wound fillers is:
A6024 — wound filler, per 6 in.

FIBRACOL PLUS Collagen Wound Dressing with Alginate

Johnson & Johnson Wound Management
Division of ETHICON, Inc.

How supplied
Pad: 2" × 2"; A6021
$\qquad$ 4" × 4⅜", 4" × 8¾"; A6022
Rope: ¾" × ¾" × 15¾"; A6024

Action
FIBRACOL PLUS Collagen Wound Dressing with Alginate combines the strength and structural support of collagen and the gel-forming properties of alginate into a soft, highly absorbent, and conformable topical wound dressing. FIBRACOL PLUS Dressing is made of 90% collagen and 10% alginate. It maintains a physiologically moist microenvironment at the wound surface that is conductive to granulation tissue formation and epithelialization and enables healing to proceed at a rapid rate. FIBRACOL PLUS Dressing is versatile as a primary wound dressing. It can be cut to the exact size of the wound, multilayered to manage deep wounds, and used in combination with either a semiocclusive or a nonocclusive secondary dressing.

Indications
To manage partial- and full-thickness wounds, including pressure ulcers, venous ulcers, ulcers caused by mixed vascular etiologies, diabetic ulcers, second-degree burns, donor sites and other bleeding surface wounds, abrasions, traumatic wounds healing by secondary intention, and dehisced surgical incisions.

FIBRACOL PLUS Dressing may be used when visible signs of infection are present in the wound area only when proper medical treatment addresses the underlying cause. FIBRACOL PLUS Dressing may be used under compression therapy with primary care provider supervision.

Contraindications
- Contraindicated for wounds with active vasculitis.
- Contraindicated for third-degree burns.
- Not recommended in patients with known senstivity to collagen or alginates.

Collagens

Application

- Debride when necessary.
- Irrigate wound site with normal saline solution.
- Cut dressing to the general size of the wound with sterile scissors.
- For heavily exuding wounds, apply to the wound bed.
- Loosely pack deep wounds.
- For wounds with minimal exudate, apply to a moistened wound bed to initiate gel-forming process.
- Cover with appropriate secondary dressing based on the amount of exudate, such as TIELLE Hydropolymer Adhesive Dressing for low to moderately exuding wounds and TIELLE PLUS Hydropolymer Adhesive Dressing for moderately to heavily exuding wounds.

Removal

- Reapply the dressing when it's saturated or whenever good wound care practice dictates a change. Wounds with heavy exudate may require daily or twice-daily dressing changes; wounds with moderate exudate require less-frequent changes (every 2 to 4 days or as directed by the primary care provider).
- Remove secondary dressing.
- Cleanse wound with normal saline.

Collagens

Kollagen-Medifil Pads
BioCore Medical Technologies, Inc.

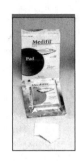

How supplied
Sterile Pad: 2″ × 3″, 3″ × 4″; A6021

Action
Kollagen-Medifil Pads are made of type I bovine collagen particles encased in a nonadherent pouch. Kollagen-Medifil Pads are highly absorbent and are excellent packing materials.

Indications
To manage pressure ulcers (stages 3 and 4), partial- and full-thickness wounds (except third-degree burns), cavity wounds, infected and noninfected wounds, wounds with drainage, red or yellow wound beds, and rimmed and undermined wounds.

Contraindications
- Contraindicated for dehydrated (dry) wounds.
- Contraindicated in patients who are sensitive to products of bovine origin.

Application
- Place the Kollagen-Medifil Pad on the wound bed.
- Allow at least ¼″ to ½″ (0.6 to 1.3 cm) space between the Kollagen-Medifil Pad and the sides of the wound to allow for expansion of the Medifil Particles. Don't pack tightly.
- Cover with an absorbent dressing, such as conventional gauze, abdominal pads, or a specialty absorbent dressing.

Removal
- Change the secondary dressing daily and the Kollagen-Medifil Pad every 1 to 3 days, depending on the amount of drainage.
- Remove the secondary dressing. If it has adhered to the wound, irrigate with sterile normal saline solution until the dressing loosens. Lift it gently.
- Remove the Kollagen-Medifil Pad.
- Irrigate the wound with sterile normal saline solution to cleanse the wound thoroughly.
- When excessive drainage has resolved, discontinue the Kollagen-Medifil Pad, and switch to Kollagen-Medifil II Particles.

Collagens

Kollagen-SkinTemp Sheets
BioCore Medical Technologies, Inc.

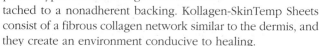

How supplied
Sheet: 2″ × 3″, 3″ × 4″; A6021
        8″ × 12″; A6023

Action
Kollagen-SkinTemp Sheets are made of a
porous type I bovine collagen membrane attached to a nonadherent backing. Kollagen-SkinTemp Sheets
consist of a fibrous collagen network similar to the dermis, and
they create an environment conducive to healing.

Indications
To manage chronic wounds (such as stage 2 pressure ulcers
and venous, arterial, and diabetic ulcers), surgical wounds (including donor sites and grafts and wounds resulting from Mohs',
laser, or podiatric surgery), surgical wound dehiscence, and
traumatic wounds (including abrasions, lacerations, partial-thickness burns, and skin tears).

Contraindications
Contraindicated in patients who are sensitive to products of
bovine origin.

Application
- For minimally draining or dehydrated wounds, hydrate
  Kollagen-SkinTemp with sterile normal saline solution before
  applying it. Also use a nonadherent secondary dressing, such
  as an impregnated gauze, a hydrocolloid, a hydrogel sheet,
  or a semipermeable film or foam.
- For moderately draining wounds, use Kollagen-SkinTemp in
  dry form.
- Apply the porous collagen side of Kollagen-SkinTemp to the
  wound. After the Kollagen-SkinTemp has been positioned on
  the wound, remove the nonadherent backing.
- If the periwound is at risk for maceration, use sterile scissors
  to cut the Kollagen-SkinTemp to fit the wound.
- Cover Kollagen-SkinTemp with a nonadherent secondary
  dressing to maintain a moist wound environment.
- Use a nonadherent secondary dressing, such as an impregnated gauze, a hydrocolloid, a hydrogel sheet, or a semipermeable film or foam.

Collagens

- Leave Kollagen-SkinTemp in place on noninfected wounds for a maximum of 7 days. This is a clinical decision based on the assessment of the patient.

Removal

- Remove the secondary dressing and any remaining Kollagen-SkinTemp.
- If Kollagen-SkinTemp has adhered to the wound, irrigate it with sterile normal saline solution. Lift it very gently.
- If Kollagen-SkinTemp adheres to the wound after irrigation, don't remove it. Rehydrate it with sterile normal saline solution and dress it with an appropriate secondary dressing.
- If the dressing has to be changed more than once a day because of excessive drainage, discontinue Kollagen-SkinTemp and switch to Kollagen-Medifil II Particles.

Collagens

Composites

Action
Composite dressings combine two or more physically distinct products and are manufactured as a single dressing with several functions. Features must include a bacterial barrier; an absorptive layer other than an alginate, foam, hydrocolloid, or hydrogel; a semiadherent or nonadherent property for covering the wound; and an adhesive border.

Indications
Composite dressings may be used as primary or secondary dressings for partial- and full-thickness wounds with minimal to heavy exudate, healthy granulation tissue, or necrotic tissue (slough or moist eschar) or mixed wounds (granulation and necrotic tissue).

Advantages
- May facilitate autolytic debridement
- Allow for exchange of moisture vapor
- Mold well
- May be used on infected wounds
- Are easy to apply and remove
- Include an adhesive border

Disadvantages
- Require a border of intact skin for anchoring the dressing

HCPCS code overview
The HCPCS codes normally assigned to composite dressings without an adhesive border are:

A6200 — pad size ≤ 16 sq. in.
A6201 — pad size > 16 sq. in., but ≤ 48 sq. in.
A6202 — pad size > 48 sq. in.

The HCPCS codes normally assigned to composite dressings with an adhesive border are:

A6203 — pad size ≤ 16 sq. in.
A6204 — pad size > 16 sq. in., but ≤ 48 sq. in.
A6205 — pad size > 48 sq. in.

Composites

Alldress
Mölnlycke Health Care

How supplied
Multilayered absorbent cover dressing: 4″ × 4″, 6″ × 6″; A6203
                        6″ × 8″; A6204

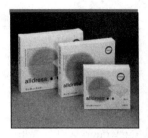

Action
Alldress is a multilayered sterile wound dressing; each layer serves a purpose. A low-adherent layer protects the wound surface. An absorbent layer wicks away excess exudate and debris, minimizing exposure of intact skin to moisture. A nonwoven adhesive tape holds the primary dressing securely in place, and a semiocclusive layer keeps external contaminants out and prevents strike-through while maintaining a moist, wound-healing environment. Alldress is waterproof.

Indications
For use as a cover dressing through all phases of healing for pressure ulcers (stages 1, 2, 3, and 4); partial- and full-thickness wounds; tunneling wounds; infected and noninfected wounds; wounds with minimal, moderate, or heavy drainage; wounds with serosanguineous or purulent drainage; and red, yellow, or black wounds.

Contraindications
None provided by the manufacturer.

Application
- If necessary, gently irrigate or flush the wound with normal saline solution or another nonirritating solution.
- Gently blot excess saline solution in the wound with sterile gauze.
- Remove one side of the dressing's backing, and place the other side on the skin. Be careful not to stretch the dressing over the wound.
- Smooth the edges to ensure secure adhesion.

Removal
- Change the dressing when it's nearly saturated (soaking is visible through the outer surface of the dressing) or as required by the product.

Composites

NEW PRODUCT
CompDress Island Dressing
Dumex Medical
Pad: 2″ × 2″, 4″ × 4″, 4″ × 6″, 6″ × 6″, 4″ × 8″, 4″ × 10″,
     6″ × 8″, 4″ × 14″

Action
CompDress is a sterile multilayer dressing combining a non-adherent gauze pad contact layer with a dressing retention tape.

Indications
For use as a primary or secondary dressing to manage acute and chronic lightly to moderately draining wounds.

Contraindications
None provided by the manufacturer.

Application
- Cleanse the wound with PrimaDerm Dermal Cleanser or solution.
- Pat dry the skin adjacent to the wound.
- Peel back the dressing's backing, and position dressing over the wound.
- Smooth the dressing edges to insure secure adhesion.

Removal
- Gently lift the edge of the dressing.
- Continue around the perimeter of the dressing until it lifts off easily.

Composites

COVADERM PLUS
DeRoyal

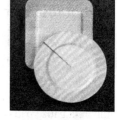

How supplied
Multilayered pad with fabric tape border: 1″ pad with 2″ tape, 1½″ pad with 2½″ tape, 2½″ pad with 4″ tape, 2″ × 7½″ pad with 4″ × 10″ tape, 4″ pad with 6″ tape, 2½″-diameter pad with 4″-diameter tape with 2″ radial slit; A6203 2″ × 11″ pad with 4″ × 14″ tape, 4″ × 6″ pad with 6″ × 8″ tape; A6204

Action
COVADERM PLUS is an adhesive barrier composite wound dressing that consists of a protective, nonadherent wound contact layer; a soft drainage absorption pad; a semiocclusive polyurethane film (to maintain moisture, prevent contamination, and allow vapor transmission); and a conformable adhesive tape border.

Indications
For use as a primary or secondary dressing to manage pressure ulcers (stages 1, 2, 3, and 4), leg ulcers, I.V. sites, chronic wounds, and surgical wounds. May also be used on partial- and full-thickness wounds, burns, tunneling wounds, infected and non-infected wounds, wounds with moderate drainage, wounds with serosanguineous or purulent drainage, and red, yellow, or black wounds. May also be used to cover orthopedic incisions and joint pins under casts.

Contraindications
None provided by the manufacturer.

Application
- Peel the dressing's backing from the center to expose the pad.
- Apply the pad over the cleansed wound, ensuring that adhesive tape doesn't touch the wound site.
- Remove the product's backing one side at a time, and smooth the dressing into place.

Removal
Carefully lift the edges of the tape, and peel off the dressing.

Composites

DuDress Film Top Island Dressing
Dumex Medical

How supplied
Pad: 4″ × 4″, 6″ × 6″, 6″ × 8″

Action
DuDress is a sterile multilayer dressing comprised of a nonadherent, gauze pad contact layer with a transparent film top layer.

Indications
For use as a primary or secondary dressing to manage acute and chronic lightly to moderately draining wounds. It's waterproof to allow bathing, reducing unnecessary dressing changes.

Contraindications
None provided by manufacturer.

Application
- Cleanse the wound with PrimaDerm Dermal Cleanser or saline solution.
- Pat dry the skin adjacent to the wound.
- Peel back the dressing's backing, and position the dressing over the wound.
- Smooth the dressing edges to insure secure adhesion.

Removal
- Lift the edge of the dressing.
- Gently stretch the dressing to facilitate removal.
- Continue around the perimeter of the dressing until it lifts off easily.

Composites

MPM Multi-Layered Dressing
MPM Medical, Inc.

How supplied
Pad: 4″ × 4″, 6″ × 6″; A6203
      6″ × 8″, 4″ × 14″; A6204

Action
MPM Multi-Layered Dressing is a nonadherent, absorbent island dressing with a protective adhesive backing that allows for moisture vapor transfer. The dressing provides a moist environment that facilitates wound healing.

Indications
To manage pressure ulcers (stages 1, 2, 3, and 4); partial- and full-thickness wounds, surgical incisions, dehisced incisions, tunneling wounds, infected and noninfected wounds, wounds with moderate to heavy serosanguineous and purulent drainage, and red, yellow, or black wounds.

Contraindications
None provided by the manufacturer.

Application
- Cleanse the wound with MPM Wound Cleanser or normal saline solution.
- Peel back and release the dressing's backing to expose the pad.
- Apply the pad over the wound, and finish removing the backing.
- Smooth the dressing into place.

Removal
Carefully lift the edge of the tape, and peel off the dressing.

Repel Wound Dressing
MPM Medical, Inc.

How supplied
Pad: 4″ × 4″; A6203
         6″ × 6″, 6″ × 8″; A6204

Action
Repel Wound Dressing is a nonadherent island dressing with a waterproof protective backing and an adhesive border that allows for moisture vapor transfer. Repel Wound Dressing maintains a moist wound environment that facilitates wound healing.

Indications
To manage pressure ulcers (stages 2, 3, and 4), venous stasis ulcers, partial- and full-thickness wounds, surgical incisions, tunneling wounds, infected and noninfected wounds, and moderately to heavily draining wounds.

Contraindications
None provided by the manufacturer.

Application
- Cleanse the wound with MPM Wound Cleanser or normal saline solution.
- Peel back the dressing's backing to expose the pad.
- Apply the pad over the wound, and finish removing the backing.
- Smooth the dressing into place.

Removal
Carefully lift the edge of the tape, and peel off the pad.

Composites

Stratasorb
Medline Industries, Inc.

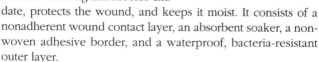

How supplied
Pad: 4″ × 4″; A6203
6″ × 6″, 6″ × 8″; A6204

Action
Stratasorb is a four-layer composite island dressing that absorbs exu-
date, protects the wound, and keeps it moist. It consists of a
nonadherent wound contact layer, an absorbent soaker, a nonwoven adhesive border, and a waterproof, bacteria-resistant
outer layer.

Indications
To manage pressure ulcers (stages 1, 2, 3, and 4), partial- and
full-thickness wounds, tunneling wounds, infected and noninfected wounds, wounds with minimal to heavy drainage,
wounds with serosanguineous or purulent drainage, and red,
yellow, or black wounds.

Contraindications
None provided by the manufacturer.

Application
- Cleanse the application site with normal saline solution or
  an appropriate cleanser. Dry the surrounding area to ensure
  that it's free from any greasy substance.
- Select the appropriate dressing size for the wound. Make sure
  the dressing extends 1¼″ to 1½″ (3.2 to 3.8 cm) beyond the
  wound so the dressing can attach to healthy tissue.
- Remove one side of the dressing's paper backing, and apply
  the exposed adhesive to the skin.
- Remove the second side of the paper backing, and apply the
  remaining adhesive, being careful not to stretch the dressing.

Removal
- Change the dressing as indicated by the wound's condition and
  the amount of exudate or as the primary dressing indicates.
- Lift the dressing by one edge and peel it back while holding
  the skin edge.
- Repeat cleansing procedure before applying a new dressing.

Composites

TELFA Adhesive Dressing
Kendall Health Care Products Company

How supplied
Pad: 2″ × 3″, 3″ × 4″

Action
TELFA Adhesive dressing is made of highly absorbent, non-woven cotton fabric on both sides. Adhesive strips keep the dressing intact. The nonadherent surface permits nontraumatic removal.

Indications
For use as a primary dressing on lightly draining wounds. May also be used on pressure ulcers (stages 1 and 2), partial-thickness wounds, infected and noninfected wounds, wounds with minimal drainage, and red wounds.

Contraindications
Contraindicated for heavily draining wounds.

Application
- Cleanse the wound with normal saline solution or a cleansing agent.
- Apply the dressing over the wound, and smooth the adhesive onto the periwound skin.

Removal
Gently remove the soiled dressing, taking care not to disturb the wound bed.

Composites

TELFA Island Dressing
Kendall Health Care Products
Company

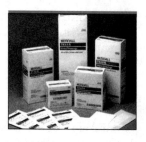

How supplied
Pad: 2″ × 3¾″, 4″ × 4″, 4″ × 5″,
       4″ × 8″, 4″ × 10″, 6″ × 6″;
       A6219
       4″ × 14″; A6220

Action
TELFA Island Dressing has a soft, nonwoven backing that conforms to the wound and seals all four sides. The dressing protects the wound from the external environment, and the nonadherent surface allows nontraumatic removal.

Indications
To manage lightly draining wounds and to act as a securing dressing for central of peripheral I.V. sites. May also be used on pressure ulcers (stages 1 and 2), infected and noninfected wounds, partial-thickness wounds, wounds with minimal drainage, and red wounds.

Contraindications
Contraindicated for heavily draining wounds.

Application
- Cleanse the wound with normal saline solution or a cleansing agent.
- Apply the dressing over the wound.
- Secure the dressing with an appropriate material, such as tape.

Removal
Gently remove the soiled dressing, taking care not to disturb the wound bed.

Composites

TELFA PLUS Island Dressing
Kendall Health Care Products Company

How supplied
Pad: 4″ × 6″; A6203
6″ × 7″, 6″ × 10″, 8″ × 8″; A6204

Action
TELFA PLUS Island Dressing absorbs moderate amounts of fluid, doesn't adhere to wounds, and provides a barrier to fluid and bacteria.

Indications
For use as a primary or secondary dressing and securing layer to manage surgical incisions, lacerations, peripheral and central I.V. line sites, pressure ulcers (stages 1, 2, and 3), partial-thickness wounds, stasis ulcers, arterial ulcers, and diabetic ulcers. May also be used for wounds with light to moderate drainage, noninfected wounds, and red wounds.

Contraindications
- Contraindicated for stage 4 pressure ulcers.
- Contraindicated for full-thickness wounds, tunneling wounds, infected wounds, and heavily draining wounds.

Application
- Cleanse the wound with a nontoxic cleansing solution, such as Constant Clens Wound Cleanser or normal saline solution.
- To remove excess cleanser or saline solution, gently pat the wound and surrounding skin with a sterile 4″ × 4″ gauze sponge. Be sure the surrounding skin is thoroughly dry to ensure a good seal between the skin and the dressing adhesive.
- Remove the dressing's release liners from the center out, position and apply the dressing over the wound, then smooth the adhesive borders to ensure contact.

Removal
Carefully peel back the island border and pad, taking care not to tear fragile skin or disturb the wound bed.

Composites

3M Medipore+Pad Soft Cloth Adhesive Wound Dressing
3M Health Care

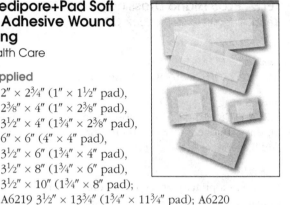

How supplied
Island: 2″ × 2¾″ (1″ × 1½″ pad),
       2⅜″ × 4″ (1″ × 2⅜″ pad),
       3½″ × 4″ (1¾″ × 2⅜″ pad),
       6″ × 6″ (4″ × 4″ pad),
       3½″ × 6″ (1¾″ × 4″ pad),
       3½″ × 8″ (1¾″ × 6″ pad),
       3½″ × 10″ (1¾″ × 8″ pad);
       A6219 3½″ × 13¾″ (1¾″ × 11¾″ pad); A6220

Action
3M Medipore+Pad Soft Cloth Adhesive Wound Dressing consists of a nonadherent pad bonded to a larger, soft cloth backing with a border of hypoallergenic, water-resistant adhesive.

Indications
To manage moderately exuding surgical incisions, lacerations, skin tears, abrasions, and burns. May also be used as a cover for I.V. catheter sites and as a secondary dressing over primary dressings, such as alginates or hydrogels. Also used to treat superficial and partial- and full-thickness chronic wounds.

Contraindications
Not for replacing sutures or other primary wound closures.

Application
- Prepare the area according to facility policy. Clip excess hair at the site, if necessary.
- Peel the paper liner from the dressing, exposing the adhesive surface.
- Position the dressing over the wound or catheter insertion site and apply it. Smooth down the edges of the dressing.
- Seal dressing securely around the catheter or wound site. Firmly smooth the adhesive border to the skin.

Removal
- Gently grasp the edge of the dressing.
- Slowly peel the dressing away from the skin in the direction of hair growth.

3M Tegaderm + Pad Transparent Dressing with Absorbent Pad
3M Health Care

How supplied
Island: 2" × 2¾" (1" × 1½" pad),
    2⅜" × 4" (1" × 2⅜" pad),
    3½" × 4" (1¾" × 2⅜" pad),
    6" × 6" (4" × 4" pad),
    3½" × 6" (1¾" × 4" pad), 3½" × 8" (1¾" × 6" pad),
    3½" × 10" (1¾" × 8" pad); A6203
    3½" × 13¾" (1¾" × 11¾" pad); A6204
Oval: 3½" × 4⅛" (1¾" × 2⅜" pad); A6203

Action
The 3M Tegaderm + Pad Transparent Dressing with Absorbent
Pad is a waterproof, bacterial barrier dressing that consists of a
nonadherent, absorbent pad bonded to a larger thin film backing with a border of hypoallergenic, water-resistant adhesive.

Indications
To manage acute wounds, cuts, burns, abrasions, I.V. catheter
sites, and surgical incisions. May also be used for superficial
and partial-thickness chronic wounds.

Contraindications
Not for replacing sutures or other primary wound closures.

Application
- Prepare the site for wound dressing or catheter insertion, according to facility policy. To ensure dressing adhesion, clip
  excess hair at the site, but don't shave. Allow all preparation
  liquids to dry completely before applying the dressing.
- Peel the paper liner from the paper-framed dressing, exposing the adhesive surface. Position the framed window over
  the wound site or catheter insertion site; apply the dressing.
- Remove the paper frame from the dressing while smoothing
  down the dressing edges and sealing them securely around
  the wound or catheter.

Removal
Grasp the edge gently and slowly peel the dressing from the
skin in the direction of hair growth.

Composites

Viasorb Wound Dressing

Kendall Health Care Products
Company

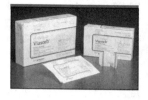

How supplied
Pad: 2" × 3" (1" × 1" pad), 4" × 6"
(2" × 4" pad), 7" × 7"
(4" × 4" pad), 3" × 10"
(1" × 8" pad); A6203 6" × 10" (3" × 7" pad); A6204

Action
Viasorb Wound Dressing is a multilayered dressing designed for highly exudating wounds. A nonadherent wound contact layer allows excess exudate to pass into the absorptive pad, permits concomitant use with topical agents, and provides for nontraumatic removal. The absorptive layer is a nonwoven rayon that will hold approximately 1.6 g of fluid per square inch, or 26 g of fluid in the 4" × 4" pad. The outer layer is a bacteria barrier that allows moisture vapor transmission; the patient may shower and bathe with the dressing in place. Because it's occlusive, the dressing reduces pain.

Indications
To manage a wide range of draining and nondraining wounds and catheter exit sites. May also be used on pressure ulcers (stages 2 and 3), partial-thickness wounds, noninfected wounds, wounds with minimal drainage, and red, yellow, or black wounds.

Contraindications
Contraindicated for infected wounds.

Application
- Cleanse the wound site with normal saline solution or Constant-Clens dermal wound cleanser.
- Pat dry the surrounding skin.
- Peel back the dressing's release paper, and position and apply the dressing to the wound.
- Smooth the dressing edges.

Removal
- Lift a corner of the dressing and stretch, releasing the dressing from the skin.
- Continue to work around the perimeter of the dressing until it is completely removed.

Composites

Contact layers

Action
Contact layers are manufactured as single layers of a woven (polyamide) net that acts as a low-adherence material when placed in contact with the base of the wound. These materials allow wound exudate to pass to a secondary dressing.

Indications
Contact layers may be used as primary dressings for partial- and full-thickness wounds; wounds with minimal, moderate, and heavy exudate; donor sites; and split-thickness skin grafts.

Advantages
- Can protect wound bases from trauma during dressing changes
- May be applied with topical medications, wound fillers, or gauze dressings.

Disadvantages
- Aren't recommended for stage 1 pressure ulcers; wounds that are shallow, dehydrated, or covered with eschar; or wounds that are draining a viscous exudate
- Require secondary dressings.

HCPCS code overview
The HCPCS codes normally assigned to contact layer dressings are:

A6206 — pad size ≤ 16 sq. in.

A6207 — pad size > 16 sq. in. but ≤ 48 sq. in.

A6208 — pad size > 48 sq. in.

Conformant 2 Wound Veil
Smith & Nephew, Inc.
Wound Management Division

How supplied
Sterile sheet: 4" × 4"; A6206
4" × 12"; A6207
12" × 12", 12" × 24", 24" × 36"; A6208
Sterile roll: 3" × 5 yd, 4" × 3 yd, 6" × 2 yd, 6" × 4 yd; A6206

Action
Conformant 2 is a single, transparent, nonadherent wound veil made of perforated high-density polyethylene. It's used to line wounds, or it's placed under packing materials. It's easy to remove and assists in the removal of other products placed over the veil. Because it's transparent, Conformant 2 allows visualization of the wound bed.

Indications
To prevent skin breakdown and to manage pressure ulcers (stages 1, 2, 3, and 4), partial- and full-thickness wounds, infected and uninfected wounds, draining wounds, and red, yellow, or black wounds. Also may be applied directly to the wound as a liner or used with any topical preparation or ointment.

Contraindications
Contraindicated for tunneling wounds.

Application
- Place the sheet over the wound and surrounding tissue.
- Affix it with tape or roll gauze.

Removal
- Remove the tape or roll gauze.
- Gently lift one corner of the sheet, and peel it back from the wound.

Contact Layers

DERMANET Wound Contact Layer
DeRoyal

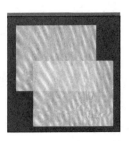

How supplied
Sheet: 3″ × 3″; A6206
      4″ × 5″; A6207
      8″ × 10″, 20″ × 15″, 24″ × 36″;
      A6208
Roll: 6″ × 72″; A6208

Action
DERMANET Wound Contact Layer is a lightweight net made from high-density polyethylene that forms a porous fine-mesh structure. It is nonlinting, inert (totally nonreactive), soft, air- and fluid-permeable, and nonadherent. It conforms to the shapes of wounds and may be used as a primary dressing, coated with ointment for burns, or used as a liner for deep wounds that need to be packed (thus allowing easy removal of packing material).

Indications
For use as a primary dressing to protect burns, graft sites, donor sites, and granulating dermal ulcers and to line deep wounds before packing.

Contraindications
Contraindicated for cleaning or debriding wounds.

Application
- Carefully apply DERMANET Wound Contact Layer to the wound after cleansing it and applying topical medications, as prescribed.
- Cover the contact layer with a secondary dressing.
- Alternatively, apply medications directly to DERMANET Wound Contact Layer, and place it over the wound before applying a cover dressing.
- For deep, open wounds, line the wound with DERMANET Wound Contact Layer, pack the wound with appropriate packing material, and then apply a cover dressing.

Removal
Gently lift the dressing off or out of the wound.

Contact Layers

Mepitel
Mölnlycke Health Care

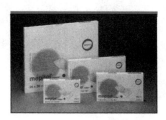

How supplied
Sheet: 2″ × 3″, 3″ × 4″; A6206
           4″ × 8″; A6207
           8″ × 12″; A6208

Action
Mepitel is a protective wound dressing.

Indications
To manage wounds resulting from trauma or surgery, graft re-
cipient sites, first- and second-degree burns, freshly debrided
wounds, wounds with friable or excoriated surrounding skin,
wounds to which current dressings adhere, and red wounds.

Contraindications
None provided by the manufacturer.

Application
- Choose a dressing size large enough to overlap the surrounding
  skin by at least ⅜″ (1 cm). If necessary, before removing the
  backing material, cut the dressing to conform to the wound.
- Clean the wound and dry the surrounding skin. If a topical
  ointment has been prescribed, apply it to the wound.
- From the side of the dressing with the two overlapping backings, remove the wider backing first, and place the exposed
  dressing surface next to the wound. Gently remove the smaller backing from underneath and then the remaining backing
  on the upper side. Lightly smooth the dressing in place. *Note*:
  For application to difficult areas, such as fingertips or toes,
  wear sterile gloves to remove all backings, then shape the
  dressing.
- If a moist, medicated compress has been prescribed, apply
  it over Mepitel.
- Cover the dressing with an absorbent dressing, or secure it
  with gauze wrap, an elastic retention bandage, or a dressing-
  fixation fabric.
- Mepitel can be left in place through several outer dressing
  changes, depending on the condition of the wound.

Removal
Peel back the dressing.

Contact Layers

N-TERFACE Interpositional Surfacing Material
Winfield Laboratories, Inc.

How supplied
Sheet: 4" × 4"; A6206
4" × 12"; A6207
12" × 12", 12" × 24"; A6208
Roll: 4" × 10"; A6208

Action
N-TERFACE Interpositional Surfacing Material is a patented, lightweight, extruded, high-density polyurethane sheeting material. It can be used as the primary wound contact layer to prevent adherence of secondary dressings or to line deep wounds for easy removal of packing material. It is nonreactive, translucent, nonlinting, air- and fluid-permeable, and nonadherent. Because it's translucent, it allows visual examination of the wound surface. The wound also can be cleansed and medicated through the material. The properties of N-TERFACE allow it to be changed daily or left in place for several days. It is useful under an Unna's boot to prevent sticking of the boot to wounds or grafts.

Indications
To manage pressure ulcers (stages 1, 2, 3, and 4), partial- and full-thickness wounds, skin graft sites, donor sites, dermatologic conditions, fungating neoplasms, burns, and tunneling wounds. May also be used for infected and noninfected wounds; wounds with serosanguineous or purulent drainage; wounds with heavy drainage; red, yellow, or black wounds; and minor lacerations. Also for use as a wet or dry dressing and postoperatively.

Contraindications
- Contraindicated for preventing skin breakdown.
- Contraindicated for third-degree burns.

Application
- Select a dressing size that covers the wound and periwound area.

Contact Layers

- Apply the desired topical agent to the wound or to the dressing before placing the dressing on the wound.
- Apply the dressing dry, or dip it in normal saline solution for better conformability.
- Apply a secondary dressing.
- Secure with stretch netting, roll gauze, or tape.

Removal
- Change the dressing as required.
- Gently lift the dressing off the wound.
- If the wound has dried or is very bloody, or if the contact layer sticks to the wound, rinse the wound with normal saline solution, leaving the contact layer in place. Then remove the contact layer, or leave this layer in place to protect fragile epithelium.
- If the contact layer is left in place for longer than 24 hours, cleanse the wound through the N-TERFACE contact layer when the secondary absorptive dressing is changed.

Profore Wound Contact Layer

Smith & Nephew, Inc.
Wound Management Division

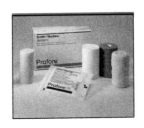

How supplied
Sheet: 4″ × 4″

Action
Profore Wound Contact Layer protects wounds from direct contact with absorbent fibers or lint and reduces trauma during dressing changes. Its natural viscose rayon monofilaments produce no lint or breakdown residues to complicate wound cleansing. Profore Wound Contact Layer won't stick to the wound surface, reducing the damage to newly formed tissue during dressing changes. The open-knit construction allows drainage to pass through to the absorbent layers.

Indications
To manage partial- and full-thickness wounds.

Contraindications
None provided by the manufacturer.

Application
- Cleanse the wound and surrounding skin according to facility policy.
- Carefully apply Profore Wound Contact Layer to the wound.
- Apply medications, as prescribed, directly over the contact layer, and cover it with an appropriate secondary dressing.

Removal
Gently lift the contact layer out of the wound.

Contact Layers

TELFA CLEAR
Kendall Health Care Products Company

How supplied
Sheet: 3″ × 3″, 4″ × 5″, 4″ × 12″, 12″ × 12″, 12″ × 24″

Action
TELFA CLEAR makes reepithelialization possible without interrupting the healing process, and it can be removed without causing pain.

Indications
For use as a primary dressing on lightly, moderately, or heavily draining wounds. Allows the freedom to choose the most appropriate absorbent secondary dressing.

Contraindications
None provided by the manufacturer.

Application
- Cleanse the wound and surrounding skin according to facility policy.
- Carefully apply the dressing to the wound.
- Apply any prescribed medications directly over the dressing.
- Cover the contact layer with an appropriate wound dressing.

Removal
- Dressing may be left in place for several days.
- Gently lift the contact layer off the wound.

3M Tegapore Wound Contact Material

3M Health Care

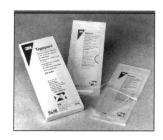

How supplied

Sheet: 3″ × 4″; A6206
3″ × 8″; A6207
8″ × 10″; A6208

Action

3M Tegapore Wound Contact Material is a woven nylon fabric with sealed edges that is a lint-free, nonadherent, nontoxic, nonirritating, and hypoallergenic material to be used on wounds along with an appropriate outer dressing. Intimate contact of the dressing's wound contact material with the wound allows the flow of exudate away from the wound, preventing pooling of fluids that can cause maceration. Maintains healthy granulation tissue, reducing or eliminating the need to debride. Nonadherence of this material minimizes disruption of healthy granulation on tissue and reepithelialized surfaces.

Indications

For use directly over wounds, including partial- and full-thickness wounds, clean closed surgical incisions, second-degree burns, donor sites, graft fixation sites, skin tears, traumatic and chronic wounds, and dermatologic lesions.

Contraindications

Not designed, sold, or intended for use except as indicated.

Application

- Debride, cleanse, or irrigate the wound and surrounding skin as necessary according to facility policy.
- Topical treatment with ointments or medicaments, if indicated, can be applied to the wound surface prior to applying the wound contact material, or they can be applied on top of the material after it has been placed on the wound.
- If the dressing material must be cut to fit, remove all frayed or loose fibers.
- When wound drainage is minimal, moisten the dressing's wound contact material with sterile saline solution to facilitate positioning and to ensure complete contact with the wound surface.

Contact Layers

- Gently position the material over the entire wound, including a margin of healthy skin. The material should extend at least ½″ beyond the edge of the wound, and the cut edges of the material should not be placed directly over the wound bed.
- Dress the wound with an outer dressing of gauze, a transparent dressing, a hydrocolloid, or another suitable wound dressing.

Removal

- Dressing may remain undisturbed on the wound for up to 7 days. If the wound is infected, change the dressing according to facility policy for infected wounds.
- Change gauze dressings as needed, or at least every 24 hours. During gauze dressing changes, moisten 3M Tegapore Wound Contact Material if necessary to maintain a moist wound environment.
- When a transparent or hydrocolloid dressing is used as the outermost dressing, follow facility policy for dressing changes.
- Gently lift 3M Tegapore Wound Contact Material off the wound. When this material is maintained in a moist environment, it's nonadherent and its removal is virtually pain-free.
- If the wound surface is dry, soak the dressing with normal saline solution and then gently remove it.

Contact Layers

NEW PRODUCT
VersaDress Wound Contact Layer
Dumex Medical

How supplied
Sheet: 3″ × 3″, 4″ × 5″, 8″ × 10″

Action
VersaDress protects the wound while allowing drainage to pass through to an appropriate secondary dressing.

Indications
For use as a primary dressing to manage partial- and full-thickness wounds.

Contraindications
None provided by the manufacturer.

Application
- Cleanse the wound with PrimaDerm Dermal Cleanser or saline solution.
- Pat dry surrounding skin.
- Apply the dressing directly to the wound.
- Cover with an appropriate secondary dressing.

Removal
- Remove the secondary dressing.
- If the wound is dry, soak the dressing with saline prior to removal.

Foams

Foams

Action

Foam dressings are nonlinting and absorbent. They vary in thickness and have a nonadherent layer, allowing nontraumatic removal. Some have an adhesive border and may have a film coating as an additional bacteria barrier. Foam dressings provide a moist environment and thermal insulation. They're manufactured as pads, sheets, and pillow (cavity) dressings.

Indications

Foam dressings may be used as primary and secondary dressings for partial- and full-thickness wounds with minimal, moderate, or heavy drainage; as primary dressings to provide absorption and insulation; or as secondary dressings for wounds with packing. They may also be used to provide additional absorption and to absorb drainage around tubes.

Advantages
- Are nonadherent
- May repel contaminants
- Are easy to apply and remove
- Absorb light to heavy amounts of exudate
- May be used under compression.

Disadvantages
- Aren't effective for wounds with dry eschar
- May macerate periwound skin if they become saturated
- May require secondary dressing, tape, wrap, or net.

HCPCS code overview

The HCPCS codes normally assigned to foam wound covers without an adhesive border are:

A6209 — pad size ≤ 16 sq. in.

A6210 — pad size > 16 sq. in. but ≤ 48 sq. in.

A6211 — pad size > 48 sq. in.

The HCPCS codes normally assigned to foam wound covers with an adhesive border are:

A6212 — pad size ≤ 16 sq. in.

A6213 — pad size > 16 sq. in. but ≤ 48 sq. in.

A6214 — pad size > 48 sq. in.

The HCPCS code normally assigned to foam wound fillers is:

A6215 — per gram.

Allevyn and Allevyn Adhesive Hydrophilic Polyurethane Foam Dressings

Smith & Nephew, Inc.
Wound Management Division

How supplied

Pad:	2″ × 2″, 4″ × 4″; A6209
	6″ × 6″; A6210
	8″ × 8″; A6211
Heel:	A6210
Adhesive dressing:	3″ × 3″, 5″ × 5″; A6212
	7″ × 7″; A6213
Sacrum:	6¾″ × 6¾″; A6212

Action

Allevyn Hydrophilic Polyurethane Foam Dressing is a sterile, absorbent foam dressing with a nonadherent wound contact layer and a semipermeable polyurethane film top layer. It maintains a moist environment and aids in preventing bacterial contamination. The dressing absorbs well under compression, conforms well in areas that are awkward to dress, and absorbs up to four times more than a hydrocolloid dressing of similar size.

Indications

To manage exudate in pressure ulcers (stages 2, 3, and 4), leg ulcers, donor sites, partial- and full-thickness wounds, wounds with moderate drainage, wounds with serosanguineous drainage, and red or yellow wounds.

Contraindications

Not intended for use on nonexuding wounds.

Application

- Apply the foam dressing directly to the wound surface.
- Secure the foam dressing with dressing retention tape, regular surgical tape, or waterproof tape.

Removal

- Soak the wound site, then remove the fixative tape.
- The dressing will come off cleanly without leaving residue in the wound.

Foams

Allevyn Cavity Wound Dressing
Smith & Nephew, Inc.
Wound Management Division

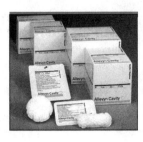

How supplied
Circular pad:
    2″, 4″; A6215
Tubular pad:
    3½″ × 1″, 4¾″ × 1½″; A6215

Action
Allevyn Cavity Wound Dressing absorbs exudate when used to pack heavily exuding cavity wounds.

Indications
To manage exudate in deep chronic wounds or separated surgical wounds. May be used on pressure ulcers (stages 2, 3, and 4), full-thickness wounds, tunneling wounds, infected (when appropriate antibiotic therapy is prescribed) and noninfected wounds, wounds with heavy drainage, wounds with purulent drainage, and red or yellow wounds.

Contraindications
Contraindicated for nonexuding wounds.

Application
- Choose the appropriate dressing size.
- Press the dressing into the wound.
- Secure the dressing with a transparent film dressing or nonwoven retention tape.

Removal
Lift the dressing out of the wound.

Biatain Adhesive Foam Dressing

Biatain Non-Adhesive Foam Dressing
Coloplast Corporation

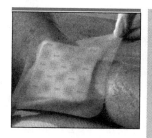

How supplied
Adhesive foam dressing
Pad: 5″ × 5″, 7″ × 7″
Non-adhesive foam dressing
Pad: 4″ × 4″, 6″ × 6″

Action
Biatain Adhesive Foam Dressing and Biatain Non-Adhesive Foam Dressing provide an exudate-handling system for wounds with light to heavy exudate. They're highly absorbent, three-dimensional (3-D) polymer dressings. Biatain Adhesive Foam Dressing has a hydrocolloid adhesive border and a central 3-D polymer absorbent pad with a waterproof, semipermeable film backing. Biatain Non-Adhesive Foam Dressing is especially suitable for use on fragile skin because it doesn't have an adhesive.

Indications
To manage leg ulcers, skin tears, and diabetic and pressure ulcers with light to heavy exudate. May be used on patients with systemic infections. Biatain Foam Dressings also may be used throughout the healing process to provide padding and protection for all types of wounds.

Contraindications
- Contraindicated for use with hypochlorite solutions or hydrogen peroxide.
- Must be removed before radiation therapy.

Application
- Rinse the wound with Sea-Clens or normal saline solution. Gently pat dry the surrounding skin.
- Choose a dressing that overlaps each side of the wound by 1″ (2.5 cm).

- Biatain Adhesive Foam Dressing may be used with Purilon Gel to encourage natural debridement of necrotic tissue.

Removal

Biatain Adhesive Foam Dressing and Biatain Non-Adhesive Foam Dressing may be left in place for up to 7 days, depending on the amount of exudate and the condition of the dressing. Change when clinically indicated or when the exudate reaches 1″ (2.5 cm) from the edge of the dressing.

CarraSmart Foam Dressing

Carrington Laboratories, Inc.

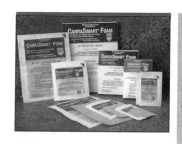

Foams

How supplied

Pad: 2" × 3", 4" × 4"; A6257
6" × 8"; A6258

Action

CarraSmart Foam Dressing is an adherent foam with a gentle adhesive backing. The foam absorbs light to moderate exudate and has a high moisture-vapor transfer rate. It maintains a moist wound environment and won't traumatize the wound or surrounding skin. It can be cut to fit a variety of wounds and is tinted for cosmetic acceptance.

Indications

To manage pressure ulcers (stages 1 and 2), venous stasis ulcers, first- and second-degree burns, cuts, abrasions, skin irritations, and partial- and full-thickness wounds with low to medium exudate as well as wounds with serosanguineous drainage and red or yellow wounds. May be used as a secondary dressing over wounds with fillers or packing or to absorb drainage from around tubes. May also be cut and applied as a primary dressing around tubes such as gastrostomy tubes.

Contraindications

Contraindicated for third-degree burns.

Application

- Flush the wound with a suitable cleanser such as UltraKlenz, CarraKlenz, or MicroKlenz.
- Apply the dressing to the wound bed by holding it and pressing it into place.

Removal

- Change the dressing as the wound condition and amount of exudate dictate or as directed by the primary care provider. Dressing may remain in place for up to 7 days.
- To remove the dressing, lift it gently.

Curafoam Plus Foam Dressing

Kendall Health Care Products Company

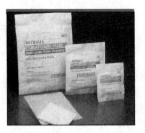

How supplied

Sterile

sheet: 2½″ × 2½″, 4″ × 4″; A6209
   4″ × 5″, 4″ × 8″, 6″ × 6″; A6210
   8″ × 8″; A6211

Action

CURAFOAM PLUS Foam Dressing provides an ideal healing environment for a variety of wounds. This highly absorbent dressing offers physical protection against external fluids and bacteria. The soft, gentle, nonadherent surface conforms to body contours.

Indications

To manage postsurgical incisions, pressure ulcers (stages 1, 2, and 3), venous stasis ulcers, diabetic foot wounds, donor sites, tubes, and drains.

Contraindications

- Contraindicated for dry wounds.
- Contraindicated for third-degree burns.

Application

- Cleanse the wound.
- Apply the dressing to the wound. For best results, leave a margin of at least 1″ (2.5 cm) around the wound. For improved fit around tubes and drains, the dressing may be cut.

Removal

Change the dressing as often as necessary.

Curafoam Wound Dressing
Kendall Health Care Products Company

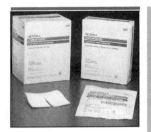

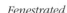

How supplied
Sterile sheet: $2'' \times 2''$, $4'' \times 4''$;
                   A6209
                   $4'' \times 5''$, $8'' \times 4''$;
                   A6210
                   $6'' \times 8''$, $8'' \times 10''$; A6211

Fenestrated drain sponge: $4'' \times 4''$; A6209

Action
CURAFOAM Wound Dressing absorbs high amounts of exudate.

Indications
To manage pressure ulcers (stages 1, 2, 3, and 4), partial- and full-thickness wounds, tunneling wounds, infected and noninfected wounds, draining wounds, and red, yellow, or black wounds.

Contraindications
- Contraindicated for dry wounds.
- Contraindicated for third-degree burns.

Application
- Apply CURAFOAM as a cover dressing.
- Secure it with a transparent dressing or tape.

Removal
Gently remove the dressing.

EPIGARD
Ormed, Inc.

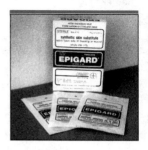

Foams

How supplied
Multilayered
pad: 3" × 4"; A6209
      3" × 9"; A6210
      5" × 12", 5" × 18"; A6211

Action
EPIGARD is a nonmedicated, nontextile, microporous, double-layered dressing used to cover wounds involving open fractures with severe soft tissue injury.

Indications
For open dressing of surface wounds and as preparation of a secondary closing of the wound.

Contraindications
- Contraindicated for wounds that have pocket formation or complex areas, such as cavities and ragged surfaces; massive infections with strong putrid secretion; restricted blood circulation; soft tissue defects with exposed bone, tendon, nerves, or vessels; and dessicated or insufficiently cleaned wound surfaces.
- Contraindicated for simultaneous use with creams or ointments.

Application
- Carefully debride the wound and create even wound boundaries. Debridement is necessary at initial wound care and may be required at secondary wound inspections.
- Irrigate the wound before applying EPIGARD.
- Cut the dressing to size and, holding it with the foam side toward the wound, fit it precisely within the wound boundaries. Don't stretch it in any direction.
- Apply a light cover wrap to secure the dressing. Don't suture or staple EPIGARD to the wound margins. It will adhere to the wound bed on its own.
- When the wound bed is sufficiently vascularized, close the wound with a split-thickness mesh graft, delayed primary suturing, or conventional dressing. Closing is usually possible after 3 to 7 days.

Removal

- Change the dressing at least once daily for maximum benefit. Never leave it on the wound for more than 24 hours. If the foam becomes saturated with exudate, change the dressing more frequently.
- Remove the dressing with sterile forceps.
- If the dressing remains on the wound too long, surgical removal may be necessary.

Foams

Flexzan Topical Wound Dressing
Bertek (Dow Hickam)
Pharmaceuticals

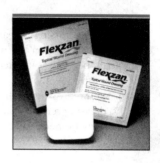

How supplied
Multilayered
pad: 2″ × 3″, 4″ × 4″; A6209
    4″ × 8″; A6210
    8″ × 8″; A6211

Action
Flexzan Topical Wound Dressing consists of an open-cell foam with a closed-cell outer surface and a patterned adhesive coating on the wound contact surface. Excess moisture from the wound passes readily through the adhesive pattern and is absorbed into the open cells of the foam. The dressing skin provides a barrier to moisture, bacteria, and contaminants but has high permeability, allowing evaporation of excess moisture from the foam to help prevent fluid accumulation under the dressing. Flexzan Topical Wound Dressing has moisture-management capabilities that make dry or moist wounds, even in areas difficult to dress, easily and comfortably managed.

Indications
To manage abrasions, lacerations, skin tears, incisions, and other dermal lesions; donor sites; and superficial burns. May also be used on pressure ulcers (stages 1, 2, 3, and 4), venous ulcers, diabetic ulcers, partial- and full-thickness wounds, tunneling wounds, noninfected wounds, wounds with minimal drainage, and red or yellow wounds. May be used as a secondary dressing over cavity-filling dressings.

Contraindications
- Contraindicated for infected wounds.
- Contraindicated for third-degree burns.

Application
- Irrigate the wound with normal saline solution or water, and dry the surrounding area.

- Remove the dressing's backing, and place the dressing over the wound as desired, leaving at least a 1″ (2.5-cm) margin over intact skin. Cut or overlap the dressing to accommodate wound size or body contour.
- Secure by applying gentle hand pressure over the dressing for approximately 20 seconds.

Removal
- Change the dressing at least every 5 days or if leakage occurs or as clinical practice dictates.
- The dressing may become discolored because of wound exudate absorption, but it doesn't need to be removed unless infection is present.

Foams

Hydrasorb Foam Wound Dressing

Kendall Health Care Products Company

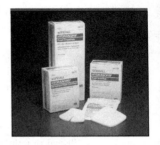

How supplied

Pad: 4" × 4", 3⅝" × 3⅛"
(fenestrated); A6209
4" × 8", 6" × 6"; A6210
8" × 8"; A6211

Action

HYDRASORB Foam Wound Dressing is a soft, nonlinting, hydrophilic polyurethane foam pad that cushions and protects the wound site. It's semi-occlusive, allowing the passage of oxygen. The dressing provides a moist healing environment, manages exudate, and protects the wound from contamination.

Indications

To manage pressure ulcers (stages 1, 2, 3, and 4), partial- and full-thickness wounds, tunneling wounds, infected and noninfected wounds, draining wounds, and red, yellow, or black wounds. May also be used as a secondary dressing for packed wounds.

Contraindications

- Contraindicated for dry wounds.
- Contraindicated for third-degree burns.

Application

- After cleansing the wound, select a dressing size that provides a minimum 1" (2.5-cm) margin around the edges of the wound.
- Place either side of the dressing directly against the wound, and secure it with gauze, elastic bandages, or adhesive tape.
- If infection develops, discontinue using the dressing and notify the primary care provider.

Removal

- Change the dressing when strike-through occurs or whenever clinical practice dictates.

- Remove securing tapes or bandages, and carefully lift the dressing off the wound.
- Heavily exudating wounds may require two or more daily changes for the first several days. In moderately exudating wounds, a daily change is usually sufficient. Changing the dressing may extend to every 3 days and then weekly as the amount of exudate decreases.
- For clean, superficial wounds with no signs of infection or dressing saturation, leave the dressing in place for several days.

Foams

NEW PRODUCT

HydroCell Adhesive Foam Dressing
Dumex Medical

How supplied
*Adhesive
foam:*   4" × 4", 6" × 6"

Action
HydroCell Adhesive Foam Dressing is a highly absorptive, non-adherent, polyurethane foam pad and an adhesive protective film covering to protect the wound from outside contaminants without the need for a secondary dressing.

Indications
To manage moderately to highly exudating wounds.

Contraindications
Contraindicated for third-degree burns.

Application
- Cleanse the wound with PrimaDerm Dermal Cleanser or saline solution. Pat dry the skin adjacent to the wound.
- Position the HydroCell Adhesive Foam Dressing pad directly on the wound.
- Smooth the edges of the adhesive border to insure secure adhesion.

Removal
- Gently remove the HydroCell Adhesive Foam Dressing.
- Removal may be facilitated by gently stretching the adhesive film border.

Foams

NEW PRODUCT
HydroCell Foam Dressing
Dumex Medical

How supplied
Nonadhesive
foam: $4'' \times 4''$, $6'' \times 6''$

Action
HydroCell Foam Dressing is a nonadherent, highly absorptive, polyurethane foam sheet with protective film covering to protect the wound from outside contaminants. A secondary dressing is required to hold this dressing in place.

Indications
To manage moderately to highly exudating wounds.

Contraindications
Contraindicated for third-degree burns.

Application
- Cleanse the wound with PrimaDerm Dermal Cleanser or saline solution. Pat dry the skin adjacent to the wound.
- Position HydroCell Foam Dressing directly on the wound.
- Secure with an appropriate secondary dressing.

Removal
- Remove the secondary dressing.
- Remove the HydroCell Foam.

NEW PRODUCT
HydroCell Thin Adhesive Foam Dressing
Dumex Medical

How supplied
*Thin adhesive
foam:* $2'' \times 3''$, $4'' \times 4''$

Action
HydroCell Thin Adhesive Foam Dressing is an absorptive polyurethane foam sheet with a nonadherent foam pad and an adhesive protective film covering to protect the wound from outside contaminants without the need for a secondary dressing.

Indications
To manage lightly exudating wounds.

Contraindications
Contraindicated for third-degree burns.

Application
- Cleanse the wound with PrimaDerm Dermal Cleanser or saline solution. Pat dry the skin adjacent to the wound.
- Position the HydroCell Thin Adhesive Foam Dressing pad directly on the wound.
- Smooth the edges of the adhesive border to insure secure adhesion.

Removal
- Gently remove the HydroCell Thin Adhesive Foam Dressing.
- Removal may be facilitated by gently stretching the adhesive film border.

LO PROFILE FOAM Wound Dressing

Gentell, Inc.

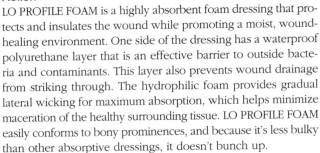

How supplied
Pad: 3" × 3", 5" × 5"

Action

LO PROFILE FOAM is a highly absorbent foam dressing that protects and insulates the wound while promoting a moist, wound-healing environment. One side of the dressing has a waterproof polyurethane layer that is an effective barrier to outside bacteria and contaminants. This layer also prevents wound drainage from striking through. The hydrophilic foam provides gradual lateral wicking for maximum absorption, which helps minimize maceration of the healthy surrounding tissue. LO PROFILE FOAM easily conforms to bony prominences, and because it's less bulky than other absorptive dressings, it doesn't bunch up.

Indications

For use as a primary dressing for minimally to moderately draining wounds and for skin tears and other superficial wounds. For use as a secondary absorptive dressing in conjunction with a primary dressing such as calcium alginate. May also be used around drainage tubes.

Contraindications

None provided by the manufacturer.

Application

- Irrigate the wound with Gentell Wound Cleanser or a similar nontoxic cleanser.
- Gently dry the skin surrounding the wound site.
- Select the dressing size that will provide a minimum margin of 1" (2.5 cm) around the edges of the wound.
- Holding the side with the green sticker away from the wound surface, place LO PROFILE FOAM dressing directly over the wound surface. Remove the green sticker.
- Secure all sides of the dressing with an appropriate fixative product.

Removal

- Gently roll back the tape strips from the skin.
- Ease the dressing from the wound.

Lyofoam Polyurethane Foam Dressing

Lyofoam A Polyurethane Foam Dressing

Lyofoam C Polyurethane Foam Dressing with Activated Carbon

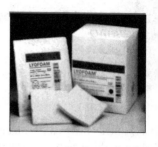

Lyofoam T Polyurethane Foam Dressing

Lyofoam Extra Polyurethane Foam Dressing
ConvaTec

How supplied

Lyofoam Polyurethane Foam Dressing
Sterile dressing: 3″ × 3″, 4″ × 4″; A6209
7″ × 4″, 10″ × 4″, 8″ × 6″; A6210
12″ × 10″, 27⅝″ × 15¾″; A6211

Lyofoam A Polyurethane Foam Dressing
Sterile dressing: 2″ × 2″, 4″ × 4″; A6212

Lyofoam C Polyurethane Foam Dressing with Activated Carbon
Sterile dressing: 4″ × 4″; A6209
8″ × 6″; A6210

Lyofoam T
Sterile dressing: 3½″ × 2½″; A6209

Lyofoam Extra Polyurethane Foam Dressing
Sterile dressing: 4″ × 4″; A6209
7″ × 4″, 8″ × 6″; A6210
12″ × 10″; A6211

Action

Lyofoam is used on cutaneous wounds with exudate, and applied directly onto clean wounds and wounds with minimal necrosis during the exuding, granulating, or epithelializing phases of healing. Lyofoam A is used as a dressing for lightly exuding wounds, such as sacral ulcers and cutaneous wounds. Lyofoam C is used in the treatment of lightly or moderately exuding wounds to absorb and neutralize offensive odors. Lyofoam

T is used as a dressing for tracheostomy and other intubation sites, cannula insertion procedures, and external bone fixators.

Indications

To manage cutaneous wounds with exudate as well as wounds with minimal necrosis during the exuding, granulating, or epithelializing stages of healing.

Contraindications

- Contraindicated for dry, superficial wounds.
- Shouldn't be left in position on shallow, drying wounds for extended periods because of the possibility of adherence.
- Despite having debriding qualities, shouldn't be applied to wounds covered by a dry scab or hard black necrotic tissue until the scab or tissue has been removed using other approved methods.

Application

- Clean and prepare the wound. For sloughy or necrotic wounds, use sterile saline solution to cleanse the wound surface before applying the dressing and at every dressing change. *Note:* Because cooling of the wound surface can delay healing, sterile saline solution should be at body temperature.
- After cleansing, dry the surrounding skin, leaving the wound surface moist. *Note:* During cleansing and dressing changes, be careful not to disturb any newly formed tissue at the edges and in the base of the wound.

    Lyofoam and Lyofoam Extra:
- Select a dressing large enough to overlap the wound area by 1″ (2.5 cm) all around. If necessary, cut the dressing to the shape required.
- Place the smooth, shiny side of the dressing directly over the wound surface.
- Where compression is required, a suitable compression bandage, such as SetoPress, may be used to retain the dressing. For other applications, Lyofoam can be retained by adhesive tape or by a suitable dressing retention bandage, such as Tubifast. *Note:* Don't fully cover Lyofoam with adhesive films or tapes because they interfere with water vapor transmission, which can reduce the dressing's effectiveness.

Foams

Foams

Lyofoam A:

- Cleanse with SAF-Clens or other appropriate cleansing solution, and dry the surrounding skin, leaving the wound surface moist.
- Peel off Lyofoam A's backing sheet from one side. Place the dressing over the wound, ensuring that the central pad of the dressing overlaps the wound by approximately 1″ (2.5 cm) on all sides. Gently smooth the exposed adhesive border into position.
- Remove the second sheet of backing paper. Smooth the other side of the adhesive border gently into position, ensuring complete contact all around the wound to avoid leakage or contamination.

Lyofoam C:

- Irrigate with SAF-Clens or other appropriate cleansing solution to remove as much necrotic material as possible. Dry the surrounding skin, leaving the wound surface moist.
- Position the appropriate size of Lyofoam C over the wound surface, allowing an overlap of approximately 1″ (2.5 cm) around wound margins.
- Secure with a conforming retention bandage, such as Tubifast.
- *Note:* Don't fully cover Lyofoam with adhesive films or tapes because they interfere with water vapor transmission, which can reduce the dressing's effectiveness.

Lyofoam T:

- Insert a tube, cannula, or pin into the tracheostomy.
- Locate the precut "cross" on Lyofoam T.
- Position the dressing carefully around the tube, cannula, or pin; then secure it.
- *Note:* Don't fully cover Lyofoam with adhesive films or tapes because they interfere with water vapor transmission, which can reduce the dressing's effectiveness.

Removal

- For lightly exuding wounds, initially change the dressing every 2 to 3 days. Extend the changing period to 4 to 7 days as the amount of exudate decreases.
- For moderately exuding wounds, changes may be needed daily or on alternate days for the first few days of treatment. After the initial period of profuse exudation, granulation should begin, and the dressing-change interval can be extended.

- The interval between dressing changes is determined by the amount of exudate and the nature and condition of the wound. The goal is to change the dressings at weekly intervals to minimize disturbance of the wound and optimize healing.
- If the absorbent surface becomes completely saturated, exudate will be visible around the edges of the dressing. This clearly indicates that the dressing should be changed, regardless of how recently it was applied.
- Dressing changes should be done as quickly as possible to avoid cooling of the wound surface, as this can delay healing. For the same reason, sterile saline solution used to cleanse the wound should be at body temperature.

Foams

Mepilex
Mölnlycke Health Care

How supplied
Pad: 4″ × 4″; A6212
4″ × 8″, 6″ × 6″; A6213
8″ × 8″; A6214

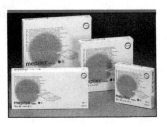

Action
Mepilex is a nonadherent absorbent foam film dressing with selective microadherent properties. Mepilex absorbs exudate even under compression. The film backing is moisture and vapor permeable.

Indications
To manage leg and foot ulcers, pressure ulcers, and shallow exuding wounds.

Contraindications
None provided by the manufacturer.

Application
- Cleanse the wound site. Ensure that the skin surrounding the wound is dry.
- Select an appropriate dressing size. For best results, Mepilex should overlap the surrounding skin by 1″ (2 cm). If necessary, cut the dressing to fit.
- Remove the release film from Mepilex, and apply the dressing with the adherent side toward the wound. Don't stretch the dressing.
- Secure the dressing with a bandage or other fixation when necessary.

Removal
- Leave Mepilex in place for up to 7 days, depending on the condition of the wound and the surrounding skin, or according to facility policy.
- To remove the dressing, simply peel it back.

Mepilex Border
Mölnlycke Health Care

How supplied
Pad: 3″ × 3″ with
    1.77″ × 1.77″ pad,
    4″ × 4″ with
    2.56″ × 2.56″ pad; A6212
    6″ × 6″ with 4.33″ × 4.33″ pad,
    6″ × 8″ with 4.33″ × 6.30″ pad; A6213

Foams

Action
Mepilex Border is an absorbent foam dressing with selective microadherent properties; it self-adheres without traditional adhesives. Mepilex Border absorbs exudate and minimizes the risk of periwound skin maceration and erosion. The film backing is moisture and vapor permeable, waterproof, and bacteria-proof.

Indications
To manage pressure ulcers, lower extremity ulcers such as diabetic ulcers, and traumatic wounds.

Contraindications
None provided by the manufacturer.

Application
- Cleanse the wound site. Ensure that the skin surrounding the wound is dry.
- Remove the release film from Mepilex Border, and apply the dressing with the adherent side toward the wound, overlapping it onto the surrounding skin. Don't stretch the dressing.

Removal
- Leave in place for 5 to 7 days, depending on the condition of the wound and surrounding skin, or according to facility policy.
- To remove the dressing, simply peel it back.

Mitraflex

Mitraflex Plus
Mölnlycke Health Care

How supplied
Mitraflex
Pad: 2″ × 2″, 4″ × 4″; A6209
       8″ × 8″; A6211
Mitraflex Plus
Pad: 2″ × 2″, 4″ × 4″; A6212

Action
Mitraflex and Mitraflex Plus are sterile, protective, semipermeable, adhesive, breathable, absorbent foam and film wound dressings. They are designed to cover and manage exudate in lightly to moderately draining partial-thickness and healing full-thickness dermal ulcers.

Indications
To manage pressure ulcers, lower extremity ulcers, donor sites, surgical incisions, superficial burns, abrasions, lacerations, and skin tears.

Contraindications
Contraindicated for infected or heavily draining wounds.

Application
- Thoroughly rinse or irrigate the wound with normal saline solution or nontoxic cleansing solution. Gently dry the skin surrounding the wound to allow secure application of the dressing.
- Ensure proper adherence to healthy skin by extending the dressing at least 1″ (2.5 cm) beyond the edge of the wound. The dressing may be overlapped or cut to accommodate the wound size. Size the dressing in such a way that the release paper split still may be used.
- Fold the dressing along the split in the release paper. Remove the release paper using minimal finger contact with the sterile dressing surface.

- Center the dressing over the wound and gently press it to the skin to smooth out any wrinkles.

Removal

- Base the frequency of dressing change on clinical judgment, leaving the dressing in place for up to 7 days.
- To remove, carefully lift an edge of the dressing while gently pressing against the skin. Continue pulling the dressing carefully from the skin.
- Cleanse the wound site before applying a new dressing.

Foams

Odor-Absorbent Dressing
Hollister Incorporated

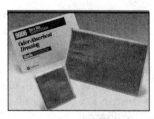

How supplied
Pad: 4″ × 4″, 6″ × 10″

Action
Odor-Absorbent Dressing, composed of carbon-impregnated foam sandwiched between fabric, effectively eliminates offending odors resulting from infection or bacterial contamination.

Indications
For use as a primary dressing for dry wounds or a secondary dressing over already dressed wounds. To control odor resulting from infection or bacterial contamination in surgical wounds, traumatic wounds, cancerous wounds, gangrenous wounds, pressure ulcers, or venous stasis ulcers. May be used on infected and noninfected wounds, wounds with minimal drainage, wounds with purulent drainage, and yellow or black wounds.

Contraindications
None provided by the manufacturer.

Application
Primary dressing over a dry wound:
- Place the dressing directly over the prepared wound surface. Dressings may overlap the wound but should never be cut to conform to wound size.
- Secure the dressing by taping its perimeter to the skin.
  Secondary dressing:
- Place the dressing directly over the primary wound dressing.
- Secure it by taping the perimeter of the dressing to the skin.

Removal
Gently remove the tape from the patient's skin and lift the dressing.

Optifoam Adhesive Foam Island Dressing
Medline Industries, Inc.

How supplied
Island dressing: 4″ × 4″ with 2.5″ × 2.5″ pad; A6212
6″ × 6″ with 4.5″ × 4.5″ pad; A6213

Action
Optifoam Adhesive Foam Island Dressing is an exudate handling system for moderately to heavily draining wounds. This hydropolymer adhesive dressing is comprised of a thin foam backing over a hydrophilic foam island. The foam backing has an adjustable MVTR from 0 to 4,500 g/m²/day, depending on the fluid level in the wound. The waterproof outer layer is coated with a medical-grade adhesive that helps maintain an optimally moist wound environment, which supports wound healing by encouraging autolytic debridement, enabling granulation to occur. The absorbent island gently expands as it takes up the exudate.

Indications
To manage chronic and acute, moderately to heavily exudating, partial- and full-thickness wounds, including superficial wounds, minor abrasions, skin tears, and second-degree burns, pressure ulcers, lower extremity ulcers (including those of venous, arterial, and mixed etiology), diabetic ulcers, and donor sites. Also suitable for use under compression bandaging. May also serve as an absorbent secondary dressing over a primary dressing, such as an alginate, to reduce frequency of dressing changes.

Contraindications
- Contraindicated for third-degree burns or lesions with active vasculitis.
- May be used in visibly infected wounds only when proper medical treatment addresses the underlying causes.

Application

- Cleanse the wound using Skintegrity Wound Cleanser or an appropriate solution. Dry the surrounding skin to allow secure adhesion of the dressing.
- Select the appropriate size dressing to allow the foam island to cover all breached or compromised skin.
- Remove the outermost release paper, and anchor the dressing at one side.
- Smooth the dressing over the wound, and remove remaining release paper. Make sure the dressing is securely adhered without wrinkles in the adhesive border or stretching of the skin.

Removal

- The dressing may be left in place for up to 7 days or until exudate is visible and nears the edge of the dressing.
- Gently press down on the skin, and lift an edge of the dressing.
- Carefully stretch the dressing laterally to the skin to promote pain-free removal.
- Repeat the cleansing procedure prior to applying a new dressing.

NEW PRODUCT

Optifoam Non-Adhesive Foam Island Dressing

Medline Industries, Inc.

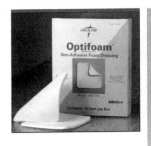

How supplied

Pad: 4″ × 4″; A6209
6″ × 6″; A6210

Action

Optifoam Non-Adhesive Foam Island Dressing is a hydropoly-mer dressing consisting of a thin foam backing over a hydrophilic foam pad. The dressing's waterproof outer layer helps to maintain an optimally moist wound environment, prevent strike-through, and aid in preventing bacterial contamination of the wound. The absorbent pad gently expands as it takes up exudate.

Indications

To manage chronic and acute, moderately to heavily exudating, partial- and full-thickness wounds, including superficial wounds, minor abrasions, skin tears, second-degree burns, pressure ulcers, lower extremity ulcers (including those of venous, arterial, and mixed etiology), diabetic ulcers, and donor sites. Also suitable for use under compression bandaging or under tracheostomies to provide cushioning. May be cut to accommodate bony prominences or smaller wound sizes or fenestrated to accommodate a gastrostomy tube or other leaking drain tubes.

Contraindications

- Contraindicated for third-degree burns or lesions with active vasculitis.
- May be used in visibly infected wounds only when proper medical treatment addresses the underlying causes.

Application

- Cleanse the wound using Skintegrity Wound Cleanser or an appropriate solution. Dry the surrounding skin.
- Select the appropriate size dressing to allow the foam to cover all breached or compromised skin.

- Apply the dressing, and secure it with elastic net, gauze roll, or tape.

Removal

- The dressing may be left in place for up to 7 days or until exudate is visible and nears the edge of the dressing.
- Gently remove the dressing.
- Repeat cleansing procedure prior to applying a new dressing.

POLYDERM BORDER Hydrophilic Polyurethane Foam Dressing
DeRoyal

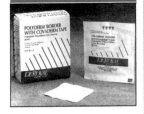

How supplied
Foam pad with border: 2¼" × 2¼" foam with 4" × 4" border, 3¾" × 3¾" foam with 6" × 6" border, circular with radial slit, 2½" foam with 4" border; A6212

Action
POLYDERM BORDER Hydrophilic Polyurethane Foam Dressing is lint-free with a stretchable fabric border that's very gentle to sensitive skin and effective for managing exuding wounds and tube sites. POLYDERM BORDER's thick foam construction provides soft, absorbent protection to painful wound sites.

Indications
For use as a primary or secondary dressing to manage pressure ulcers (stages 2, 3, and 4), partial- and full-thickness wounds, tube sites, donor sites, tunneling wounds, infected and noninfected wounds, and draining wounds. May also be used for red, yellow, and black wounds and for exudate management.

Contraindications
None provided by the manufacturer.

Application
- Cleanse the wound site with normal saline solution.
- Peel back the release liner from the dressing's center to expose the foam.
- Center the foam over the wound and press it into place.
- Secure the border with tape.

Removal
Gently lift the edges of the border, then peel off the dressing.

Polyderm Hydrophilic Polyurethane Foam Dressing
DeRoyal

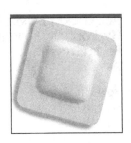

How supplied
*Foam pad
with border:* 2¼″ × 2¼″, 3¾″ × 3¾″

Action
Polyderm is a nonadherent, highly absorbent, lint-free foam dressing for the management of heavily exudating wounds.

Indications
For use as a primary or secondary dressing to manage pressure ulcers (stages 2, 3, and 4), partial- and full-thickness wounds, donor sites, second-degree burns, lacerations, cuts, abrasions, and draining wounds. May also be used for red, yellow, or black wounds and for exudate management.

Contraindications
None provided by the manufacturer.

Application
- Cleanse the wound site with normal saline solution.
- Center the foam over the wound.
- Secure the dressing.

Removal
- Remove any secondary dressing.
- Gently lift the foam dressing from the wound.

Polyderm Plus Barrier Foam Dressing
DeRoyal

How supplied
Foam pad
with border: 2¼" × 2¼" foam with 4" × 4" border,
3¾" × 3¾" foam with 6" × 6" border

Action
Polyderm Plus is a nonadherent, highly absorbent, semi-occlusive, lint-free foam dressing with a nonwoven tape border. It maintains a moist wound environment conducive to healing and resists external contaminants and blood or drainage strike-through.

Indications
For use as a primary or secondary dressing to manage pressure ulcers (stages 2, 3, and 4), partial- and full-thickness wounds, donor sites, tunneling wounds, infected and noninfected wounds, and draining wounds. May also be used for red, yellow, or black wounds and for exudate management.

Contraindications
None provided by the manufacturer.

Application
- Cleanse the wound with normal saline solution.
- Peel back the release liner from the dressing's center to expose the foam.
- Center the foam over the wound and press into place.
- Secure the border with tape.

Removal
Gently lift the edges of the border, then peel off the dressing.

PolyMem Adhesive Film Dressings

PolyMem Adhesive Cloth Dressings

PolyMem Non-Adhesive Dressings

Ferris Manufacturing Corp.

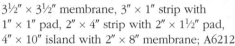

How supplied

PolyMem Adhesive Film Dressings
Sterile pad: 2″ × 2″ dot with 1″ × 1″ membrane, 4″ × 5″ island with 2″ × 3″ membrane, 6″ × 6″ island with 3½″ × 3½″ membrane, 3″ × 1″ strip with 1″ × 1″ pad, 2″ × 4″ strip with 2″ × 1½″ pad, 4″ × 10″ island with 2″ × 8″ membrane; A6212

PolyMem Adhesive Cloth Dressings
Sterile pad: 2″ × 2″ dot with 1″ × 1″ membrane, 4″ × 5″ island with 2″ × 3″ membrane, 6″ × 6″ island with 3½″ × 3½″ membrane, 3″ × 1″ strip with 1″ × 1″ pad, 2″ × 4″ strip with 2″ × 1½″ pad, 4″ × 8″ strip with 2″ × 8″ pad, 4″ × 10″ strip with 2″ × 8″ pad; A6212

PolyMem Non-Adhesive Dressings
Sterile pad: 3″ × 3″, 4″ × 4″; A6209
5″ × 5″; A6210
6½″ × 7½″; A6211
Sterile roll: 4″ × 12½″, 4″ × 24″; A6211

Action

Ferris PolyMem contains three wound-healing agents: a wound cleanser (F68 surfactant) to loosen debris and facilitate movement of fluid, a moisturizer (glycerin) to soften necrotic tissue and prevent the dressing from adhering to the wound, and an absorbent (superabsorbent polymer) to draw fluids away from the wound bed. This formulation allows autolytic debridement and stimulates cell regeneration. PolyMem's semipermeable polyurethane film also offers a balanced exchange of gas necessary to advance the wound-healing process.

Indications
To manage pressure ulcers (stages 1, 2, 3, and 4), partial- and full-thickness wounds, tunneling wounds, infected and noninfected wounds, wounds with all types of drainage, and red, yellow, or black wounds.

Contraindications
Contraindicated for use with hypochlorite solutions (bleach) and other strong oxidizing agents.

Application
- Initial application: Prepare the wound according to facility policy or as directed by the primary care provider. With subsequent dressing changes, cleansing is not recommended unless infection or gross contamination is present.
- Select a PolyMem dressing of appropriate size. The pink membrane should be ¼″ to ½″ (0.6 to 1.3 cm) larger than the wound area.
- Apply the PolyMem dressing film-side/printed-side out.

Removal
- A dramatic increase in wound fluid may be observed during the first few days.
- Keep the dressing dry when bathing the patient. Change the dressing if it gets wet.
- Change the dressing before exudate reaches the periwound area. Change it daily if the patient has a compromised immune system, diabetes, or an infection at the wound site. For a mildly exudating wound in an otherwise healthy patient, the dressing may remain in place for a recommended maximum of 5 days.
- Gently remove the PolyMem dressing from the wound site. It won't adhere to the wound.
- Don't disturb the wound bed. Don't cleanse the wound or flush with saline or water unless the wound is infected or contaminated. PolyMem dressings contain a wound cleanser and leave no residue. Additional cleansing of the wound may delay the wound-healing process.
- Apply a new PolyMem dressing.

Foams

PolyMem Calcium Alginate

Ferris Manufacturing Corp.

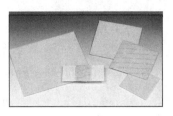

How supplied

Pad: 3″ × 3″, 4″ × 4″; A6209

5″ × 5″; A6210

6.5″ × 7.5″; A6211

Strip: 2″ × 4″ (2″ × 1.5″ pad); A6212

Action

The Ferris PolyMem Calcium Alginate Pad is the only dressing that is infused with calcium alginate and contains a safe wound cleanser (F68 surfactant) to loosen debris and facilitate movement of fluid, moisturizer (glycerin) to soften necrotic or dead tissue and prevent the dressing from adhering to the wound, and a superabsorbent (starch copolymer) to draw fluids away from the wound bed. This formulation allows the wound to autolytically debride and stimulate cell regeneration while healing. PolyMem Calcium Alginate does not contain any toxic drugs or irritants. Ferris' Alginate pad's semipermeable polyurethane film and adhesive (on some of its dressings) offer a balanced exchange of gas (oxygen and carbon dioxide) necessary to advance the wound healing process.

In testing, PolyMem's 3″ × 3″ Alginate pad has been shown to absorb more than 35 cc or grams of exudate from a wound. (The larger-sized Alginate dressings absorb the same percentage in correlation with their size; for example, the 4″ × 4″ pad absorbs more than the 3″ × 3″ pad.) Because of this unique absorbency, PolyMem Calcium Alginate allows extended time between dressing changes, reduces dressings required for wounds with some depth (but less than a tunneling or deep cavity wound) but significant drainage, and saves time and money with fewer changes.

Indications

PolyMem Calcium Alginate is a primary dressing designed to manage pressure ulcers (stages 3 and 4), partial- and full-thickness wounds, exudating wounds, and infected and noninfected wounds.

Contraindications

Contraindicated for use with hypochlorite solutions (bleach) and other strong oxidizing agents.

Application

- Initial application: Prepare the wound according to facility policy or as directed by the primary care provider. With subsequent dressing changes, cleansing is not recommended unless infection or gross contamination is present.
- Select a PolyMem dressing of appropriate size. The pink membrane should be ¼″ to ½″ (0.6 to 1.3 cm) larger than the wound area.
- Apply the PolyMem dressing film-side/printed-side out.

Removal

- A dramatic increase in wound fluid may be observed during the first few days.
- Keep the dressing dry when bathing the patient. Change the dressing if it gets wet.
- Change the dressing before exudate reaches the periwound area. Change it daily if the patient has a compromised immune system, diabetes, or an infection at the wound site. For a mildly exudating wound in an otherwise healthy patient, the dressing may remain in place for a recommended maximum of 5 days.
- Gently remove the PolyMem dressing from the wound site. It won't adhere to the wound.
- Don't disturb the wound bed. Don't cleanse the wound or flush with saline or water unless the wound is infected or contaminated. PolyMem dressings contain a wound cleanser and leave no residue. Additional cleansing of the wound may delay the wound-healing process.
- Apply a new PolyMem Calcium Alginate dressing.

PolyTube Tube-Site Dressing

Ferris Manufacturing Corp.

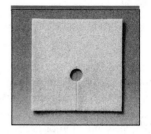

How supplied
Sterile tube-site dressing:
  3½″ × 3½″; A6209

Action
The PolyTube Tube-Site Dressing
is a hydrophilic polyurethane membrane with a precut design
for tube sites, such as tracheotomies, colostomies, colectomies,
and other ostomies. PolyTube contains a wound cleanser to reduce site odor, irritation, and inflammation; a superabsorbent
polymer that wicks fluids from the wound bed; and a moisturizer that prevents the dressing from adhering to the wound.

Indications
For use as a primary dressing around tube sites to continuous-
ly clean the site and reduce unpleasant wound odors.

Contraindications
Contraindicated for use with hypochlorite solutions (bleach) or
other strong oxidizing agents.

Application
- Prior to initial PolyTube application, clean and prepare the
  wound according to facility policy or as directed by the primary care provider.
- Apply the PolyTube dressing film side out, using the precut
  slit to wrap the dressing around the tube area.

Removal
- Change PolyTube when drainage becomes heavy or wound
  odors increase.
- The dressing may be worn for up to 5 days if no exudate is
  present. Change it more often if the patient is diabetic or has
  a reduced immune condition or infection. Change it immediately if the wound area becomes contaminated or the dressing becomes wet.

PolyWic Cavity Wound Filler

Ferris Manufacturing Corp.

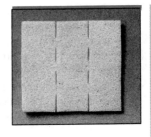

How supplied
Sterile pad: 3″ × 3″; A6215

Action
PolyWic Cavity Wound Filler is a hydrophilic polyurethane membrane with a preslit, perforated design that can be easily separated into three 1″ strips to accommodate the wound bed size. It is designed to be placed into open wounds to eliminate dead space, absorb exudate, and maintain a moist wound environment. PolyWic contains three wound-healing agents: a wound cleanser (F68 surfactant) to loosen debris and facilitate movement of fluid, a moisturizer (glycerin) to soften necrotic tissue and prevent the dressing from adhering to the wound, and an absorbent (superabsorbent polymer) to draw fluids away from the wound bed. This formulation allows autolytic debridement while healing. As it absorbs fluid, PolyWic expands to fill dead space.

Indications
To manage moderately to heavily exuding wounds; partial- and full-thickness wounds; wounds with undermining; infected and noninfected wounds; and red, yellow, or black wounds—types of wounds that are often associated with pressure ulcers (stages 3 and 4), acute wounds, vascular ulcers, and diabetic ulcers. PolyWic requires a secondary dressing.

Contraindications
Contraindicated for use with hypochlorite solutions (bleach) or other strong oxidizing agents.

Application
- Initial PolyWic application: Prepare the wound according to facility policy or as directed by the primary care provider. With subsequent dressing changes, cleansing is not recommended unless infection or gross contamination is present.
- Ensure that PolyWic is 30% smaller than the wound diameter. PolyWic will expand as it wicks and absorbs fluid. Avoid

overfilling the wound, as overfilling may increase pressure on the tissue in the wound bed, potentially causing additional damage.

- Lightly place the wound filler in the middle of the wound, either side up. PolyWic is perforated so that 1"-wide strips can be detached, cut, folded, or placed as is into the cavity.
- Cover the wound and PolyWic with a PolyMem dressing or suitable secondary dressing.

Removal

- Change PolyWic and secondary dressing when the exudate reaches the periwound area. Change daily if the patient has a compromised immune system, diabetes, or an infection at the wound site.
- Gently remove the wound filler in one piece. It won't adhere to the wound.
- Don't disturb the wound bed. Don't cleanse the wound or flush with saline or water unless the wound is infected or contaminated. Additional cleansing may delay the wound-healing process.
- Discontinue use if PolyWic is not fully saturated upon dressing change.

SOF-FOAM Dressing
Johnson & Johnson Wound
Management
Division of ETHICON, Inc.

How supplied
Pad: 3″ × 3″; A6209
                    4″ × 5″, 4″ × 8″; A6210
Fenestrated pad: 3⅝″ × 3⅛″; A6209

Action
SOF-FOAM Dressing is a hydrophilic, polyurethane foam that is a soft, nonlinting dressing designed to cushion and protect the wound site. When used as a primary dressing, the hydrophilic foam absorbs exudate and provides a moist wound environment. The nonadherent foam pad won't break down, making dressing changes easier. Fenestrated SOF-FOAM cushions the wound site and reduces the risk of particulate contamination.

Indications
To manage drainage around surgically induced drainage sites, such as tracheostomy and gastrostomy tubes. SOF-FOAM Dressing also can be used for partial-thickness wounds, such as abrasions, lacerations, donor sites, and superficial burns. It's also appropriate for partial- and full-thickness, moderately to heavily exuding wounds, such as venous ulcers, diabetic ulcers, pressure ulcers, and surgical incisions.

Contraindications
Contraindicated for third-degree burns.

Application
- Cleanse the wound with normal saline solution. Remove any loose necrotic tissue.
- Choose the appropriate dressing size to allow a 1″ (2.5-cm) overlap around the wound margin.
- Apply the dressing; secure it with adhesive tape or a bandage.

Removal
- Check the dressing for saturation and for strike-through at least once every 8 hours. Change the dressing when strike-through occurs or according to facility policy.
- Gently release the tape or wrap and lift up the dressing.

Foams

NEW PRODUCT

SorbaCell Foam Dressing
Dumex Medical

How supplied
Sheet: 2" × 2", 4" × 4"
Strip: 1" × 8"

Action
SorbaCell Foam Dressing is a nonadherent, highly absorptive polyurethane foam sheet that cushions and protects the wound. A secondary dressing is required to protect the wound from outside contaminants and hold the dressing in place.

Indications
To manage moderately to highly exudating wounds.

Contraindications
Contraindicated for third-degree burns.

Application
- Cleanse the wound with PrimaDerm Dermal Cleanser or saline solution. Pat dry the skin adjacent to the wound.
- Position SorbaCell Foam Dressing directly on the wound.
- Secure with an appropriate secondary dressing.

Removal
- Remove the secondary dressing.
- Remove the SorbaCell Foam.

TIELLE Hydropolymer Adhesive Dressing
Johnson & Johnson Wound Management
Division of ETHICON, Inc.

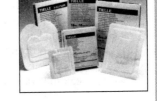

Foams

How supplied
Sterile island dressing: 2¾″ × 3½″, 4¼″ × 4¼″; A6212
5⅞″ × 7¾″, 7″ × 7″, 7″ × 7″ (sacrum); A6213

Action
TIELLE Hydropolymer Adhesive Dressing is a fluid-handling system. As exudate is absorbed by the dressing, the hydropolymer central island swells and fills any irregular contours in the wound, minimizing exudate build-up and the chance of maceration. Evaporation of excess moisture through the vapor-permeable polyurethane backing allows the dressing to manage additional exudate, a continuous process during wound healing.

Indications
To manage chronic and acute, low to moderately exuding, partial- and full-thickness wounds, pressure ulcers (stages 2, 3, and 4), lower extremity ulcers (venous, arterial, and mixed etiology), diabetic ulcers, and donor sites. Also suitable for use under compression bandaging.

Contraindications
- Contraindicated for third-degree burns and for lesions with active vasculitis.
- May be used in visibly infected wounds only when proper medical treatment addresses the underlying cause.

Application
- Position the dressing over the wound site, ensuring that the foam pad covers the wound and the smooth center portion is in place.
- One at a time, peel away the side backing papers while smoothing the film onto the intact periwound skin.

Foams

Removal

- Change the dressing when fluid is present at the edges of the hydropolymer central island. Do not allow exudate to accumulate under the backing.
- Lift one corner, and carefully peel back.
- On fragile or friable skin, water or saline solution may be used to break the adhesive seal.

TIELLE PLUS Hydropolymer Dressing
Johnson & Johnson Wound Management
Division of ETHICON, Inc.

How supplied
Pad: 4¼″ × 4¼″; A6212
5⅞″ × 5⅞″, 5⅞″ × 7¾″; A6213

Action
TIELLE PLUS Hydropolymer Dressing is an exudate-handling system for moderately to heavily exuding wounds. This island dressing maintains a moist wound environment, encouraging autolytic debridement and enabling granulation to proceed under optimal conditions. Autolytic debridement may initially increase the wound size, which is normal and is expected before wound granulation. During use, the absorbent island gently expands as it takes up exudate.

Indications
To manage chronic and acute, moderately to heavily exuding, partial- and full-thickness wounds, including superficial wounds, such as minor abrasions, skin tears, and second-degree burns. May be used under the direction of a health care professional to manage pressure ulcers, lower extremity ulcers (venous, arterial, and mixed etiology), diabetic ulcers, and donor sites. Also suitable for use under compression bandaging. May be used when visible signs of infection are present in the wound area only when proper medical treatment addresses the underlying cause.

Contraindications
- Contraindicated for third-degree burns
- Contraindicated for lesions with active vasculitis.

Application
- Prepare the wound according to facility policy. *Note*: If the wound appears healthy and clean of necrotic debris, cleansing may not be required.
- Ensure that the skin surrounding the wound is dry.
- Position the dressing over the wound site, ensuring that the foam pad covers the wound, and smooth the center portion in place.

■ One at a time, peel away the side backing papers while smoothing the adhesive border onto intact skin.

Removal

■ Change the dressing when wound fluid is present at the edges of the foam pad. Don't allow exudate to accumulate under the backing. The dressing may be left in place up to 7 days, depending on the amount of exudate.

■ Lift one corner of the dressing, and carefully peel it back, avoiding trauma to the intact skin.

■ On fragile or friable skin, use water or normal saline solution to break the adhesive seal.

Foams

VigiFOAM Dressing
Bard Medical Division, C.R. Bard, Inc.

How supplied
Pad: 4″ × 4″, 4″ × 8″ (individual sterile packages
   for single use)

Action
VigiFOAM Dressing, constructed of soft, nonlinting polyurethane
and nonadhesive, is designed to create a moist wound environment and to absorb moderate to heavy amounts of drainage.
The dressing can be cut to fit.

Indications
To manage partial- and full-thickness wounds, leg ulcers, and
superficial wounds, such as abrasions, donor sites, and second-
degree burns. Also may be used in the management of postsurgical incisions and as a cover dressing.

Contraindications
Contraindicated for third-degree burns.

Application
- Cleanse the wound with Biolex Wound Cleanser or another
  appropriate product such as saline solution.
- Pat dry the surrounding skin.
- Choose a dressing size that overlaps the edges of the wound
  by 1″ (2.5 cm).
- Apply either side of the dressing to the wound, and secure
  it with tape, such as Scanpor tape, or transparent film.

Removal
- Change VigiFOAM Dressing when strike-through exudate sat-
  urates the dressing or after a maximum of 7 days.
- Carefully lift the secondary dressing or tape, then gently remove the VigiFOAM Dressing. No adherence should occur.

Hydrocolloids

Hydrocolloids

Action

Hydrocolloids are occlusive or semiocclusive dressings composed of materials such as gelatin, pectin, and carboxymethylcellulose. The composition of the wound contact layer may differ considerably among dressings. These dressing provide a moist healing environment that allows clean wounds to granulate and necrotic wounds to debride autolytically. Some hydrocolloids may leave a residue in the wound, and others may adhere to the skin around the wound. Hydrocolloids are manufactured in a variety of shapes, sizes, adhesive properties, and forms, including wafers, pastes, and powders.

Indications

Hydrocolloid dressings may be used as primary or secondary dressings to manage select pressure ulcers, partial- and full-thickness wounds, wounds with necrosis or slough, and wounds with light to moderate exudate.

Advantages

- Are impermeable to bacteria and other contaminants
- Facilitate autolytic debridement
- Are self-adherent and mold well
- Provide slight to moderate absorption
- Minimize skin trauma and disruption of healing
- Allow observation of the healing process, if transparent
- May be used under compression products (compression stockings, wraps, pumps, and Unna's boot).

Disadvantages

- Aren't recommended for wounds with heavy exudate, sinus tracts, or infections; wounds surrounded by fragile skin; or wounds with exposed tendon or bone
- Can be opaque, making wound assessment difficult
- May be dislodged if the wound produces heavy exudate
- Provide an occlusive property that limits gas exchange between the wound and the environment
- May curl at edges
- May injure fragile skin upon removal.

HCPCS Code Overview

The HCPCS codes normally assigned to hydrocolloid wound covers without an adhesive border are:

A6234 — pad size ≤ 16 sq. in.

A6235 — pad size > 16 sq. in. but ≤ 48 sq. in.

A6236 — pad size > 48 sq. in.

The HCPCS codes normally assigned to hydrocolloid wound covers with an adhesive border are:

A6237 — pad size ≤ 16 sq. in.

A6238 — pad size > 16 sq. in. but ≤ 48 sq. in.

A6239 — pad size > 48 sq. in.

The HCPCS codes normally assigned to hydrocolloid wound fillers are:

A6240 — paste, per fluid ounce

A6241 — dry form, per gram.

CarraSmart Hydrocolloid with Acemannan Hydrogel
Carrington Laboratories, Inc.

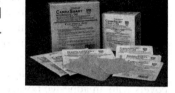

How supplied
Pad: 4" × 4"; A6234
         6" × 6"; A6235

Action
CarraSmart Hydrocolloid wound dressing is a hydrocolloid with a high moisture vapor transfer rate and Acemannan Hydrogel. The "smart" film backing allows moisture to transpire through the hydrocolloid dressing. The hydrocolloid material reacts with the wound exudate to form a gelatinous mass, which provides for a moist wound-healing environment and reduces the potential for tissue damage during dressing changes.

Indications
To manage minimally to moderately exuding wounds, donor sites, partial- to full-thickness wounds, trauma wounds, postoperative surgical wounds, and dermal lesions. Also used as a protective dressing.

Contraindications
Contraindicated for dermal ulcers involving muscle, tendon, or bone; ulcers resulting from infection; and lesions in patients with active vasculitis.

Application
- Gently cleanse the wound with a suitable wound cleanser, such as CarraKlenz, UltraKlenz, or MicroKlenz. Dry the surrounding skin.
- Select the correct dressing size to allow 1¼" (3.2 cm) overlap at the wound margins; trim as desired.
- Remove the release paper from the dressing, minimizing contact with the adhesive surface.
- Apply dressing with a rolling motion; don't stretch it. When applying to a sacral ulcer, press well down into the anal fold.
- Smooth and press into place.

Removal
- Dressings may be changed up to every 7 days as indicated.
- Press down on the skin, and carefully lift the dressing edges.

CombiDERM ACD Absorbent Cover Dressing
ConvaTec

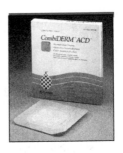

How supplied
Pad: 4″ × 4″, 5¼″ × 5¼″, 6″ × 7″;
    A6237
    6″ × 10″, 8″ × 8″, 8″ × 9″; A6238

Action
CombiDERM ACD Absorbent Cover Dressing is a sterile dressing with a hydrocolloid adhesive and an absorbent pad. This absorbent pad wicks exudate and doesn't damage tissue.

Indications
To manage exuding, chronic dermal ulcers, such as pressure ulcers, leg ulcers, and diabetic ulcers, as well as acute wounds, such as abrasions, lacerations, biopsies, and open and closed surgical wounds.

Contraindications
Contraindicated in patients with a known sensitivity to the dressing or its components.

Application
- Cleanse wound surface and surrounding skin with an appropriate cleansing solution. Dry surrounding skin thoroughly.
- Debride if necessary.
- Determine the ideal dressing size, allowing a minimum 1¼″ (3.2-cm) margin beyond the reddened skin.
- If a filler or exudate management product is required, apply AQUACEL Hydrofiber, KALTOSTAT alginate dressing, or other appropriate dressing.
- Remove Combiderm ACD's release paper, and place the dressing directly over the wound.
- Press and smooth the dressing edges to ensure adherence and a firm seal.

Removal
- Gently press down on the skin, and carefully lift the blue tab on the corner of the dressing. Continue until all edges are free.
- Carefully lift away the dressing.

Hydrocolloids

CombiDERM Non-Adhesive
ConvaTec

How supplied
Pad: 3″ × 3″, 6″ × 10″
    5¼″ × 5¼″; A6235

Action
CombiDERM Non-Adhesive is a sterile nonadhesive wound dressing that consists of absorbent hydrocolloids that provide a moist environment and absorb exudate without damaging tissue. The product may be used alone or in combination with other primary dressings to manage wound exudate.

Indications
To manage exuding chronic wounds, such as pressure ulcers, leg ulcers, and diabetic ulcers, as well as acute exuding wounds, such as abrasions, lacerations, biopsies, and open and closed surgical wounds.

Contraindications
Contraindicated in patients with known sensitivity to the dressing or its components.

Application
- Cleanse the wound site, rinse well, and dry the surrounding skin. For highly exuding wounds, the use of Aquacel or Kaltostat in combination with CombiDERM Non-Adhesive is recommended.
- Chose a dressing that extends 1″ (2.5 cm) beyond the wound.
- Place the dressing white-side-down directly over the wound.
- Secure the dressing with hypoallergenic tape or with the use of a secondary bandage or wrap.

Removal
- Change the dressing when clinically indicated or as the softened area approaches the edge of the dressing. The dressing can be left in place for up to 7 days.
- Carefully lift the dressing away from the wound.

Comfeel Plus Hydrocolloid Contour Dressing

Comfeel Plus Hydrocolloid Pressure Relief Dressing

Comfeel Plus Hydrocolloid Triangle Dressing

Comfeel Hydrocolloid Paste and Powder
Coloplast Corporation

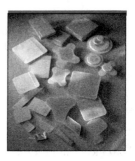

How supplied
Comfeel Plus Hydrocolloid Contour Dressing
Wafer: 24 in^2, 42 in^2; A6238
Comfeel Plus Hydrocolloid Pressure Relief Dressing
Wafer: 3″ butterfly, 4″ round; A6237
                  6″ round; A6238
Comfeel Plus Hydrocolloid Triangle Dressing
Wafer: 7″ × 8″; A6239
Comfeel Hydrocolloid Paste
Tube: 1.76 oz (50 g); A6240
Single-dose Tube: 0.42 oz (12 g); A6240
Comfeel Hydrocolloid Powder
Capsule: 0.21 oz (6 g); A6241

Action
The range of Comfeel hydrocolloid dressings provides an optimal, moist wound-healing environment. Comfeel Hydrocolloid Paste and Comfeel Hydrocolloid Powder are supplements to the chosen wound dressing. Comfeel Hydrocolloid Paste provides filling of the wound cavity, which prevents collapse of undermined wounds. Comfeel Hydrocolloid Powder is highly absorbent and can therefore prolong the wear time of the wound dressing.

Indications
Comfeel Plus Hydrocolloid Contour Dressing is primarily used to manage pressure ulcers in difficult-to-dress sites. Comfeel Plus Hydrocolloid Pressure Relief Dressing is primarily used to

Hydrocolloids

manage and prevent pressure ulcers. Comfeel Plus Hydrocolloid Triangle Dressing is primarily used to manage pressure ulcers in the sacral or hard-to-dress areas. Comfeel Hydrocolloid Paste is used for filling cavity wounds to give the wound extra support and create a contact between the wound bed and the dressing. Comfeel Hydrocolloid Paste should always be used in combination with a Comfeel Plus Hydrocolloid dressing to ensure a moist wound environment. Comfeel Hydrocolloid Powder is used on superficial, highly exuding wounds. These Comfeel products can be used for diabetic or infected wounds under the supervision of a health care professional.

Contraindications

- Continued use may be contraindicated if a wound becomes infected.
- Must be removed prior to radiation therapy.

Application

- Rinse the wound with Sea-Clens or normal saline solution. Gently pat dry the skin around the wound.
- Choose a dressing that allows for ⅜″ to 1″ (1- to 2.5-cm) overlap of the wound.

  Comfeel Plus Hydrocolloid Contour Dressing:
- Remove the protective paper from the center of the dressing, and place the dressing on the wound.
- Remove the protective paper from the wings, and gently press the wings one at a time to ensure that the dressing adheres to the skin.

  Comfeel Plus Hydrocolloid Pressure Relief Dressing:
- Remove the number of foam rings with orange print to get a foam-free area about ⅜″ to 1″ (1 to 2.5 cm) larger than the wound.
- Remove the protective paper from the dressing, and roll the dressing on from one side.
- Remove the protective paper from the microporous tape, and gently apply it to the skin.

  Comfeel Plus Hydrocolloid Triangle Dressing:
- Remove the protective paper from the center of the dressing.
- Spread the gluteal fold, place the dressing's narrow end into the deepest depression of the gluteal fold, and secure it in

place. Ensure that the wound has 1″ (2.5 cm) of intact peri-
wound skin and that the dressing adheres to the skin.
- Remove the second protective paper from the dressing, and
secure it into place.
  Comfeel Hydrocolloid Paste:
- Fill the wound with the paste to approximately one-third of
the wound depth.
- Use the tube key to empty the tube completely. When using
the single dose, squeeze the paste out from one corner.
  Comfeel Hydrocolloid Powder:
- Gently press the capsule to direct the powder into the wound
bed.

Removal

- As Comfeel dressings absorb wound exudate, they turn white
or lighten. Change the dressing when the color-change indicator spreads to ⅜″ (1 cm) from the border. Change Comfeel
Hydrocolloid Paste and Powder when changing the wound
dressing.
- In case of leakage or nonadherence, change the dressing immediately.
- Although Comfeel dressings are odorproof, the wound itself
may have a characteristic odor. This is normal, and the odor
should resolve once the wound is rinsed. If the odor persists,
contact a health care professional.

Hydrocolloids

Comfeel Plus Hydrocolloid Ulcer Dressing

Comfeel Hydrocolloid Ulcer Care Dressing

Comfeel Plus Hydrocolloid Clear Dressing
Coloplast Corporation

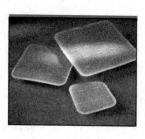

How supplied
Comfeel Plus Hydrocolloid Ulcer Dressing
Wafer: 4″ × 4″; A6234
6″ × 6″; A6235
8″ × 8″; A6236
Comfeel Hydrocolloid Ulcer Care Dressing
Wafer: 1½″ × 2½″, 4″ × 4″; A6234
6″ × 6″; A6235
8″ × 8″; A6236
Comfeel Plus Hydrocolloid Clear Dressing
Wafer: 2″ × 2¾″, 4″ × 4″; A6234
3½″ × 5½″, 6″ × 6″, 2″ × 10″, 6″ × 8″; A6235
8″ × 8″; A6236

Action
Comfeel hydrocolloid dressings provide an optimal, moist, wound-healing environment.

Indications
Primarily to manage minimally to moderately exuding leg ulcers and pressure ulcers. May be used for superficial burns, partial-thickness burns, donor sites, postoperative wounds, and skin abrasions. May also be used for diabetic or infected wounds under the supervision of a health care professional.

Contraindications
- Continued use may be contraindicated if a wound becomes infected.
- Must be removed prior to radiation therapy.

Application
- Rinse the wound with Comfeel Sea-Clens or normal saline solution. Gently pat dry the skin around the wound.
- Choose a dressing that allows for $\frac{3}{8}$" to 1" (1- to 2.5-cm) overlap of the wound.
- Use the handles on the dressing to ensure aseptic application. Remove the protective paper.
- Place the adhesive side to the wound. Remove the handle.

Removal
- As Comfeel dressings absorb wound exudate, a gel forms. When the gel reaches the upper film surface of the dressing, it turns white or lightens. Change the dressing when the white gel spreads to $\frac{3}{8}$" (1 cm) from the border.
- In case of leakage or nonadherence, change the dressing immediately.
- Although Comfeel dressings are odorproof, the wound itself may have a characteristic odor. This is normal, and the odor should resolve once the wound is rinsed. If the odor persists, contact a health care professional.

Hydrocolloids

Comfeel TRIAD Hydrophilic Wound Dressing
Coloplast Corporation

How supplied
Tube: 2.5 oz, 6 oz; A6240

Action
Comfeel TRIAD Hydrophilic Wound Dressing gently adheres to moist, exuding wounds and spreads evenly over areas inaccessible to conventional dressings. It's noncytotoxic and promotes autolytic debridement.

Indications
To manage pressure ulcers (stages 2, 3, and 4), venous stasis ulcers, partial- and full-thickness wounds, superficial wounds, scrapes, and first- and second-degree burns. May be used on tunneling wounds; wounds with minimal, moderate, or heavy drainage; wounds with serosanguineous drainage; and red, yellow, or black wounds.

Contraindications
Contraindicated for third-degree burns and infected wounds.

Application
- Cleanse the wound using a wound cleanser or normal saline solution.
- Fill the wound bed with the dressing, and apply a lighter layer on the periwound area. Cover this with a secondary dressing.
- For an open skin tear, apply a thin layer of dressing over it, then cover it with petroleum-impregnated gauze or a nonadherent dressing and secure.
- For necrotic tissue, cover all the tissue and periwound skin with a thin layer of the dressing. Use a cover dressing if desired.

Removal
- If the dressing has dried out, spray with a wound cleanser or normal saline solution. Then, cover with gauze moistened with cleanser or normal saline solution, and allow it to remain for 2 to 3 minutes before removing the dressing.
- If the dressing is moist, spray with a wound cleanser or normal saline solution. Then, gently remove the dressing.

DermaFilm HD

DermaFilm Thin
DermaRite Industries

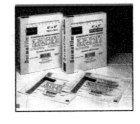

How supplied
DermaFilm HD
Film: 4″ × 4″
DermaFilm Thin
Film: 4″ × 4″

Action
DermaFilm is a pressure-sensitive dressing that interacts with wound exudates to form a soft gel. It helps isolate the wound against bacterial and other external contamination. The thin formula allows visibility and maintenance of the wound bed through course treatment.

Indications
To manage pressure ulcers (stages 1, 2, 3, and 4), partial- and full thickness wounds, clinically infected wounds, minor abrasions, and second-degree burns. Also used to prevent skin breakdown associated with urine and fecal breakdown.

Contraindications
- Contraindicated for third-degree burns.
- Contraindicated for ulcers involving muscle, tendon, or bone.

Application
- Cleanse the wound area, and dry the periwound skin.
- Choose a dressing that overlaps the wound by at least 1″ (2.5 cm). Apply the dressing without stretching it.
- Press the dressing gently around the perimeter, forming it to the wound site.

Removal
- Change the dressing when the exudate extends to the edges. Dressing may be left in place for a maximum of 7 days.
- Press down on the skin, and carefully lift an edge of the dressing. Continue lifting around the dressing until all edges are free.
- Repeat the cleansing procedure.

Hydrocolloids

DERMATELL

DERMATELL SECURE
Gentell, Inc.

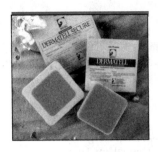

How supplied
DERMATELL
Wafer: 4½″ × 4½″; A6235
DERMATELL SECURE
Wafer: 5½″ × 5½″; A6238

(side tab) Hydrocolloids

Action
DERMATELL wafers absorb minimal to moderate wound exudate and interact with it to form a soft, protective gel. The dressing promotes autolysis, prevents secondary infection, and reduces pain. It also provides protection from urine, stool, and other contaminants.

Indications
To manage venous ulcers in conjunction with compression therapy, pressure ulcers (stages 1, 2, and 3), first- and second-degree burns, and granulating wounds with minimal to moderate exudate.

Contraindications
Contraindicated for heavily exuding wounds, stage 4 pressure ulcers, infected wounds, and third-degree burns.

Application
- Cleanse the wound with a wound cleanser. Gently dry the periwound skin.
- Remove the paper carrier from the dressing, and apply the dressing, allowing 2″ (5 cm) of the wafer to extend beyond the wound margin.
- For proper placement, center the wafer and gently adhere the dressing to the site, especially around the edges.

Removal
- Gently press down on skin, and carefully lift an edge of the dressing. Continue until all edges are free.
- Repeat cleansing procedure.

DuoDERM CGF
ConvaTec

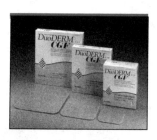

How supplied
Wafer: 4"x 4"; A6234
6" × 6", 6" × 8"; A6235
8" × 8", 8" × 12"; A6236

Action
DuoDerm CGF Control Gel Formula Dressing is an adhesive hydrocolloid wound contact dressing. The self-adherent dressing absorbs wound fluid and provides a moist environment, which supports the body's healing process and aids in autolytic debridement without damaging new tissue. The dressing acts as a barrier against bacterial, viral, and other external contamination.

Indications
To manage minor abrasions, lacerations, minor cuts, minor scalds and burns, leg ulcers (venous stasis ulcers, arterial ulcers, and leg ulcers of mixed etiology), diabetic ulcers and pressure ulcers (partial- and full-thickness). Also used for surgical wounds (wounds left to heal by secondary intention, donor sites, and dermatological excisions), second-degree burns, and traumatic wounds.

Contraindications
Contraindicated in patients with a known sensitivity to any of the dressing's components.

Application
- Choose a dressing size that is 1¼" inches (3.2 cm) larger than the wound.
- Remove the release paper from the back, minimizing finger contact with the adhesive surface.
- Hold the dressing over the wound, line up the center of the dressing with the center of the wound, and place the dressing directly over the wound.
- For difficult-to-dress sites, such as heel or sacrum, a supplementary securing device, such as tape, may be required.

Hydrocolloids

Removal

- Change the dressing when clinically indicated or when strike-through occurs. Otherwise, it may be left in place for up to 7 days.
- Press down gently on the skin, and carefully lift one corner of the dressing until it no longer adheres to the skin. Continue until all edges are free.

Hydrocolloids

DuoDERM CGF Border
ConvaTec

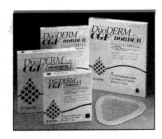

How supplied
Pad: 2½″ × 2½″ (¾″ adhesive
border), 4″ × 4″ (¾″ ad-
hesive border), 6″ × 6″
(1″ adhesive border),
4″ × 5″ (1″ adhesive bor-
der), 6″ × 7″ (1″ adhesive border); A6237

Action
DuoDERM CGF Border interacts with wound exudate to produce a soft mass that allows removal of the dressing with little
or no damage to newly formed tissue. It helps isolate the wound
against bacterial and other external contamination.

Indications
To manage dermal ulcers, diabetic foot ulcers, and leg ulcers.
May also be used on pressure ulcers (stages 1, 2, 3, and 4), full-
thickness wounds, minor abrasions, second-degree burns, and
donor sites.

Contraindications
Contraindicated in patients with a known sensitivity to the dressing or its components.

Application
- Cleanse the wound according to facility policy. Irrigate with
  normal saline solution, then dry the surrounding skin to ensure that it's grease-free.
- Before applying the dressing, remove eschar that's particularly thick or fused to the wound margins.
- Choose a dressing size that's at least 1¼″ (3.2 cm) larger than
  the wound margins.
- Remove the top backing paper only, and apply the dressing
  over the wound. Smooth into place, especially at the edges
  of the center adhesive. *Note:* The triangle-shaped dressing
  can be applied in several directions, depending on the location of the ulcer. For sacral ulcers, fold the dressing in half
  lengthwise to make it easy to apply in the sacral folds.

Hydrocolloids

- Fold back the border, remove the release papers, and press the borders into place. Additional taping isn't required.
- If infection develops, continue using the dressing as directed by the primary care provider.
- Using an occlusive dressing when necrotic tissue is present may initially increase wound size and depth when debris is cleaned away. In some wounds, using an occlusive dressing may cause hypergranulation tissue to develop and prevent wound closure. If this occurs, notify the primary care provider.

Removal

- Leave the dressing in place for up to 7 days unless it's uncomfortable or leaking or infection develops.
- Press down on the skin, and carefully lift an edge of the dressing. Continue lifting around the dressing until all edges are free.
- Repeat the cleansing procedure. It's unnecessary to remove all residual dressing material from the surrounding skin.

DuoDERM Extra Thin
ConvaTec

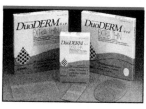

How supplied
Wafer: 1¼″ × 1½″ (spots),
        2″ × 4″, 2″ × 8″,
        3″ × 3″, 4″ × 4″; A6234
        4″ × 6″, 6″ × 6″, 6″ × 7″; A6235

Action
DuoDERM Extra Thin interacts with wound exudate to produce
a soft mass that allows dressing removal with little or no damage to newly formed tissue. It helps isolate the wound against
bacterial and other external contamination. This dressing is particularly suitable for areas subject to friction or those requiring
contouring, such as elbows or heels.

Indications
For use as a protective dressing and to manage superficial, dry-
to lightly exuding dermal ulcers and postoperative wounds.

Contraindications
Contraindicated in patients with a known sensitivity to the dressings or their components.

Application
- Cleanse the wound. Irrigate with normal saline solution, and
  dry the surrounding skin to ensure that it's grease-free.
- Choose a dressing size that extends beyond the wound mar-
  gin at least 1¼″ (3.2 cm).
- Apply in a rolling motion, avoiding stretching and minimiz-
  ing finger contact with the adhesive surface.
- Smooth into place, especially around the edges.
- Use hypoallergenic tape to secure the edges.
- For a heel or elbow, cut a slit approximately one-third across
  each side of the dressing to make application easier.
- For a sacral ulcer, press the dressing into the gluteal fold. The
  triangle-shaped dressing can be applied in different directions, depending on the location and depth of the ulcer.
- Using an occlusive dressing in the presence of necrotic material may initially increase wound size and depth when the
  necrotic debris is cleaned away.

Hydrocolloids

- If infection develops, continue using the dressing as directed by the primary care provider.

Removal
- Leave the dressing in place for up to 7 days unless it's uncomfortable or leaking or infection develops.
- Press down on the skin, and carefully lift an edge of the dressing. Continue lifting around the dressing until all edges are free.
- Repeat the cleansing procedure. It's unnecessary to remove all residual dressing material from the surrounding skin.

DuoDERM Hydroactive Paste
ConvaTec

How supplied
Tube: 30 g; A6240

Action
DuoDERM Hydroactive Paste is a hypoallergenic paste that's composed of natural hydrocolloids in a dermatologically approved vehicle.

Indications
For local management of exuding dermal ulcers to extend the life of the dressings.

Contraindications
Contraindicated in patients with a known sensitivity to the dressing or its components.

Application
- Cleanse the wound according to facility policy. Irrigate with normal saline solution, and carefully dry the surrounding skin to remove any greasy substances that may interfere with the dressing's adherence.
- Use alcohol to swab the piercing spike on the cap of the tube.
- Remove the cap and puncture the tube's opening by inverting the cap and pressing it on the metal membrane. *Note:* A small amount of clear liquid may be expelled when the tube is opened. This is normal and doesn't indicate deterioration.
- Squeeze the paste into the wound. Smooth the paste, if necessary, using a sterile spatula or a sterile glove finger. Keep the paste at the level of surrounding skin, and remove any excess from the skin. *Note:* The presence of paste on the surrounding healthy skin will impair adherence.
- Select a cover dressing that overlaps the healthy periwound skin by at least 1¼" (3.2 cm). Apply the dressing in a rolling motion, and hold it gently in place to ensure good adherence.
- Using an occlusive cover dressing may cause hypergranulation tissue to develop, preventing wound closure. If this occurs, notify the primary care provider.

Hydrocolloids

- Using an occlusive dressing may initially increase wound size and depth when the debris is cleaned away. This isn't a contraindication for further use of the paste.

Removal
- If infection develops and is verified, discontinue use of the paste until the infection has been eradicated.
- The paste will gradually form a gel-like substance in the presence of moisture. It can be removed with normal saline solution during dressing changes.
- It's unnecessary to completely remove material adhering to the wound margins before applying a new dressing.

Exuderm

Exuderm LP

Exuderm RCD

Exuderm Sacrum

Exuderm Ultra
Medline Industries, Inc.

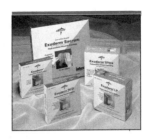

How supplied

Exuderm
Wafer: 4″ × 4″; A6234
       8″ × 8″; A6236

Exuderm LP
Wafer: 4″ × 4″; A6234
       6″ × 6″; A6235

Exuderm RCD
Wafer: 4″ × 4″; A6234
       6″ × 6″; A6235
       8″ × 8″; A6236

Exuderm Sacrum
Wafer: 3½″ × 4″; A6234
       6″ × 6½″; A6235

Exuderm Ultra
Wafer: 4″ × 4″; A6234

Action

Traditional Exuderm reacts with wound exudate to create a moist, healing environment while absorbing wound exudate. Exuderm LP's low-profile design is used to protect against skin breakdown or to dress superficial wounds. Exuderm Regulated Colloidal Dispersion (RCD) is used to manage and absorb exudate with minimal meltdown. Exuderm Sacrum's butterfly design is anatomically shaped to conform to the natural shape of the body and features a hinged center for a flush fit. Exuderm Sacrum has a low-residue formula and a tapered edge, facilitating longer wear time. Exuderm Ultra features an intelligent film backing that responds to the exudate level, adjusting the rate of exhaustion to provide an optimally moist wound bed;

its low-profile, conformable design resists roll-up. All Exuderm dressings provide a protective, occlusive barrier, facilitating granulation or autolytic debridement if necessary.

Indications

To manage dermal ulcers, leg ulcers, pressure ulcers (stages 2, 3, and 4), partial-thickness wounds, minor abrasions, second-degree burns, donor sites, wounds with slough or necrosis, and red, yellow, or black wounds. Exuderm Sacrum manages such wounds as sacral pressure ulcers (stages 2 and 4) and incontinence-induced denuded areas; it's also useful for postoperative wounds, superficial wounds, and abrasions. Exuderm LP manages wounds with light drainage. Exuderm, Exuderm Sacrum, Exuderm RCD, and Exuderm Ultra manage wounds with light to moderate drainage.

Contraindications

Contraindicated for third-degree burns.

Application

- Cleanse the application site with normal saline solution or another appropriate cleanser, such as Skintegrity Wound Cleanser. Dry the surrounding area to ensure that it's free of any greasy substance.
- Select the appropriate-sized dressing to allow 1¼″ to 1½″ (3.2 to 3.8 cm) for attachment to healthy periwound skin.
    Exuderm, Exuderm LP, Exuderm RCD, and Exuderm Ultra:
- Remove the paper carrier from the dressing.
- Center Exuderm over the site, and apply to skin using a rolling motion.
- Smooth the dressing into place, especially around the edges, and hold for 5 seconds to maximize adhesive qualities.
- For traditional hydrocolloids like Exuderm and Exuderm RCD, picture-framing (taping down all sides) with a skin-friendly tape such as Medfix can help prevent roll-up.
    Exuderm Sacrum:
- Remove one side of the paper carrier from the dressing. Place the dressing's "hinge" into the gluteal fold, and apply the exposed adhesive portion to the buttocks.
- Remove the last part of the protective paper, and apply the second half of the adhesive portion to the skin.

- Inspect the dressing, making sure that the edges adhere well.
- Place your hand on top of the dressing for about 1 minute, warming the dressing to body temperature to enhance adherence.

Removal

- Dressing may remain in place for 2 to 7 days, depending upon the amount of wound drainage. If the dressing begins to lift or leak, change it immediately.
- An adhesive remover may be used to loosen the dressing.
- Carefully press down on the skin, and lift an edge of the dressing. Continue around the dressing until all edges are free.
- Repeat the cleansing procedure.

Hydrocolloids

Hydrocol

Hydrocol Thin
Bertek (Dow Hickam)
Pharmaceuticals

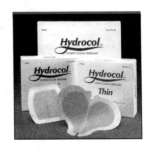

How supplied
Hydrocol
Wafer: 3" × 3", 4" × 4"; A6234
      6" × 6", 6" × 8"; A6235
      8" × 8"; A6236
Wafer (sacral): 6" × 7"; A6235
Hydrocol Thin
Wafer: 3" × 3", 4" × 4"; A6234
      6" × 6", 6" × 8"; A6235

Action
These Hydrocol products provide a moist, wound-healing environment by absorbing excess exudate and interacting with it to form a soft gel. These dressings also protect the wound from exogenous bacteria, urine, feces, and other contaminants.

Indications
To manage dermal wounds, including full-thickness wounds, pressure ulcers (stages 1, 2, 3, and 4), leg ulcers, superficial wounds and abrasions, trauma wounds, and surgical wounds. Hydrocol manages light to moderately heavy exudate. Hydrocol sacral dressing manages sacral ulcers and breakdown. Hydrocol Thin manages superficial wounds and abrasions where maximum dressing wear time is desired.

Contraindications
Contraindicated for third-degree burns.
Contraindicated in patients with a known sensitivity to the dressing or its components.

Application
- Break open the backing paper by folding the dressing back over itself along the cut in the back.
- Hold the dressing by the side that has the smaller release backing. With your other hand, separate the backing paper

from the hydrocolloid on the protruding ear tab. Remove the larger backing paper first, pulling it back over the dressing

- Avoid touching the dressing's wound contact surface.
- With the smaller release backing still on the dressing, center the dressing over the wound site and apply. Avoid touching the dressing's wound contact surface.
- Remove the remaining backing paper by grasping the ear tab and peeling the backing paper back under itself.
- Smooth out all wrinkles. Place your hand over the dressing, and apply slight pressure for 30 to 40 seconds to warm the dressing and promote adherence.

Removal
- Hydrocol dressings may remain in place for up to 7 days. However, change them immediately if they reach full absorbency or leak.
- Starting at one corner of the dressing, press down on the skin and carefully peel back the dressing. Continue this process around the dressing until all edges are free.
- Carefully wash or irrigate the wound to remove any residue.

Hydrocolloids

Hydrocolloids

NEW PRODUCT

Hyperion Hydrocolloid Dressing
Hyperion Medical, Inc.

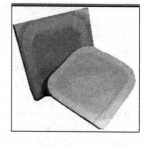

How supplied
Thin pad: 4″ × 4″
Bordered pad: 4″ × 4″

Action
Hyperion Hydrocolloid Dressings provide a moist, healing environment and assist with granulation and autolytic debridement.

Indications
To manage superficial or partial-thickness wounds, wounds with necrosis and slough, and wounds with light-to-moderate exudate.

Contraindications
- Contraindicated for wounds with heavy exudate, sinus tracts, or infections or wounds with exposed bone or tendon.
- Contraindicated for third-degree burns.

Application
- Cleanse the wound with a suitable wound cleanser.
- Choose the appropriate size dressing.
- Apply the dressing with a rolling motion; don't stretch. When applying to a sacral ulcer, press well down into the gluteal fold.
- Smooth and press into place.

Removal
- Gently remove the dressing from the wound bed.
- Irrigate with wound cleanser.

NEW PRODUCT
MPM Excel Hydrocolloid Wound Dressing
MPM Medical, Inc.

How supplied
Pad: 2″ × 2″, 3.6″ × 4″, 4″ × 5″, 6″ × 6.5″, 8″ × 4″

Action
MPM Excel Hydrocolloid Wound Dressings are thin with a foam top. They protect the wound from the outside environment and assist the body in healing by maintaining a moist wound environment.

Indications
To manage pressure ulcers (stages 1, 2, and 3) and leg ulcers.

Contraindications
- Contraindicated for infected wounds.
- Contraindicated for stage 4 wounds.
- Contraindicated for third-degree burns.

Application
- Select a dressing that overlaps the wound by 1″.
- Cleanse the wound and dry the periwound skin.
- Apply the dressing directly over the wound. The dressing is self-adherent.

Removal
- Change the dressing every 2 to 5 days, when exudate begins to leak from the edges.
- Lift one corner, then gently remove entire dressing.

Hydrocolloids

PrimaCol Bordered Hydrocolloid Dressing
Dumex Medical

How supplied
Wafer: 2″ × 2″, 4″ × 4″, 6″ × 6″, 8″ × 8″

Action
PrimaCol Bordered Hydrocolloid Dressing provides a moist, wound-healing environment and protects the wound from outside contaminants. In contact with wound fluid, it produces a soft mass, allowing nontraumatic removal. PrimaCol Bordered Hydrocolloids do not require a secondary dressing.

Indications
To manage minimally to moderately exudating, partial-thickness wounds.

Contraindications
Contraindicated for third-degree burns.

Application
- Cleanse the wound with PrimaDerm Dermal Cleanser or saline solution. Dry the skin adjacent to the wound.
- Choose a dressing that allows the hydrocolloid pad to extend 1″ beyond the wound margins.
- Place the dressing directly on the wound without stretching the dressing.
- Smooth the film border to insure secure adherence.

Removal
Carefully lift an edge of the dressing, and continue lifting around the entire perimeter of the dressing until all of the adhesive edge is free.

NEW PRODUCT
PrimaCol Hydrocolloid Dressing
Dumex Medical

How supplied
Wafer: 4″ × 4″, 6″ × 6″, 8″ × 8″

Action
PrimaCol Hydrocolloid Dressing provides a moist, wound-healing environment and protects the wound from outside contaminants. In contact with wound fluid, it produces a soft mass, allowing nontraumatic removal.

Indications
To manage minimally to moderately exudating partial- and full-thickness wounds.

Contraindications
Contraindicated for third-degree burns.

Application
- Cleanse the wound with PrimaDerm Dermal Cleanser or saline solution. Dry the skin adjacent to the wound.
- Choose a dressing that extends 1″ beyond the wound margins.
- Place the dressing directly on the wound while avoiding stretching the dressing.

Removal
Carefully lift an edge of the dressing, and continue lifting around the entire perimeter of the dressing until all of the adhesive edge is free.

Hydrocolloids

PrimaCol Specialty Hydrocolloid Dressing
Dumex Medical

How supplied
Wafer: Heel and elbow, sacrum

Action
PrimaCol Specialty Hydrocolloid Dressing provides a moist, wound-healing environment and protects the wound from outside contaminants. In contact with wound fluid, it produces a soft mass, allowing nontraumatic removal. PrimaCol Specialty Hydrocolloids are designed for difficult-to-dress areas, such as the sacral area, heel, and elbow.

Indications
To manage minimally to moderately exudating, partial-thickness wounds. Also used for difficult-to-dress areas, such as bony prominences.

Contraindications
Contraindicated for third-degree burns.

Application
- Cleanse the wound with PrimaDerm Dermal Cleanser or saline solution. Dry the skin adjacent to the wound.
- Choose a dressing that allows the hydrocolloid pad to extend 1″ beyond the wound margins.
- Place the dressing directly on the wound without stretching the dressing.
- Smooth the film border to ensure secure adherence.

Removal
Carefully lift an edge of the dressing, and continue lifting around the entire perimeter of the dressing until all of the adhesive edge is free.

Hydrocolloids

NEW PRODUCT
PrimaCol Thin Hydrocolloid Dressing
Dumex Medical

How supplied
Wafer: 2″ × 2″, 4″ × 4″, 6″ × 6″

Action
PrimaCol Thin Hydrocolloid Dressing provides a moist, wound-healing environment and protects the wound from outside contaminants. In contact with wound fluid, it produces a soft mass, allowing nontraumatic removal. PrimaCol Thin is a transparent hydrocolloid, which facilitates wound inspection.

Indications
To manage superficial and minimally exudating, partial-thickness wounds. Also used for difficult-to-dress areas, such as bony prominences.

Contraindications
Contraindicated for third-degree burns.

Application
- Cleanse the wound with PrimaDerm Dermal Cleanser or saline solution. Dry the skin adjacent to the wound.
- Choose a dressing that extends 1″ beyond the wound margins.
- Place the dressing directly on the wound without stretching the dressing.

Removal
Carefully lift an edge of the dressing, and continue lifting around the entire perimeter of the dressing until all of the adhesive edge is free.

Hydrocolloids

Procol Hydrocolloid Dressing
DeRoyal

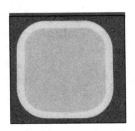

Hydrocolloids

How supplied
Wafer: 2″ × 2″, 4″ × 4″; A6237
6″ × 6″; A6238

Action
Procol is a self-adherent, hydrocolloid wound dressing that creates a moist wound environment conducive to local wound healing. It protects against wound dehydration, acts as a bacterial barrier, and helps to control wound drainage. Procol's matrix formulation helps reduce the residue left in the wound and also helps avoid damaging newly formed tissue during dressing changes.

Indications
For use as a primary or secondary dressing to manage dermal ulcers, superficial wounds, lacerations, abrasions, first- and second-degree burns, donor sites, and postoperative wounds.

Contraindications
Contraindicated for third-degree burns.

Application
- Cleanse the wound site with normal saline solution.
- If necessary, cut Procol to desired size.
- Remove the dressing's release liner, and apply the exposed side to the wound.
- Because Procol adheres to the skin around the wound, extra tape isn't necessary.

Removal
Gently lift edges, and peel the dressing off.

RepliCare

RepliCare Thin
Smith & Nephew, Inc.
Wound Management Division

How supplied
RepliCare
Wafer: $1\frac{1}{2}'' \times 2\frac{1}{2}''$, $4'' \times 4''$; A6234
    $6'' \times 6''$; A6235
    $8'' \times 8''$; A6236
RepliCare Thin
Wafer: $2'' \times 2\frac{3}{4}''$; A6234
    $3\frac{1}{2}'' \times 5\frac{1}{2}''$, $6'' \times 8''$; A6235

Action
RepliCare is a semitransparent dressing, and RepliCare Thin is a transparent dressing; both allow observation of the wound. The dressings' outer component, a waterproof polyurethane film, aids in preventing bacterial contamination.

Indications
Both products are used to manage pressure ulcers (stages 1 and 2), partial-thickness wounds, lightly exuding wounds, and skin tears and abrasions. RepliCare is also used for stages 3 and 4 pressure ulcers, full-thickness wounds, and red or yellow wounds.

Contraindications
- Contraindicated for ulcers involving muscle, tendon, or bone.
- Contraindicated in patients with active vasculitis, deep systemic infections, or signs of local infection at the wound site.

Application
- Make sure the surrounding skin is clean and dry.
- Select a dressing size that overlaps the periwound skin by $\frac{1}{2}''$ to $1''$ (1.3 to 2.5 cm) for proper adherence.
- Spend 1 to $1\frac{1}{2}$ minutes pressing the dressing into place. Work from the center out, concentrating on adhering the tapered edges.
- Tape edges in moist or high-friction areas.

Hydrocolloids

Removal

- Change the dressing every 4 days or when it becomes transparent or leaks.
- Support the dressing with one hand while using the other hand to pull the edges laterally (parallel to the skin surface) away from the center.

Restore Cx Wound Care Dressing
Hollister Incorporated

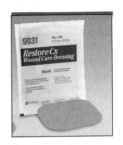

How supplied
Wafer: 4″ × 4″; A6234
6″ × 8″; A6235
8″ × 8″; A6236

Action
Restore Cx Wound Care Dressing is a sterile, occlusive dressing. The flexible outer layer protects wounds from microorganisms, urine and feces, and the external environment. The self-adherent inner layer maintains a moist environment while absorbing excess exudate.

Indications
To manage venous stasis ulcers and partial-thickness wounds with moderate to heavy exudate in difficult-to-manage sites, such as the sacrum and coccyx. May also be used on pressure ulcers (stages 1 and 2), noninfected wounds, wounds with moderate drainage, and red or yellow wounds.

Contraindications
- Contraindicated for ulcers involving muscle, tendon, or bone.
- Contraindicated in patients with active vasculitis, deep systemic infections, or signs of local infection at the wound site.

Application
- Prepare the wound area according to facility policy. For secure application, make sure the periwound skin is clean and dry.
- To ensure adherence, select a dressing that extends at least 1″ (2.5 cm) beyond the wound edge. Overlap or cut the dressing to size.
- Remove the printed release paper from the dressing.
- Center the dressing over the wound site, and press it against the skin. Smooth to remove wrinkles.

Removal
- Carefully lift the edge of the dressing while pressing against the skin.
- Continue around the wound bed until all edges are free.

Hydrocolloids

Restore Extra Thin Dressing
Hollister Incorporated

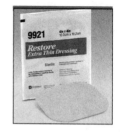

How supplied:
Wafer: 4″ × 4″; A6234
6″ × 8″; A6235
8″ × 8″; A6236

Action
Restore Extra Thin Dressing is a sterile, extrathin occlusive dressing. The flexible film backing acts as a barrier to urine and feces and protects wounds from the external environment. The self-adherent dressing helps maintain a moist, wound-healing environment. Transparency allows for wound observation.

Indications
To protect the skin, prevent skin breakdown, and manage superficial wounds with little or no exudate, especially those at risk for friction injury. May be used on stage 1 pressure ulcers, partial-thickness wounds, noninfected wounds, wounds with minimal drainage, and red wounds.

Contraindications
- Contraindicated for ulcers involving muscle, tendon, or bone.
- Contraindicated in patients with active vasculitis, deep systemic infections, or signs of local infection at the wound site.

Application
- Prepare the wound area according to facility policy. Make sure the skin is clean, dry, and free from oily residue.
- To ensure adherence, select a dressing that extends at least 1″ (2.5 cm) beyond the wound edge. Overlap or cut the dressing to size.
- Remove the printed release paper from the dressing.
- Center the dressing over the wound site and press it against the skin. Smooth out the wrinkles.

Removal
Carefully lift the dressing edge, and peel gently away from the skin.

Hydrocolloids

Restore Plus Wound Care Dressing
Hollister Incorporated

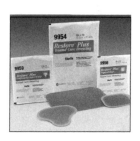

How supplied
Wafer: 4" × 4"; A6234
                6" × 6", 6" × 8"; A6235
                8" × 8"; A6236

Tapered-edge
wafer: 4" × 4"; A6234
                6" × 8"; A6235
                8" × 8"; A6236
                triangle (17 sq. in.), triangle (26.5 sq. in.); A6238

Action
Restore Plus Wound Care Dressing provides a moist, wound-healing environment for noninfected dermal ulcers, including full-thickness wounds. It also isolates the wound against bacteria and viruses (such as hepatitis B and C and human immunodeficiency virus infection).

Indications
To manage dermal ulcers, including full-thickness wounds, pressure ulcers (stages 1, 2, 3, and 4), leg ulcers, superficial wounds (minor abrasions), second-degree burns, and donor sites.

Contraindications
Contraindicated for third-degree burns.

Application
- Clean and dry the skin according to facility policy.
- Measure the wound using the wound-measuring guide.
- Choose a dressing that extends 1" (2.5 cm) beyond the wound edges on all sides.
- Grasp the dressing tab and remove the release paper, touching the adhesive side of the dressing as little as possible.
- Center the dressing over the wound site, then gently press the dressing to the skin and smooth out the wrinkles.

Removal
- Carefully lift edges of dressing while pressing down on the skin.
- Continue this procedure around the wound bed until all edges are free.

Hydrocolloids

Restore Wound Care Dressing

Hollister Incorporated

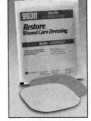

How supplied

Wafer: 4″ × 4″; A6234
       6″ × 8″; A6235
       8″ × 8″; A6236

Action

Restore Wound Care Dressing is a sterile, occlusive dressing. The flexible foam outer layer protects wounds from microorganisms, urine and feces, and the external environment. The self-adherent inner layer maintains a moist environment while absorbing excess exudate to prevent fluid pooling.

Indications

To manage partial-thickness wounds with moderate to heavy exudate. May also be used on pressure ulcers (stages 1 and 2), noninfected wounds, and red or yellow wounds.

Contraindications

Contraindicated for infected wounds or ulcers involving muscle, tendon, or bone. It should not be used in patients with active vasculitis or systemic infections.

Application

- Prepare the wound area according to facility policy. The skin should be clean and dry for secure application.
- Measure the wound, using the wound-measuring guide.
- Overlap or cut the dressing to accommodate the size of the wound. The dressing should extend at least 1″ (2.5 cm) beyond the wound edge to adhere properly.
- Remove the backing from the wound side of the dressing. Center the dressing over the wound site, press it to the skin, and smooth out the wrinkles.

Removal

- Carefully lift the edges of the dressing while pressing down on the skin.
- Continue around the wound bed until all the edges are free.

Hydrocolloids

SignaDRESS Hydrocolloid Dressing
ConvaTec

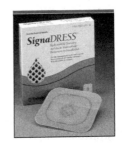

How supplied
Pad: 3" × 4"; A6234
5" × 5"; A6235
7" × 8"; A6236

Action
SignaDRESS is a moisture-retentive dressing that adheres to slightly moist skin. It provides a microbial barrier and promotes healing by creating a moist environment, which facilitates autolytic debridement of devitalized tissue.

Indications
To manage partial- and full-thickness wounds, wounds with or without necrotic tissue or fibrin slough, and lightly to moderately exuding wounds.

Contraindications
Contraindicated for individuals with a known sensitivity to the dressing or its components.

Application
- Cleanse the wound and surrounding skin with SAF-Clens, normal saline solution, or another nontoxic wound cleanser. Debride if necessary.
- Hold the dressing's clear plastic cover over the wound. The wound should fit in the raised box, and the dressing should extend at least 1¼" (3.2 cm) beyond the wound edges.
- Hold the dressing by its corner, and pull back the release paper about halfway.
- Apply the dressing from the outside edge toward the wound, completely removing the paper backing.
- Mold the entire dressing gently but firmly into place.

Removal
- Gently press down on the skin with one hand.
- Carefully peel up one edge of dressing with the other hand.
- Continue until all edges are free.

Hydrocolloids

Hydrocolloids

Sorbex

Sorbexthin
Bard Medical Division
C.R. Bard, Inc.

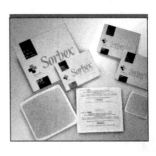

How supplied
Sorbex
Wafer: 4″ × 4″, 6″ × 6″, 8″ × 8″
Sorbexthin
Wafer: 4″ × 4″

Action
Sorbex and Sorbexthin hydrocolloid dressings are designed to create a moist environment. Sorbex dressings absorb moderate amounts of exudate. Sorbexthin dressings absorb light amounts of exudate and are particularly suitable for areas that require contouring, such as sacral and heel ulcers. Both products are one-step, waterproof, adhesive dressings. They're sterile and packaged individually for single use.

Indications
Sorbex hydrocolloid dressing is used for local management of partial- and full-thickness wounds, including pressure ulcers (stages 1, 2, 3, and 4), dermal ulcers, donor sites, incisions, superficial partial-thickness burns, abrasions, and lacerations. Sorbexthin hydrocolloid dressing is used for local management of superficial burns, pressure ulcers, dermal ulcers, postoperative wounds or suture sites, abrasions, and lacerations; it may also be used as a protective cover dressing.

Contraindications
- Contraindicated for infected wounds. A primary care provider should be consulted prior to using either dressing on a wound with high risk of infection.
- Contraindicated for third-degree burns.
- Contraindicated in patients with a known sensitivity to the dressing or its components.

Application
- Cleanse the wound with a wound cleanser or another appropriate product, such as normal saline solution.

- Pat dry surrounding skin to help ensure proper dressing adherence.
- Choose a dressing size that allows for a 1″ (2.5 cm) overlap from wound edges. It may be cut to fit oddly shaped wounds.
- Apply the dressing, pressing around the perimeter to secure it to periwound skin. For extra security, Sorbex and Sorbexthin dressings may be window-paned with tape, such as Scanpor tape.

Removal

- Change the dressing when exudate has saturated the dressing or after a maximum of 7 days.
- Carefully lift an edge of the dressing, and gently lift around the entire dressing while holding skin in place.

Hydrocolloids

3M Tegasorb Hydrocolloid Dressing

3M Tegasorb THIN Hydrocolloid Dressing
3M Health Care

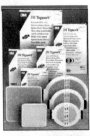

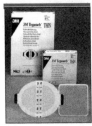

How supplied
3M Tegasorb Hydrocolloid Dressing
Oval wafer: 2¾" × 3½", 4" × 4¾"; A6237
5½" × 6¾"; A6238
Square wafer: 4" × 4"; A6234
6" × 6"; A6235
Sacral wafer: 5" × 5½"; A6238
3M Tegasorb THIN Hydrocolloid Dressing
Oval wafer: 2¾" × 3½", 4" × 4¾"; A6237
5½" × 6¾"; A6238
Square wafer: 4" × 4"; A6234
6" × 6"; A6235
Sacral wafer: 5" × 5½"; A6238

Action
3M Tegasorb hydrocolloid dressings are sterile wound dressings. They consist of a hypoallergenic, hydrocolloid adhesive with an outer clear adhesive cover film and an inner layer of hydrocolloid adhesive that rapidly absorbs exudate. The breathable outer film layer provides a consistently high rate of moisture-vapor transmission. These features ensure an optimal moist wound environment, minimize the risk of damage to healthy periwound skin, and provide extended wear for up to 7 days.

Indications
To manage partial-thickness dermal ulcers, superficial wounds, abrasions, first- and second-degree burns, and donor sites. 3M Tegasorb Hydrocolloid Dressing may also be used to manage full-thickness dermal ulcers. 3M Tegasorb THIN Hydrocolloid Dressing may also be used to manage leg ulcers and as a protective dressing on at-risk, undamaged skin or on skin beginning to show signs of damage from friction or shear.

Contraindications

None supplied by the manufacturer.

Application

- Clip excess hair at the wound site, thoroughly clean the wound and surrounding skin, and allow the skin to dry.
- If the patient's skin is easily damaged or drainage is expected to go beyond the wound edge, a skin protectant or a skin barrier film may be applied.
- Select a dressing that extends 1″ (2.5 cm) beyond the wound edge.

    Oval dressing:
- Remove the paper liner from the dressing by lifting and pulling one of the square end tabs marked "1," exposing the adhesive surface. Minimize contact with the border or the adhesive side of the dressing.
- Center the dressing over the wound. Then, gently press the adhesive side against the wound. Press from the center outward, and avoid stretching the dressing or the skin.
- Smooth the film edges to ensure good adherence.
- Remove the top delivery film by lifting one of the center tabs marked "2" and pulling it toward the edge of the dressing. Smooth down the dressing edges as you remove the film. Remove the other side of the top film in the same way.
- Gently tear off the square end tabs marked "1" at the perforations in a downward direction and discard. Avoid lifting the film edge while removing the tabs. Secure the entire film edge by pressing firmly.

    Square dressing:
- Remove the top liner from the back of the dressing. *Note:* 3M Tegasorb THIN Hydrocolloid Dressing may be cut to size before removing its top liner.
- Peel the dressing from its paper liner, minimizing contact with the dressing adhesive surface.
- Center the dressing over the wound, and gently press the adhesive side against the wound. Press from the center outward, and avoid stretching the dressing or the skin.
- Apply tape firmly around the edges of the dressing.

    Sacral dressing:
- Before removing the printed liner, fold the dressing in half.

Hydrocolloids

- Hold the tabs together, and remove the printed liner on one half of the dressing until the adhesive is exposed.
- Continue to remove the printed liner from the other half until the adhesive surface is completely exposed.
- While still holding both tabs, position the dressing over the wound, tilting the dressing toward the anal area. Spread the buttocks to get better placement. Secure the dressing notch in the anal region first to minimize risk of incontinence contamination or wrinkling.
- Gently press the adhesive side of the dressing down from the center outward. Avoid stretching the dressing or the skin.
- Remove the dressing frame, starting at the top and pulling down. Don't lift the film edge. Reinforce and smooth the dressing from the center outward.
- Repeat until all sections of the frame are removed.

Removal

- The dressing should be changed if it's leaking, falling off, or has been on the wound for 7 days.
- Carefully lift the dressing edges from the skin. For easy removal, apply tape to the edge of the dressing and use the tape to lift.
- Continue lifting the edges until all are free from the skin surface.
- Remove the dressing slowly, folding it over itself. Pull carefully in the direction of hair growth.
- *Note:* It's not unusual for wounds to have an odor. This may be noticed when the dressing is removed or when leakage occurs. The odor should disappear after the wound is cleaned.

Ultec Hydrocolloid Dressing

Ultec Pro Alginate Hydrocolloid Dressing
Kendall Health Care Products Company

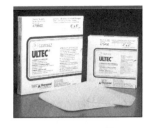

How supplied
Ultec Hydrocolloid Dressing
Wafer: 4″ × 4″; A6234
  6″ × 6″, 6″ × 8″; A6235
  8″ × 8″; A6236
Ultec Pro Alginate Hydrocolloid Dresing
Wafer: 4″ × 4″, 6″ × 6″, 8″ × 8″
  2½″ × 2½″ with adhesive island, 4″ × 4″ with adhesive island, 4″ × 5″ sacral with adhesive island; A6237
  6″ × 6″ with adhesive island, 6″ × 7″ sacral with adhesive island; A6238

Action
Ultec Hydrocolloid Dressings are pressure-sensitive adhesive dressings that absorb exudate and interact with it to form a soft gel. The gel helps form and maintain a seal against bacterial contamination, which allows the dressings to remain in place for up to 7 days and to minimize potential contamination from urine and feces. Ultec Pro Alginate Hydrocolloid Dressing's alginate/hydrocolloid formulation also helps prevent exudate from macerating periwound skin.

Indications
To manage a wide range of wound types, to relieve pressure at potential ulcer sites, and to prevent skin breakdown. May be used on pressure ulcers (stages 1, 2, 3, and 4); partial- and full-thickness wounds; infected and noninfected wounds; wounds with minimal drainage; wounds with serosanguineous drainage; surgical sites; and red, yellow, or black wounds. May also be used as a secondary dressing over hydrocolloid fillers.

Contraindications
Contraindicated for ulcers involving muscle, tendon, or bone.

Application

- Cleanse the wound site.
- Choose a dressing that overlaps the wound by at least 1″ (2.5 cm), and apply it using a clean technique. Avoid stretching the dressing.
- Press the dressing gently, forming it to the wound area and to any skin folds or creases.

Removal

- Change the dressing weekly. Change it more often if there's exudate leakage or if the occlusive seal breaks.
- Lift and slowly pull in the direction of hair growth.
- If removal is difficult, soak the edges with sterile water.

Hydrogels

Action
Hydrogels are water- or glycerin-based amorphous gels, impregnated gauzes, or sheet dressings. Because of their high water content, some can't absorb large amounts of exudate. Hydrogels help maintain a moist wound environment, promote granulation and epithelialization, and facilitate autolytic debridement.

Indications
For use as primary dressings (amorphous and impregnated gauzes) or as primary or secondary dressings (sheets); to manage partial- and full-thickness wounds, deep wounds (amorphous, impregnated gauzes), wounds with necrosis or slough, minor burns, and tissue damaged by radiation.

Advantages
- Are soothing and reduce pain
- Rehydrate the wound bed
- Facilitate autolytic debridement
- Fill in dead space (amorphous, impregnated gauzes)
- Provide minimal to moderate absorption
- Applied and removed easily from the wound
- Can be used when infection is present.

Disadvantages
- Aren't usually recommended for wounds with heavy exudate
- Dehydrate easily if not covered
- Some require secondary dressing
- Some may be difficult to secure
- Some may cause maceration.

HCPCS code overview
The HCPCS codes normally assigned to hydrogel wound covers without an adhesive border are:
A6242—pad size ≤16 sq. in.
A6243—pad size >16 sq. in., but ≤48 sq. in.
A6244—pad size >48 sq. in.

The HCPCS codes normally assigned to hydrogel wound covers with an adhesive border are:

A6245—pad size ≤16 sq. in.

A6246—pad size >16 sq. in., but ≤48 sq. in.

A6247—pad size >48 sq. in.

The HCPCS code normally assigned to hydrogel wound fillers is:

A6248—gel, per fluid oz.

The HCPCS codes normally assigned to gauze dressings impregnated with hydrogel without an adhesive border are:

A6231—pad size ≤16 sq. in.

A6232—pad size >16 sq. in., but ≤48 sq. in.

A6233—pad size >48 sq. in.

NEW PRODUCT

AcryDerm Moist Hydrophilic Wound Dressing

AcryMed, Inc.

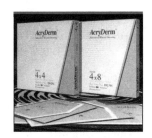

How supplied
Sheet: 2″ × 2″, 4″ × 4″; A6242
    4″ × 8″; A6243

Action
AcryDerm Moist Hydrophilic Wound Dressing creates a semipermeable environment to manage moisture levels, promote moist wound healing and debridement, and protect new granulation and epithelial tissue.

Indications
To manage pressure ulcers (stages 1, 2, and 3), partial-thickness wounds, infected wounds (with appropriate antibiotic treatment), uninfected wounds, wounds without drainage, wounds with light or moderate drainage, and red, yellow, or black wounds. May also be used to prevent skin breakdown.

Contraindications
Contraindicated for stage 4 pressure ulcers, full-thickness wounds, tunneling wounds, and heavily draining wounds.

Application
- Cleanse the wound according to facility policy.
- Cut the dressing to size if needed.
- Ensure that the dressing extends at least 1″ (2.5 cm) beyond wound edges.
- Apply the dressing using a rolling motion.
- Secure with hypoallergenic tape, nonwoven breathable tape, or transparent film.

Removal
Carefully lift the edge of the dressing and gently peel away from the skin.

Hydrogels

NEW PRODUCT
Amerigel Ointment
Amerx Health Care Corporation

How supplied
Tube: 1 oz

Action
Amerigel Ointment is a nonsterile, thick, pale gel that liquefies at body temperature. It contains oak extract, meadowsweet extract, zinc acetate, polyethylene glycol 400 and 3350, and water. It's an astringent, derived from tannins, which proliferates proteins to the wound site, decreases cell membrane permeability, and promotes wound contracture. Oak bark extract shows broad-range bacteriostatic action on 49 gram-positive and gram-negative microbes. The ointment is antimicrobial, antifungal, anti-inflammatory, and a unique autolytic debrider.

Indications
To manage pressure ulcers (stages 1, 2, 3, and 4), diabetic skin ulcers, stasis (insufficiency) ulcers, postsurgical incisions, and first- and second-degree burns.

Contraindications
Contraindicated in patients with an allergy to oak or oak pollen.

Application
- Cleanse the wound with saline solution.
- Apply a thin layer of Amerigel Ointment over the wound bed and ½″ of the periwound skin.
- Cover with moist saline gauze and secure.

Removal
Change dressing daily after irrigating with saline solution.

Hydrogels

Aquaflo
Kendall Health Care
Products Company

How supplied
Disc: 1.5", 3.0", 4.75"

Action
Aquaflo hydrogel wound dressings offer superior fluid management and can be used on mildly to moderately exuding wounds. These dressings maintain an optimal moist wound-healing environment.

Indications
To manage partial- and full-thickness wounds, dermal ulcers (stages 1, 2, and 3), diabetic leg ulcers, donor sites, first- and second-degree burns, and incisions.

Contraindications
Contraindicated for heavily draining wounds.

Application
- Cleanse the wound with normal saline solution or an appropriate wound cleanser.
- Cut the dressing to shape if desired.
- Apply the dressing and secure it.

Removal
Gently lift edge and peel dressing away.

Hydrogels

AquaGauze Hydrogel Impregnated Gauze Dressing
DeRoyal

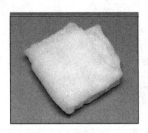

How supplied
Pads: 2″ × 2″, 4″ × 4″, 4″ × 8″

Action
AquaGauze dressings provide and maintain a moist wound environment conducive to healing and protect against wound dehydration. These dressings don't adhere to wound beds.

Indications
For use as a primary dressing for pressure ulcers (stages 2, 3, and 4), partial- and full-thickness wounds, dermal ulcers, leg ulcers, diabetic ulcers, minor burns, lacerations, cuts, and abrasions.

Contraindications
Contraindicated for third-degree burns.

Application
- Cleanse the wound site with normal saline solution.
- Cover or pack the wound loosely with AquaGauze.
- Apply an appropriate cover or secondary dressing.

Removal
- Remove any secondary dressing.
- Gently lift the dressing from the wound.

Hydrogels

NEW PRODUCT
Aquasite Amorphous Hydrogel
Dumex Medical

How supplied
Amorphous
hydrogel: 1 fluid oz, 3 fluid oz

Action
Aquasite Amorphous Hydrogels are clear, preserved hydrogels used to fill wound space and provide a moist environment. These products are capable of absorbing small to moderate amounts of exudate and provide a soothing, cooling, pain-reducing effect. A secondary dressing is required to secure the dressing in place.

Indications
For use on partial- and full-thickness wounds with minimal to moderate drainage.

Contraindications
Contraindicated for third-degree burns.

Application
- Cleanse the wound with PrimaDerm Dermal Cleanser or saline solution.
- Dry the skin adjacent to the wound.
- Squeeze the desired amount of Aquasite Amorphous Hydrogel into the wound bed.
- Cover with an appropriate secondary dressing.

Removal
- Remove the secondary dressing.
- Remove remaining Aquasite Amorphous Hydrogel.
- Cleanse the wound according to facility policy.

Hydrogels

Aquasite Impregnated Gauze Hydrogel
Dumex Medical

How supplied
Gauze: 2" × 2", 4" × 4", 4" × 8"

Action
Aquasite Impregnated Gauze Hydrogels are sterile hydrogels impregnated into 100% cotton sponges. These products are used to fill wound space and provide a moist environment. They are capable of absorbing small to moderate amounts of exudate and provide a soothing, cooling, pain-reducing effect. A secondary dressing is required to secure the dressing in place.

Indications
For use on partial- and full-thickness wounds with minimal to moderate drainage.

Contraindications
Contraindicated for third-degree burns.

Application
- Cleanse the wound with PrimaDerm Dermal Cleanser or saline solution. Dry the skin adjacent to the wound.
- Place Aquasite Impregnated Gauze Hydrogel into the wound bed. Pack deeper wounds loosely to avoid excess pressure on delicate wound tissue.
- Cover with an appropriate secondary dressing.

Removal
- Remove the secondary dressing.
- Remove the gauze and remaining hydrogel.
- Cleanse the wound according to facility policy.

Hydrogels

NEW PRODUCT
Aquasite Impregnated Non-Woven Hydrogel
Dumex Medical

How supplied
Gauze: 2″ × 2″, 4″ × 4″, 4″ × 8″

Action
Aquasite Impregnated Non-Woven Hydrogel, a sterile hydrogel impregnated into a special nonwoven sponge, is used to fill wound space and provide a moist environment. It's capable of absorbing small to moderate amounts of exudate and provides a soothing, cooling, pain-reducing effect. A secondary dressing is required to secure the dressing in place.

Indications
For use on partial- and full-thickness wounds with minimal to moderate drainage.

Contraindications
Contraindicated for third-degree burns.

Application
- Cleanse the wound with PrimaDerm Dermal Cleanser or saline solution. Dry the skin adjacent to the wound.
- Place Aquasite Impregnated Non-Woven Hydrogel into the wound bed. Pack deeper wounds loosely to avoid excess pressure on delicate wound tissue
- Cover with an appropriate secondary dressing.

Removal
- Remove the secondary dressing.
- Remove the gauze and remaining hydrogel.
- Cleanse the wound according to facility policy

Hydrogels

NEW PRODUCT

Aquasite Sheet Hydrogel
Dumex Medical

How supplied
Sheet: 2″ × 2″, 2″ × 3″, 4″ × 4″, 6″ × 8″, 12″ × 12″, 12″ × 24″

Action
Aquasite Sheet Hydrogels are clear sheets of sterile hydrogel used to provide a moist environment and absorb small to moderate amounts of exudate. The products provide a soothing, cooling, pain-reducing effect. A secondary dressing is required to secure the dressing in place.

Indications
For use on partial and full-thickness wounds with minimal to moderate drainage.

Contraindications
Contraindicated for third-degree burns or deep, tunneling wounds.

Application
- Cleanse the wound with PrimaDerm Dermal Cleanser or saline solution. Dry the skin adjacent to the wound.
- Choose a dressing that extends at least 1″ (2.5 cm) beyond the wound margins.
- Position Aquasite Sheet Hydrogel directly on the wound.
- Secure with an appropriate secondary dressing.

Removal
- Remove the secondary dressing.
- Remove the Aquasite Sheet Hydrogel.

Hydrogels

Aquasorb Hydrogel Wound Dressing
DeRoyal

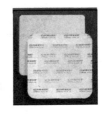

How supplied
Sheet: $2\frac{1}{2}'' \times 2\frac{1}{2}''$, $3\frac{3}{4}'' \times 3\frac{3}{4}''$; A6242
$3\frac{3}{4} \times 4\frac{1}{2}''$, $3\frac{3}{4}'' \times 6''$; A6243
$7\frac{1}{2}'' \times 7\frac{1}{2}''$, $7\frac{1}{2}'' \times 18''$; A6244

Sheet
with border: $2\frac{1}{2}'' \times 2\frac{1}{2}''$ gel, $\frac{5}{8}''$ film or tape border; A6245
$3\frac{3}{4}'' \times 4\frac{1}{2}''$ gel, $1\frac{1}{8}''$ film or tape border; A6246
$2\frac{1}{4}'' \times 1\frac{1}{4}''$gel, oval, $\frac{5}{8}''$ tape border; A6245

Action
Aquasorb Hydrogel Wound Dressings are nonadherent, transparent dressings that incorporate a gel matrix with a semipermeable film. They allow for moisture vapor transmission, which provides a moist environment and protects against wound dehydration. The products act as a bacterial barrier, absorb drainage from the wound, and provide a cool, pain-relieving cover.

Indications
For use as primary dressings to manage leg ulcers, pressure ulcers (stages 1, 2, 3, and 4), superficial wounds, lacerations, cuts, abrasions, donor sites, and first- and second-degree burns. May also be used on partial- and full-thickness wounds, infected and noninfected wounds, wounds with moderate to heavy drainage, and red, yellow, or black wounds.

Contraindications
Contraindicated for third-degree burns.

Application
- Cleanse excess exudate from the wound.
- Cut the sheet to the desired size if necessary.
- Remove the release liner and apply the dressing to the wound.
- Secure the dressing if necessary.

Removal
- Leave the dressing in place for up to 7 days, unless patient discomfort, exudate leakage, or infection occurs.
- Lift the edge of the dressing carefully; then peel off.

Hydrogels

Biolex Wound Gel
Bard Medical Division
C.R. Bard, Inc.

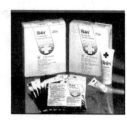

How supplied
Tube: ½ oz, 3 oz; A6248

Action
Biolex Wound Gel adds moisture to the wound and maintains a moist wound environment. Its slightly acidic nature promotes healing.

Indications
To manage first- and second-degree burns, dermal ulcers, cuts, abrasions, postoperative incisions, pressure ulcers (stages 2, 3, and 4), and partial- and full-thickness wounds. May be used on tunneling and undermined wounds, infected and noninfected wounds, and red, yellow, or black wounds.

Contraindications
- Contraindicated in patients with known hypersensitivity to Biolex components.
- Not recommended for third-degree burns.

Application
- Cleanse the wound.
- Apply a layer of Biolex Wound Gel, approximately ⅛″ to ¼″ (0.3 to 0.6 cm) deep, directly to the wound bed. For deep wounds, saturate gauze with the gel and loosely pack it into the wound.
- Cover with an appropriate cover dressing.

Removal
- Change the dressing when the gel has been absorbed, moisture must be added to wound, or exudate has saturated the dressing. Don't disturb the wound bed for at least 12 hours because this may interfere with the healing process.
- Remove the cover dressing.
- Irrigate and cleanse the wound. *Note:* Because the gel won't harm healthy tissue, complete removal is unnecessary.

Hydrogels

CarraDres Clear Hydrogel Sheet

Carrington Laboratories, Inc.

How supplied
Sheet: 4″ × 4″; A6242

Action

CarraDres Clear Hydrogel Sheets
consist of 89.5% water combined with a cross-linked polyethylene matrix in sterile hydrogel polymer sheets especially formulated for managing partial- and full-thickness wounds. The hydrophilic dressings absorb at least three times their weight in water, serum, or blood. The products have a high specific heat to provide a cooling effect; the sheets may be refrigerated for maximum cooling.

Indications

To dress and manage pressure ulcers (stages 1, 2, 3, and 4), venous stasis ulcers, first- and second-degree burns, cuts, abrasions, skin irritations, radiation dermatitis, diabetic ulcers, foot ulcers, postsurgical incisions, and skin conditions associated with peristomal care. May also be used on partial- and full-thickness wounds, tunneling wounds, infected and noninfected wounds, wounds with moderate exudate, wounds with serosanguineous drainage, and red, yellow, or black wounds.

Contraindications

None provided by the manufacturer.

Application

- Flush the wound with a suitable cleanser, such as UltraKlenz, CarraKlenz, or MicroKlenz.
- Remove dressing's blue backing and apply moist side of the dressing to the wound bed.
- Cover with a secondary dressing, such as CarraFilm or CarraSmart Film.

Removal

- Change dressing according to the wound condition and amount of exudate or as directed by the primary care provider.
- The dressing may remain in place 3 to 5 days.
- Gently lift to remove.

Hydrogels

CarraGauze Pads and Strips with Acemannan Hydrogel
Carrington Laboratories, Inc.

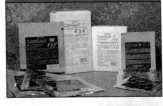

How supplied
Pad: 2" × 2", 4" × 4"; A6231
Strip: 1½" × 5 yards

Action
CarraGauze Pads and Strips are impregnated with Carrasyn Gel Wound Dressing containing Acemannan Hydrogel. They provide a primary cover or filler for wounds, absorb exudate, and create a moist wound environment.

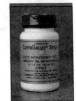

Indications
To manage pressure ulcers (stages 1, 2, 3, and 4), stasis ulcers, first- and second-degree burns, cuts, abrasions, skin conditions associated with peristomal skin, diabetic ulcers, foot ulcers, radiation dermatitis, postoperative incisions, and trauma wounds.

Contraindications
Contraindicated in patients with known hypersensitivity to Acemannan Hydrogel or other components of the dressing.

Application
- Flush wound with a suitable cleanser, such as CarraKlenz, UltraKlenz, or MicroKlenz.
- Pack the wound loosely with CarraGauze Pads. For CarraGauze Packing Strips, an applicator may be used to guide the strip into small tunnels or crevices in the wound.
- Cover with a secondary dressing of CarraFilm, CarraSmart Film, or gauze. If using gauze and the wound bed is dry, moisten the gauze.

Removal
- Change all hydrogel dressings as often as needed, usually daily.
- Remove the secondary dressing.
- Gently remove the gauze pad or strip from the wound bed.

Hydrogels

CarraSmart Gel Wound Dressing with Acemannan Hydrogel
Carrington Laboratories, Inc.

How supplied
Tube: 1 oz, 3 oz

Action
CarraSmart Gel is a nonadherent, smooth, colorless wound dressing containing Acemannan Hydrogel, specially formulated to create and maintain the moist environment vital to wound healing. The gel has the unique property of donating moisture to dry wounds and absorbing moisture from wet wounds; it also relieves pain by cooling, coating, and protecting the wound.

Indications
To manage pressure ulcers (stages 1, 2, 3, and 4), stasis ulcers, foot ulcers, first- and second-degree burns, minor cuts and abrasions, and skin conditions associated with peristomal care.

Contraindications
Contraindicated in patients with known hypersensitivity to Acemannan Hydrogel or other components of the dressing.

Application
- Cleanse the wound with a suitable cleanser, such as CarraKlenz, UltraKlenz, or MicroKlenz, by spraying the affected area.
- Gently dry the surrounding skin with soft gauze. No rinsing is required.
- Apply a ⅛″ to ¼″ (0.3- to 0.6-cm) thick layer of CarraSmart Gel to areas of ulceration.
- Cover with an appropriate nonadherent secondary dressing.

Removal
- Change dressing according to the wound condition and amount of exudate or as directed by the primary care provider.
- Rinse away any remaining gel with gentle irrigation.

Hydrogels

Carrasyn Gel Wound Dressing with Acemannan Hydrogel

Carrasyn Spray Gel Wound Dressing with Acemannan Hydrogel

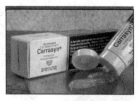

Carrasyn V with Acemannan Hydrogel
Carrington Laboratories, Inc.

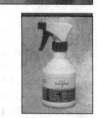

How supplied
Carrasyn Gel Wound Dressing
Tube: ½ oz, 1 oz, 3 oz; A6248
Carrasyn Spray Gel Wound Dressing
Bottle: 8 oz; A6248
Carrasyn V
Tube: ½ oz, 3 oz; A6248

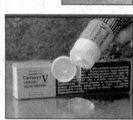

Action
All three products provide the moist environment necessary for healing and facilitate autolytic debridement. All three are nonoily hydrogels containing Acemannan Hydrogel. Carrasyn V is a thicker, more viscous version of Carrasyn Gel Wound Dressing.

Indications
All three products manage pressure ulcers (stages 1, 2, 3, and 4), venous stasis ulcers, first- and second-degree burns, cuts, abrasions, skin irritations, and skin conditions associated with peristomal care. They may also be used on partial- and full-thickness wounds, tunneling wounds, infected and noninfected wounds, wounds with serosanguineous drainage, and red, yellow, or black wounds. Carrasyn Spray Gel Wound Dressing may be used on wounds with moderate drainage. Carrasyn Gel Wound Dressing and Carrasyn V also manage radiation dermatitis, diabetic ulcers, foot ulcers, postsurgical incisions, and wounds with low exudate.

Contraindications
Contraindicated in patients with known sensitivity to aloe vera extract or to Acemannan Hydrogel.

Hydrogels

Application

- Flush the wound with a suitable wound cleanser, such as CarraKlenz, UltraKlenz, or MicroKlenz.

  Carrasyn Gel Wound Dressing and Carrasyn V (when a thicker formulation of gel is desired):

- Apply a generous amount of gel to the wound area in a layer approximately ¼″ (0.6 cm) thick.
- If using gauze as a secondary dressing, moisten it first.
- If using CarraSmart Film Transparent Dressing as the secondary dressing, dry the periwound tissue first. Use a skin barrier wipe on any intact skin under the film.

  Carrasyn Spray Gel Wound Dressing:

- Adjust the nozzle setting on the bottle to either spray or stream.
- Apply a generous amount of gel, approximately ¼″ (0.6-cm) thick, to the wound and wound margins.
- Apply spray gel as often as needed, usually daily.
- If using gauze as a cover dressing, moisten it first.

Removal

- Change all hydrogel dressings as often as needed, usually daily.
- Flush wound with normal saline solution or an appropriate wound cleanser, such as CarraKlenz, UltraKlenz, or Micro-Klenz.

Hydrogels

Comfort-Aid
Southwest Technologies, Inc.

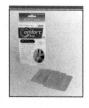

How supplied
*Sheet with
adhesive border:* $1\frac{1}{2}'' \times 2\frac{1}{2}''$, $4'' \times 4''$; A6245

Action
Comfort-Aid is designed to provide effective management of a wide variety of wounds and to protect the skin and newly formed tissue. The gel's high glycerin content assists the natural wound-healing process. Glycerin is a main component in every fat molecule and is a natural moisturizing agent. Comfort-Aid provides cool, soothing relief when applied to an open wound, will not dry out, and is bacteriostatic and fungistatic.

Indications
To manage first- and second-degree burns, cuts, abrasions, rashes, radiation skin reactions, surgical incisions, foot and leg ulcers, pressure ulcers (stages 1, 2, 3, and 4), partial- and full-thickness wounds, wounds with moderate drainage, wounds with serosanguineous drainage, and red, yellow, or black wounds.

Contraindications
- Contraindicated for highly exuding wounds that may require packing with additional dressing or other highly absorbent material.
- Use caution when applying to an infected wound.

Application
- Cleanse the wound with normal saline solution or an appropriate wound cleanser.
- Select the appropriate size dressing or cut one to the desired size or shape. It should extend $1''$ to $2''$ (2.5 to 5 cm) beyond the wound opening. Leave the clear plastic film on the gel while cutting.
- Remove the clear plastic film and apply the exposed gel directly on the wound. Don't remove the white fabric backing.
- Secure dressing with tape, elastic or gauze wrap, or stretch netting.
- Protect the dressing from contamination with a waterproof covering, such as the tape supplied with the dressing.

Removal
Change the dressing when it's saturated with exudate.

Hydrogels

Curafil Gel Wound Dressing and Impregnated Strips

Kendall Health Care Products Company

How supplied

Tube: 0.5 oz, 1 oz, 3 oz; A6248

Impregnated pad: 2" × 2", 4" × 4" , 4" × 8", 1" × 36"

Action

Curafil Gel Wound Dressing and Impregnated Strips help maintain a moist wound environment, promote granulation and epithelialization, and facilitate autolytic debridement.

Indications

To manage pressure ulcers (stages 2, 3, and 4), partial- and full-thickness wounds, tunneling wounds, uninfected wounds, wounds with light drainage, and red, yellow, or black wounds.

Contraindications

None provided by the manufacturer.

Application

- Apply hydrogel dressing or hydrogel gauze to wound, gently filling in dead space.
- Secure in place with hydrogel wafer or transparent dressing.

Removal

- Gently remove dressing.
- For gel dressing, flush out remaining gel with cleanser or saline solution.

Hydrogels

Curagel
Kendall Health Care Products
Company

How supplied
Borderless
dressing: 2" × 3", 4" × 4"; A6242
            8" × 8"; A6244
Island
dressing: 3" × 4" (2" × 3" pad),
            5" × 5" (4" × 4" pad), 8½" × 9½" (8" × 8" pad);
            A6245

Action
Curagel hydrogel dressings offer balanced hydration in a soothing, clear gel. The polyurethane layer maintains dressing integrity and controls fluid management.

Indications
To manage partial- and full-thickness wounds, dermal ulcers
(stages 1, 2, and 3), diabetic leg ulcers, donor sites, abrasions,
and first- and second-degree burns.

Contraindications
Contraindicated for heavily draining wounds.

Application
- Cleanse the wound.
- Select the appropriate size dressing.
- Allow 1" (2.5 cm) overlap around wound margins for best fit.
  If necessary, cut the dressing.
- Secure the dressing.

Removal
Change the dressing ecery 3 to 5 days.

Hydrogels

CURASOL Gel Wound Dressing
Healthpoint

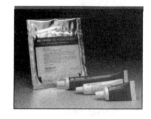

How supplied
Nonsterile tube: 1 oz, 3 oz; A6248
Sterile pad: 4″ × 4″

Action
CURASOL Gel Wound Dressing is a clear, viscous hydrogel that protects the wound from foreign contaminants and provides a moist wound-healing environment.

Indications
To manage pressure ulcers (stages 1, 2, 3, and 4), stasis ulcers, diabetic ulcers, foot ulcers, postoperative wounds, first- and second-degree burns, cuts, abrasions, and minor irritations of the skin.

Contraindications
None provided by the manufacturer.

Application
- Cleanse the wound with ALLCLENZ Wound Cleanser.
- Apply ⅛″ to ¼″ (0.3 to 0.6 cm) of CURASOL Gel onto the wound bed. If using CURASOL Gel Wound Dressing, loosely pack it into the wound.
- Cover with a secondary dressing.

Removal
- Remove secondary dressing.
- Flush CURASOL Gel from the wound bed with ALLCLENZ Wound Cleanser during each dressing change.

Hydrogels

DermaGel Hydrogel Sheet
Medline Industries, Inc.

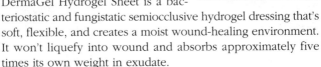

How supplied
Sheet: 4″ × 4″; A6242

Action
DermaGel Hydrogel Sheet is a bacteriostatic and fungistatic semiocclusive hydrogel dressing that's soft, flexible, and creates a moist wound-healing environment. It won't liquefy into wound and absorbs approximately five times its own weight in exudate.

Indications
To manage leg ulcers, pressure ulcers (stages 1, 2, 3, and 4), superficial wounds, lacerations, cuts, abrasions, donor sites, partial- and full-thickness wounds, infected and noninfected wounds, wounds with light to moderate drainage, and red, yellow, or black wounds.

Contraindications
- Contraindicated as a primary dressing for highly exudating-wounds.
- Contraindicated for deep, tunneling wounds.

Application
- Cleanse the application site with normal saline solution or an appropriate wound cleanser such as Skintegrity Wound Cleanser. Dry the surrounding area to ensure that it's free of greasy substances.
- Select the appropriate size dressing for the wound. Be sure it will cover the entire wound area.
- Remove the clear plastic cover from the dressing and apply the pad to the wound. Leave the cloth backing in place.
- Tape the edges of the dressing to keep it in place, or use elastic net for nonadhesive securement.
- If waterproofing is desired, cover with a transparent film.

Removal
- Change dressing every 2 to 5 days, depending on drainage.
- Carefully press down on the skin and lift an edge of the dressing. Continue around the dressing until all edges are free.
- Repeat cleansing procedure.

Hydrogels

Dermagran Hydrophilic Wound Dressing

Derma Sciences, Inc.

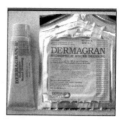

How supplied

Tube: 3 oz (amorphous);
        A6248

Sterile impregnated
gauze: 2″ × 2″, 4″ × 4″; A6231
        4″ × 8″; A6232

Action

Dermagran Hydrophilic Wound Dressing contains a zinc-nutrient formulation and provides a primary cover or filler, absorbs mild exudate, and creates a mildly acidic environment that is conducive to wound healing.

Indications

To manage skin ulcers (diabetic, venous stasis), pressure ulcers (stages 1, 2, 3, and 4), surgical incisions, and superficial injuries such as partial-thickness burns, superficial lacerations, cuts, or abrasions.

Contraindications

None provided by the manufacturer.

Application

- Cleanse the wound.
- Choose an appropriate size Dermagran Hydrophilic Wound Dressing.
- Place dressing directly into the wound.
- Cover with an appropriate dressing and secure in place.

Removal

- Change dressing once daily or as directed by the primary care provider.
- Remove the dressing and cleanse the wound.

Dermagran Zinc-Saline Hydrogel

Derma Sciences, Inc.

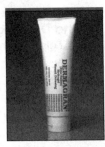

How supplied
Tube: 3 oz; A6248

Action
Dermagran Zinc-Saline Hydrogel is an amorphous hydrogel that contains zinc-nutrient formulation and balanced pH technology. It provides a primary cover or filler for wound deficiencies that absorbs wound exudate and creates a moist environment for granulation tissue formation.

Indications
To manage pressure ulcers (stages 1, 2, 3, and 4), venous stasis ulcers, partial-thickness thermal burns, surgical incisions, skin irritations, abrasions, and conditions associated with peristomal care.

Contraindications
None provided by the manufacturer.

Application
- Obtain surgical consult or consider sharp debridement of necrotic tissue.
- Cleanse the wound, then wick out excessive moisture using a gauze sponge.
- Apply a generous layer of Dermagran Zinc-Saline Hydrogel to entire wound bed.
- Cover with an appropriate secondary dressing, such as DermaSite or DermaFilm.

Removal
- Change once daily or as directed by a primary care provider.
- Remove the dressing.
- Cleanse the area with Dermagran Wound Cleanser or other appropriate wound cleanser.

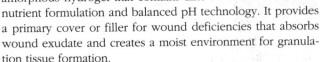

Hydrogels

DermaSyn

DermaGauze
DermaRite Industries

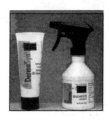

How supplied
DermaSyn
Tube: 3 oz
Spray: 8oz
DermaGauze
Sterile pad: 4″ × 4″

Action
DermaSyn hydrogel dressings and DermaGauze hydrogel-impregnated gauze dressings provide a primary cover or filler for wounds and promote a moist wound-healing environment. Their primary purpose is to fill in dead space associated with sinus tracts and undermining or deep wounds.

Indications
To manage partial-thickness dermal wounds, including pressure ulcers, venous ulcers, diabetic ulcers, and arterial ulcers. Used for tunneling wounds, infected and noninfected wounds, and wounds with minimal or moderate drainage.

Contraindications
Contraindicated for third-degree burns.

Application
- Cleanse the wound.
- Using either the tube or the spray, apply a layer of DermaSyn hydrogel directly into the wound bed. For deep wounds and packing material, use DermaGauze and pack it loosely into the wound.
- Cover with appropriate secondary dressing.

Removal
- Remove the secondary dressing.
- During each dressing change, irrigate the wound bed with DermaKlenz.

Hydrogels

DiaB Gel with Acemannan Hydrogel

Carrington Laboratories, Inc.

How supplied

Tube: 3 oz

Action

DiaB Gel is a hydrogel wound dressing containing Acemannan Hydrogel in a nonoily preparation, specially targeted for wound care in diabetic foot ulcers.

Indications

To manage diabetic ulcers.

Contraindications

Contraindicated for patients with known hypersensitivity to Acemannan Hydrogel or any components of the dressing.

Application

- Cleanse the wound with a suitable cleanser, such as DiaB Klenz, by spraying the affected area.
- Gently dry the surrounding skin with soft gauze. No rinsing is required.
- Follow with a layer of DiaB Gel ⅛" to ¼" (0.3- to 0.6-cm) thick on areas of ulceration.
- Cover with an appropriate nonadherent secondary dressing.

Removal

- Change dressing according to the wound condition and amount of exudate or as directed by a primary care provider.
- Rinse away any remaining gel with gentle irrigation.

Hydrogels

Elasto-Gel

Elasto-Gel Plus
Southwest Technologies, Inc.

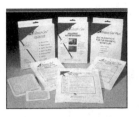

How supplied
Elasto-Gel
Sheet without tape: 2″ × 3″, 4″ × 4″;
                  A6242
                  5″ × 5″; A6243
                  6″ × 8″; A6248
                  8″ × 16″, 12″ × 12″; A6244

Elasto-Gel
*Horseshoe shape with
adhesive border:* 8″ × 8″
ElastoGel Plus
Sheet with tape: 2″ × 3″, 4″ × 4″; A6242
                5″ × 5″; A6243
                6″ × 8″; A6248
                8″ × 16″, 12″ × 12″; A6244

Action
Elasto-Gel absorbs exudate and seals, protects, and cushions the wound. It permits water vapor transmission and is bacteriostatic and fungistatic. It also reduces odor, acts as a thermal barrier, and reduces pressure.

Indications
To manage first- and second-degree burns, cuts, abrasions, rash, radiation skin reactions, surgical incisions, foot and leg ulcers, pressure ulcers (stages 1, 2, 3, and 4), partial- and full-thickness wounds, wounds with moderate drainage, wounds with serosanguineous drainage, and red, yellow, or black wounds. Also used to prevent skin breakdown, to pad tracheostomy and pressure ulcer sites, under casts and splints, and on heels and elbows.

Contraindications
- Contraindicated for highly exuding wounds that may require packing with additional dressing or other highly absorbent material.

Hydrogels

- Use caution when applying to an infected wound. Consult a primary care provider first.

Application
- Cleanse the wound with normal saline solution or an appropriate wound cleanser.
- Select the appropriate size dressing or cut one to the desired size or shape. It should extend 1″ to 2″ (2.5 to 5 cm) beyond the wound opening. Leave the clear plastic film on the gel while cutting.
- Remove the clear plastic film and apply the exposed gel directly on the wound. Don't remove the white fabric backing.
- Secure dressing with tape, elastic or gauze wrap, or stretch netting.
- If the dressing is exposed to moisture, protect it from contamination with a waterproof covering, such as the tape supplied with the dressing.

Removal
- Change the dressing when it is saturated with exudate.

Hydrogels

Elta Hydrogel Impregnated Gauze
Swiss-American Products, Inc.

How supplied
Sterile foil pouch: 2″ × 2″, 4″ × 4″; A6231
4″ × 8″; A6232
8″ × 8″; A6233

Action
Elta Hydrogel Impregnated Gauze maintains a moist wound environment for 24 hours and absorbs moderate exudate. The dressings are kept in place by their viscous glycerin base.

Indications
For use on wounds (stage 1, 2, 3, and 4), dry to moderately exudative. May also be helpful in tunneling wounds.

Contraindications
None provided by the manufacturer.

Application
- Apply dressing appropriate to the size of the wound bed.
- Cover with an appropriate dressing.

Removal
- Gently lift the dressing away from the wound.
- Cleanse the wound with saline solution or wound cleanser.

Hydrogels

Elta Hydrovase Wound Gel
Swiss-American Products, Inc.

How supplied
Bellows bottle: 1 oz; A6248

Action
Elta Hydrovase Wound Gel controls moisture delivery by maintaining a moist wound environment without macerating the wound. The product contains 10% glycerin for moisture retention, and its high viscosity allows it to stay in place. Absorbs dry to moderate exudate.

Indications
To keep the wound bed moist for 24 hours.

Contraindications
None provided by the manufacturer.

Application
- Apply ¼″ (0.6 cm) layer of gel to wound bed.
- Cover with an appropriate dressing.

Removal
- Gently lift the dressing away from the wound site.
- Spray the wound with wound cleanser to lift away necrotic tissue and cleanse the wound.

Hydrogels

Elta Wound Gel
Swiss-American Products, Inc.

How supplied
Bellows bottle: 1 oz; A6248
Squeeze tube: 4 oz; A6248

Action
Elta Wound Gel maintains a moist wound environment for 24 hours. It is kept in place by its viscous glycerin base.

Indications
For use on stage 1, 2, 3, and 4 wounds with dry to moderate exudate.

Contraindications
None provided by the manufacturer.

Application
- Apply ¼″ (0.6 cm) layer of gel to wound bed.
- Cover with appropriate dressing.

Removal
- Gently lift the dressing away from the wound site.
- Spray the wound with wound cleanser to lift away necrotic tissue and cleanse the wound.

Hydrogels

FlexiGel
Smith & Nephew, Inc.
Wound Management Division

How supplied
Sheet: 2" × 2", 4" × 4"; A6242
     4" × 8"; A6243

Action
FlexiGel is a moist, waterproof, latex-free, wound-healing gel sheet dressing made of a polyacrylamide matrix with embedded hydrophilic polysaccharide particles. FlexiGel has a moisture vapor transfer rate greater than 2,000 g/m²/24 hours. This dressing can absorb and evaporate exudate. Some of the exudate absorbed by FlexiGel can evaporate from the upper surface of the dressing, increasing the moisture-handling capacity of the dressing and extending the time between dressing changes.

Indications
To manage partial-thickness wounds and minor wounds, including skin tears, abrasions, lacerations, minor burns, and scalds. Moderately exuding, full-thickness wounds that can be managed by FlexiGel, on the recommendation and under the supervision of a primary care provider, include pressure ulcers (stages 2, 3, and 4), venous leg ulcers, diabetic foot ulcers, and surgical wounds.

Contraindications
Contraindicated for third-degree burns.

Application
- Cleanse wound with normal saline solution or an appropriate wound cleanser. Be sure periwound area is as dry as possible before applying the dressing.
- Select a dressing that is at least ¼" to ½"(0.6 to 1.2 cm) larger than the wound. Dressing may be cut to the desired size; this will be easier to do while the dressing is still in the package.
- Place one edge of the dressing on one side of the wound, then use a rolling motion to complete placement.
- For dry wounds, secure the dressing with a thin film, which will enhance the ability to create a moist environment.

Hydrogels

- For lightly or moderately exuding wounds, apply a porous cover dressing. Secure the cover dressing by taping completely over the dressing or by taping only the dressing edges.

Removal
- The dressing is nonadherent and easily removed.
- To change, lift at one side or corner and gently peel back the dressing.

Hydrogels

Gentell Hydrogel
Gentell, Inc.

How supplied
Impregnated
2-ply gauze pads: 2″ × 2″, 4″ × 4″;
A6231
4″ × 8″; A6232
Spray gel: 8-oz adjustable spray; A6248
Tube: 4 oz; A6248

Action
Gentell Hydrogel is an aloe vera-based hydrogel that protects the wound bed and promotes the moist environment essential to the natural healing process.

Indications
To manage pressure ulcers (stages 2, 3, and 4), venous ulcers, first- and second-degree burns, and nondraining wounds.

Contraindications
None provided by the manufacturer.

Application
- Cleanse the wound with an appropriate cleanser.
- Choose and apply the appropriate size Gentell Hydrogel dressing.
- Cover with a secondary dressing and secure with the appropriate fixative product.

Removal
Change the dressing every 24 hours or as indicated.

Hydrogels

Hypergel
Mölnlycke Health Care

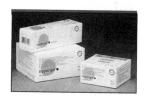

How supplied
Tube: 5-g, 15-g, 85-g multidose;
     A6248

Action
Hypergel's 20% sodium chloride hydrates and penetrates necrotic tissue to create a hypertonic environment and promote autolytic debridement. It naturally pulls drainage, debris, edema, and bacteria out of the wound and into the dressing while maintaining a moist wound-healing environment.

Indications
To soften and remove dry necrotic eschar on pressure ulcers (stages 3 and 4), partial- and full-thickness wounds, tunneling wounds, noninfected wounds, wounds with minimal drainage (if eschar is still present), wounds with serosanguineous or purulent drainage (if eschar is still present), and black wounds. Treatment is discontinued when the wound is covered with less than 25% eschar.

Contraindications
Not recommended for ulcers with no devitalized (dead) tissue or for wounds that have compromised arterial blood supply.

Application
- Gently irrigate or flush the wound with normal saline solution, if necessary, and blot excess saline solution with absorbent gauze.
- Apply a light coating (dime thickness) to the dry necrotic eschar. Avoid applying it to intact skin. *Note:* Hypergel isn't a wound filler; it's designed to coat the wound surface.
- Pack deep wounds with suitable material.
- Cover with Alldress or other cover dressing.

Removal
Change the dressing every 24 hours or when drainage is visible through the cover dressing.

Hydrogels

NEW PRODUCT
Hyperion Hydrogel Gauze Dressing
Hyperion Medical, Inc.

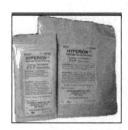

How supplied
Pad: 2″ × 2″, 4″ × 4″; A6231

Action
Hyperion Hydrogel Gauze Dressing features a glycerin-based hydrogel impregnated in a nonwoven gauze sponge. It's designed to provide a moist wound-healing environment for full-thickness wounds. The high glycerin content provides a level of assurance against maceration, should the product inadvertently contact intact skin.

Indications
To manage pressure ulcers (stages 1, 2, 3, and 4), stasis ulcers, first- and second-degree burns, cuts, and minor skin irritations.

Contraindications
- Contraindicated for wounds with moderate to heavy exudate.
- May require secondary dressing.

Application
- Cleanse the wound with a suitable wound cleanser.
- Pack the wound loosely with the pad. To prevent maceration, don't apply to intact skin.
- Apply secondary dressing of choice.

Removal
- Gently remove dressing from wound bed.
- Irrigate the wound with wound cleanser.

Hydrogels

Hyperion Hydrophilic Wound Gel

Hyperion Hydrophilic Wound Dressing
Hyperion Medical, Inc.

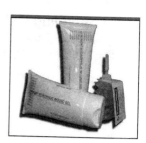

How supplied
Hyperion Hydrophilic Wound Gel
Tube (unit dose-accordion): 1 oz, 3 oz; A6248
Hyperion Hydrophilic Wound Dressing
Impregnated gauze: 2″ × 2″, 4″ × 4″; A6231
                         4″ × 8″

Action
Hyperion Hydrophilic Wound Gel and Wound Dressing hydrate the wound bed to maintain a moist wound environment, and promote an osmotic gradient.

Indications
To manage pressure ulcers (stages 1, 2, 3, and 4), stasis ulcers, first- and second-degree burns, cuts, and minor skin irritations.

Contraindications
Contraindicated for wounds with moderate to heavy exudate.

Application
- Cleanse the wound with a suitable wound cleanser.
  Hyperion Hydrophilic Wound Gel:
- Apply gel to wound area. To prevent maceration, don't apply to intact skin.
- Cover with appropriate dressing.
  Hyperion Hydrophilic Wound Dressing:
- Cover or pack wound loosely with pad. To prevent maceration, don't apply to intact skin.
- Apply appropriate secondary dressing.

Removal
Hyperion Hydrophilic Wound Gel:
- Flush or irrigate wound with an appropriate wound cleanser.
  Hyperion Hydrophilic Wound Dressing:
- Gently remove gauze pad.
- Flush wound with an appropriate wound cleanser.

Hydrogels

Iamin Hydrating Gel
Bard Medical Division
C.R. Bard, Inc.

How supplied
Tube (containing copper peptide): ½ oz (15 g), 3 oz (90 g);

Action
Iamin Hydrating Gel provides a moist environment for wounds or burns.

Indications
To manage pressure ulcers (stages 1, 2, 3, and 4), partial- and full-thickness wounds, diabetic ulcers, stasis ulcers, first- and second-degree burns, arterial ulcers, donor sites, postoperative incisions, cuts, abrasions, skin irritations, and skin conditions associated with peristomal care.

Contraindications
Contraindicated for third-degree burns.

Application
- Cleanse the wound with a suitable wound cleanser.
- Apply Iamin Hydrating Gel wound dressing once daily or with each dressing change, making sure to sufficiently cover the entire area of the wound.
- If using gauze as a wound covering, moisten gauze before applying.

Removal
Cleanse the wound as needed with a suitable wound cleanser, normal saline solution, or moistened gauze.

Hydrogels

IntraSite Gel
Smith & Nephew, Inc.
Wound Management Division

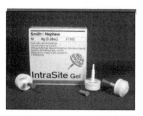

How supplied
Applipaks: 8 g, 15 g, 25 g; A6248

Action
IntraSite Gel is a sterile, nonadherent, amorphous hydrogel containing water, propylene, glycol, and starch. It hydrates granulation tissue and rehydrates dry eschar and slough, liquefying the necrotic tissue for easy removal.

Indications
To facilitate autolysis and to create a moist environment at the wound bed. May be used on pressure ulcers (stages 2, 3, and 4), partial- and full-thickness wounds, tunneling wounds, infected wounds (with concomitant antibiotic therapy), noninfected wounds, wounds with minimal drainage, wounds with purulent drainage, and red, yellow, or black wounds.

Contraindications
Contraindicated for third-degree burns.

Application
- Squeeze the gel onto the wound surface to a depth of ¼″ (0.6 cm).
- Cover with a transparent film (if the wound is noninfected), gauze and tape, or a polyurethane foam dressing (if the wound is moderately to heavily exuding).

Removal
- Remove the cover dressing.
- Irrigate the wound with normal saline solution or an appropriate wound cleanser.

Hydrogels

MPM Excel Gel

MPM Hydrogel
MPM Medical, Inc.

How supplied
MPM Excel Gel
Tube: 3 oz
MPM Hydrogel
Tube: ½ oz, 1 oz

Action
MPM Excel Gel is an aloe vera- and glycerin-based hydrogel that maintains a moist wound environment, promotes healing, and facilitates autolytic debridement.

Indications
To manage pressure ulcers (stages 2, 3, and 4), venous stasis ulcers, partial- and full-thickness wounds, superficial wounds, first- and second-degree burns, and tunneling wounds.

Contraindications
Not recommended for draining wounds.

Application
- Cleanse wound with normal saline solution or MPM wound cleanser.
- Apply MPM Excel Gel or Hydrogel to the wound in a layer ⅛" to ¼" (0.3 to 0.6 cm) thick.
- Cover with a secondary dressing.

Removal
- Change dressing daily.
- Flush the wound with normal saline solution or another appropriate wound cleanser.
- Gently remove the dressing.

Hydrogels

MPM GelPad Hydrogel Saturated Dressing

MPM Medical, Inc.

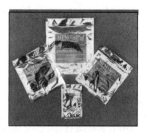

How supplied
Sterile pad: 2″ × 2″, 4″ × 4″; A6231
       8″ × 4″; A6232
       10″ × 6″; A6233

Action
MPM GelPad Hydrogel Saturated Dressing is saturated with stabilized aloe vera hydrogel and provides a primary cover for wounds. It creates a moist environment that facilitates wound healing and autolytic debridement, using Johnson & Johnson NuGauze to assist in elimination of fibers and to maintain moisture.

Indications
To manage pressure ulcers (stages 1, 2, 3, and 4), partial- and full-thickness wounds, first- and second-degree burns, tunneling wounds, infected and noninfected wounds, and red, yellow, or black wounds. Manages wounds with moderate drainage.

Contraindications
Not recommended for draining wounds.

Application
- Cleanse the wound with normal saline solution or MPM wound cleanser.
- Apply the dressing to the wound, or loosely pack the wound with the dressing.
- Secure with an appropriate secondary dressing.

Removal
- Change the dressing daily.
- Remove the secondary dressing.
- Flush the wound with normal saline solution or another appropriate wound cleanser.

Hydrogels

MPM Regenecare
MPM Medical, Inc.

How supplied
Tube: 3 oz

Action
MPM Regenecare wound gel is a collagen-, aloe vera-, and vitamin E-based gel that maintains a moist wound environment, promotes healing, and facilitates autolytic debridement.

Indications
To manage pressure ulcers (stages 2, 3, and 4), venous stasis ulcers, partial- and full-thickness wounds, secreting dermal lesions, superficial wounds, first- and second-degree burns, and tunneling wounds.

Contraindications
None provided by the manufacturer.

Application
- Cleanse the wound with normal saline solution or an appropriate wound cleanser.
- Apply MPM Regenecare to the wound in a layer ¼" (0.6 cm) thick.
- Cover with a secondary dressing.

Removal
- Change dressing daily.
- Remove the dressing.
- Flush the wound with normal saline solution or an appropriate wound cleanser.

Hydrogels

Normlgel
Mölnlycke Health Care

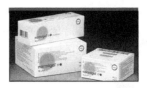

How supplied
Sterile tube: 5 g, 15 g single dose,
3 oz multidose; A6248

Action
Normlgel protects the wound and maintains a moist, natural wound-healing environment over the granulating wound.

Indications
To manage pressure ulcers (stages 2, 3, and 4), partial- and full-thickness wounds, tunneling wounds, noninfected wounds, wounds with minimal drainage, wounds with fibrin, and red wounds.

Contraindications
Contraindicated for infected wounds.

Application
- Irrigate or flush the wound gently with normal saline solution or a nonirritating solution, if necessary. Gently blot excess moisture with absorbent gauze.
- Choose appropriate-sized tube.
- Apply a light coating (dime thickness) to the wound surface. *Note:* Normlgel is designed to coat, not fill, the wound surface. Don't oversaturate the wound bed with Normlgel.
- If the wound is deep, pack it with Normlgel-impregnated gauze.
- Cover with Alldress or another cover dressing.

Removal
Change the dressing every 48 hours or when drainage is visible through the cover dressing.

Hydrogels

NU-GEL Collagen Wound Gel
Johnson & Johnson Wound
Management
Division of ETHICON, Inc.

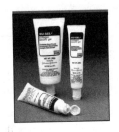

How supplied
Tube: 30 g (1.06 oz), 90 g (3.17 oz);
A6248

Action
NU-GEL Collagen Wound Gel is a hydrogel containing collagen. It's designed to maintain a moist wound environment and encourage autolytic debridement.

Indications
To manage pressure ulcers (stages 2, 3, and 4), first- and second-degree burns, venous stasis ulcers, minor injuries, and partial- and full-thickness wounds.

Contraindications
Contraindicated for third-degree burns.

Application
- Cleanse the wound thoroughly using normal saline solution.
- Apply gel directly to the wound.
- Cover with a secondary wound dressing.

Removal
- Remove dressing when appropriate, and repeat procedure.

Hydrogels

PanoPlex Hydrogel Wound Dressing

PanoGauze Non Woven Hydrogel Dressing
Sage Pharmaceuticals

How supplied
PanoPlex Hydrogel Wound Dressing
Syringe: 1 oz
Tube: 3.5 oz
PanoGauze Non Woven Hydrogel Dressing
Impregnated Gauze Pad: 2″ × 2″, 4″ × 4″, 4″ × 8″, 6″ × 10″

Action
PanoPlex Hydrogel Wound Dressing and PanoGauze Non Woven Hydrogel Dressing help create and maintain a moist wound-healing environment and prevent contaminants from entering the wound area.

Indications
To manage pressure ulcers (stages 1, 2, 3, and 4), dermal ulcers, first- and second-degree burns, postoperative incisions, skin conditions associated with peristomal care, and partial- and full-thickness wounds. May also be used on tunneling wounds, infected and noninfected wounds, and red, yellow, or black wounds.

Contraindications
None provided by the manufacturer.

Application
- Cleanse the wound thoroughly with a suitable wound cleanser, such as ClinsWound or SeptiCare.
- Apply dressing generously onto the wound.
- Cover with appropriate dressing.

Removal
- Change dressing as needed.
- Remove PanoPlex Hydrogel Wound Dressing or PanoGauze Non Woven Hydrogel Dressing with a wound cleanser, such as ClinsWound or SeptiCare.

Hydrogels

Phyto Derma Wound Gel
Aloe Life International

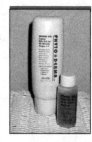

How supplied
Squeeze bottle: 1 oz, 4 oz

Action
Phyto Derma Wound Gel is a topical healing aid designed to create a moist and mildly acidic environment to facilitate wound healing.

Indications
To manage all wounds, including pressure ulcers (stages 1, 2, 3, and 4).

Contraindications
None provided by the manufacturer.

Application
- Gently cleanse the wound with normal saline solution, and pat dry with sterile gauze.
- Perform a patch test to assess compatibility on healthy skin before applying the wound gel.
- Apply a *small amount* of Phyto Derma Wound Gel to the entire wound bed.
- Cover with a poly-mem-type membrane dressing over pad.

Removal
- If the wound has a large amount of exudate, perform wound care daily.
- If the wound has a deep ecchymotic tissue with blistered tissue, change the dressing every other day or two times a week.
- If the tissue surrounding the wound bed becomes macerated, apply less wound gel.

Hydrogels

Purilon Gel
Coloplast Corporation

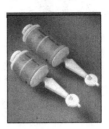

How supplied
Accordion pack: 8 g, 15 g, 25 g

Action
Purilon Gel is a sterile, clear, cohesive, amorphous hydrogel for effective autolytic debridement of necrotic tissue.

Indications
To treat necrotic and sloughy wounds, such as leg ulcers and pressure ulcers. May also be used throughout the healing process to provide a moist wound-healing environment in all types of wounds. May be used on infected wounds under medical supervision.

Contraindications
Contraindicated for third-degree burns.

Application
- Cleanse the wound with Sea-Clens wound cleanser or normal saline solution. Gently dry the skin around the wound.
- Remove the label from the accordion pack by pulling the corner, as indicated on the package. Swab the nozzle below the snap-off tip with a suitable antiseptic; remove the tip.
- Gently press the base of the accordion pack to apply Purilon Gel to the wound, in a layer no higher than the periwound skin.
- Cover with a secondary dressing.

Removal
- For necrotic and sloughy wounds, change Purilon Gel at least every 3 days. In clean wounds, change Purilon Gel according to the amount of exudate.
- To remove the gel from the wound, rinse with a wound cleanser or normal saline solution.

RadiaGel with Acemannan Hydrogel

RadiaDres Gel Sheet
Carrington Laboratories, Inc.

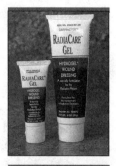

How supplied
RadiaGel
Tube: ½ oz, 3 oz
RadiaDres Gel Sheet
Sheet: 4" × 4"

Action
RadiaGel is a hydrogel wound dressing containing Acemannan Hydrogel in a nonoily preparation, specially formulated for the management of radiation dermatitis. RadiaDres Gel Sheet dressings are sterile, hydrogel polymer sheets consisting of 89.5% water and a hydrogel

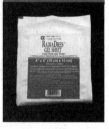

combined with a 10.5% cross-linked polyethylene oxide matrix in 4" × 4" gel sheets, specially targeted for the management of radiation-induced dermatitis. These dressings have a high specific heat to provide a cooling effect, are hydrophilic, and will absorb at least three times their own weight in water, serum, or blood. RadiaDres Gel Sheets may be refrigerated for maximum cooling effect.

Indications
To condition the skin before radiation therapy and to manage skin reactions after radiation therapy. RadiaDres Gel Sheet dressings may also be used to manage radiation-induced dermatitis.

Contraindications
Contraindicated in patients with known hypersensitivity to Acemannan Hydrogel or other components of the dressing.

Application
Pretherapy:
- Cleanse the skin with a suitable cleanser, such as RadiaKlenz.

Hydrogels

- Massage a small amount of RadiaGel into the skin two or three times daily to condition the skin. Begin as far in advance of therapy as possible.

    During therapy:

- Continue to massage a small amount of RadiaGel into the skin three or four times daily throughout the entire treatment period.
- Cleanse the affected area with a suitable cleanser, such as RadiaKlenz, by spraying it onto the desired area.
- Gently pat affected area with a soft gauze. No rinsing is required.
- Follow with the appropriate topical preparation, such as a thin layer of RadiaGel to intact skin, or a ⅛″ to ¼″ (0.3- to 0.6-cm) layer of gel to areas of ulceration.
- Cover with appropriate nonadhering dressing, such as RadiaDres Gel Sheet. Remove the red film backing from the sheet and gently press it in place over the area of ulceration or reaction.

Removal

- Change dressing according to the wound condition and amount of exudate or as directed by the primary care provider.
- Gently lift RadiaDres Gel Sheet to remove.
- Rinse away any remaining gel with gentle irrigation.

Hydrogels

Restore Hydrogel Dressing
Hollister Incorporated

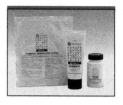

How supplied
Amorphous tube: 3 oz
Impregnated gauze sponge: 4″ × 4″
*Impregnated gauze
packing strip:*   2″ × 2½ yd

Action
Amorphous Restore Hydrogel Dressing maintains a moist wound environment. Restore Hydrogel Impregnated Gauze Sponges and Packing Strips fill in dead space associated with sinus tracts and undermining or deep wounds.

Indications
To maintain a moist environment in pressure ulcers (stages 1, 2, 3, and 4), arterial stasis ulcers, first- and second-degree burns, skin tears, cuts, abrasions, and conditions associated with peristomal care.

Contraindications
None provided by the manufacturer.

Application
- Cleanse and dry the skin according to facility policy.
  Amorphous Restore Hydrogel Dressing:
- Apply to the wound to a minimum depth of ¼″ (0.6 cm).
- Cover with a secondary dressing, and secure with tape or other appropriate material.
  Restore Hydrogel Sponge or Packing Strip:
- Apply sponge or strip to the wound.
- Cover with a secondary dressing, and secure with tape or other appropriate material.

Removal
- Remove the secondary dressing.
- Gently remove Restore hydrogel dressing.
- Rinse away remaining gel using Restore Wound Cleanser or normal saline solution.

Hydrogels

SAF-Gel Hydrating Dermal Wound Dressing
ConvaTec

How supplied
Tube: 3 oz; A6248

Action
SAF-Gel Hydrating Dermal Wound Dressing is an alginate-containing wound gel designed to promote an optimal, moist environment for the wound-healing process.

Indications
To manage chronic wounds, pressure ulcers (stages 1, 2, 3, and 4), stasis ulcers, first- and second-degree burns, cuts, abrasions, and skin tears.

Contraindications
None provided by the manufacturer.

Application
- Cleanse the wound with normal saline solution or an appropriate cleansing solution, such as SAF-Clens Chronic Wound Cleanser or Shur Clens Skin Wound Cleansing Solution.
- Apply a ⅛″ to ¼″ (0.3 to 0.6 cm) layer of SAF-Gel Hydrating Dermal Wound Dressing to cover the entire wound surface.
- Cover with an appropriate secondary cover dressing.

Removal
Change the dressing daily or when the wound begins to dry out.

Hydrogels

Skintegrity Amorphous Hydrogel

Skintegrity Hydrogel Impregnated Gauze
Medline Industries, Inc.

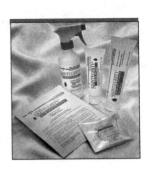

How supplied
Bellows bottle: 1 oz; A6248
Tube: 4 oz; A6248
Impregnated gauze: 4″ × 4″; A6231

Action
Skintegrity Hydrogel dressings are greaseless and maintain a moist wound environment. Skintegrity Hydrogel Impregnated Gauze is compression-saturated gauze sponge, which ensures thorough hydration. A special formulation balances viscosity and hydration, added aloe vera aids healing, and the greaseless formulation irrigates easily from the wound bed.

Indications
To manage pressure ulcers (stages 2, 3, and 4), partial- or full-thickness wounds, venous stasis ulcers, first- and second-degree burns, cuts, abrasions, skin irritations, postoperative incisions, infected and noninfected wounds, wounds with light drainage, and red, yellow, or black wounds.

Contraindications
Contraindicated in patients with known hypersensitivity to components of the gel.

Application
- Cleanse the wound with normal saline solution or appropriate wound cleanser, such as Skintegrity Wound Cleanser. Dry the periwound skin.
- If the wound has large amounts of drainage, it may be appropriate to consider use of a more absorbent product in the wound.
  Skintegrity Amorphous Hydrogel:
- Apply a generous layer of hydrogel to all wound surfaces.
- Cover with an appropriate secondary dressing, such as Stratasorb composite dressing or bordered gauze.

- Repeat every 72 hours or as necessary to maintain a moist wound bed.

  Skintegrity Hydrogel Impregnated Gauze:
- Unfold the hydrogel gauze pad and loosely pack it in the wound bed, being sure to fill undermining and tunneling areas.

Removal

- Carefully remove the secondary dressing and irrigate the wound bed with normal saline solution or appropriate wound cleanser, such as Skintegrity Wound Cleanser. Dry the peri-wound skin.
- If the dressing has dried to the wound edge or the base of the wound, moisten with Skintegrity Wound Cleanser or normal saline solution until it loosens, then remove it.
- Cover with an appropriate secondary dressing, such as Stratasorb composite dressing or bordered gauze.

Hydrogels

SoloSite Wound Gel

SoloSite Gel Conformable Wound Dressing
Smith & Nephew, Inc.
Wound Management Division

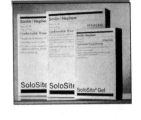

How supplied
SoloSite Wound Gel
Tube: 3 oz; A6248
Push-button applicators: 2 oz, 7 oz; A6248
SoloSite Gel Conformable Wound Dressing
Gel pad: 2″ × 2″, 4″ × 4″; A6242

Action
SoloSite Wound Gel hydrates granulation tissue and rehydrates eschar and slough, liquefying the necrotic tissue for easy removal. SoloSite Gel Conformable Wound Dressing is a clean, latex-free wound dressing made of nonwoven gauze that is impregnated or thoroughly saturated with SoloSite Wound Gel. Preservatives are added to the product to help prevent bacterial growth. The dressing will keep gel in contact with the wound surface, absorb excess exudate, and create a moist wound-healing environment that supports autolytic debridement. It meets United States Pharmacopeia requirements for cytotoxicity and is nonsensitizing, systemically nontoxic, nonmutagenic, and nonhemolytic.

Indications
To manage partial- and full-thickness acute and chronic wounds, such as skin tears, pressure ulcers, and venous leg ulcers. SoloSite Gel Conformable Wound Dressing is also indicated for minor burns.

Contraindications
Contraindicated for third-degree burns.

Application
- Cleanse the wound with saline solution or an appropriate wound cleanser.

Hydrogels

SoloSite Wound Gel:

- Apply SoloSite Wound Gel to cover the wound surface, and smooth the gel to a depth of ⅛″ to ¼″ (0.3 to 0.6 cm).
- Cover the primary dressing with an appropriate secondary dressing.

SoloSite Gel Conformable Wound Dressing:

- Choose a dressing size that is slightly larger than the wound. Press the dressing into the wound so that it makes contact with the wound bed. The dressing should cover the entire wound surface; however, it shouldn't extend beyond the edges.
- Cover the primary dressing with an appropriate secondary dressing.

Removal

- Change SoloSite Wound Gel at least daily if wound is covered with necrotic or sloughy debris. Change dressing every 2 days for wounds that are granulating or epithelializing because these wounds have significantly less drainage.
- Change SoloSite Gel Conformable Wound Dressing when necessary.

Hydrogels

NEW PRODUCT
TenderWet Gel Pad
Medline Industries, Inc.

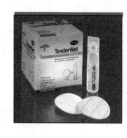

How supplied

TenderWet
System: 8-30 ml Ringer's activation solution plus 1.6″ rounds, 2.2″ rounds, or 3″ × 3″ squares, A6242

TenderWet
Cavity System: 16-30 ml Ringer's activation solution plus 4″ × 4″ squares; A6242

Action

TenderWet is a multilayer wound dressing pad whose central component is an absorbent polymer gel. The covering layer is composed of a hydrophobic knitted fabric that allows wound exudate to pass through to the absorptive gel layer while helping to prevent the dressing from adhering to the wound. The gel holds a significant amount of TenderWet (Ringer's) solution, which provides a moist wound environment. The solution is released into the wound bed while the wound exudate is absorbed, providing an autolytic debriding process that helps remove necrotic tissue and debris while allowing tissue granulation to occur in an optimal, moist wound environment.

The side of the Tender Wet dressing with green stripes (placed away from the patient) has a water-repellent layer, making this dressing appropriate for flat wounds or wounds with superficial depth.

The cavity dressings have a symmetrical structure without a water-repellent layer. Both sides function equally and, therefore, make it particularly suitable for packing deeper wounds.

Indications

To manage dry, light to moderately exudating, and partial- and full-thickness wounds, such as minor burns, superficial injuries, lacerations, cuts, abrasions, incisions or surgical wounds, and skin tears. Also for chronic wounds, such as pressure ulcers (stages 2, 3, and 4), lower extremity ulcers, venous ulcers, arterial ulcers, diabetic ulcers, and ulcers of mixed etiology. May also be used on infected wounds.

Hydrogels

Contraindications

Contraindicated for third-degree burns unless otherwise advised by the primary care provider.

Application

- Before application, open the dressing's peel-pack and activate the dressing with the appropriate amount of Ringer's solution:
  - 1.6″ or 2.2″ round dressing: about 15 ml (1 vial)
  - 3″ × 3″ square dressing: about 30 ml (1 vial)
  - 4″ × 4″ square dressing: about 60 ml (2- to 30-ml vials).

  TenderWet is completely activated after 2 to 3 minutes of soaking.
- Extra Ringer's solution may be used to irrigate the wound bed before the dressing is applied. Oversaturation of the dressing is not a concern because the dressing will only absorb a set amount of solution.
- Apply the white side of the TenderWet dressing to the entire surface of the wound. Make sure that the green stripes face away from the patient.
- Pack deeper wounds with TenderWet Cavity, which doesn't feature a water-repellent layer; it then can be covered with regular TenderWet.
- *Note:* TenderWet must cover the edge of the wound. The white, soft tissue that forms around the wound edges and is sometimes mistaken for maceration of the epidermis is a layer of squames or corneocytes. These harmless cells are nonviable and are usually sloughed off by the daily activities of bathing, scratching, or changing clothes.
- Secure TenderWet by using a roll gauze, such as Sof-Form Conforming Gauze, or a six-ply roll bandage, such as Bulkee II. Or use a self-adherent cohesive bandage; an elastic net for adhesive-sensitive patients; a dressing retention tape such as Medfix; a bordered gauze; or a waterproof, composite island dressing, such as Stratasorb.
- If the dressing dries out, rewet using Ringer's solution.
- *Note:* Use TenderWet only after activating with Ringer's solution. Don't reuse TenderWet; product is intended for single use only. Don't mechanically damage the TenderWet covering layer.

Hydrogels

Removal

- Change TenderWet within 24 hours. Depending on drainage, TenderWet Cavity dressings may need to be changed twice daily.
- Gently remove the secondary dressing and lift TenderWet out of the wound bed.

3M Tegagel Hydrogel Wound Fillers

3M Health Care

How supplied
Pad: 4″ × 4″(0.88 oz hydrogel); A6242
Tube: 3 oz; A6248

Action
3M Tegagel Hydrogel Wound Fillers are amorphous hydrogel dressings that help provide a moist wound-healing environment and help prevent wound desiccation. The products assist with autolytic debridement by hydrating devitalized tissue, and they fill dead space in full-thickness wounds.

Indications
To manage partial-thickness dermal wounds, including pressure ulcers, venous insufficiency ulcers, diabetic ulcers, and arterial ulcers. Also used to manage postsurgical incisions, dehisced surgical wounds, first- and second-degree burns, donor sites, skin tears, lacerations, abrasions, minor skin irritations, peristomal skin irritations, radiation dermatitis, cancerous lesions, and wounds exhibiting dry eschar and fibrinous slough. May be used with gauze to lightly pack tunneling or undermined chronic wounds.

Contraindications
- Contraindicated for third-degree burns.
- Contraindicated in patients who have a known sensitivity to any product ingredient.
- If infection develops, consult the primary care provider and implement appropriate medical treatment.

Application
- Cleanse skin and wound thoroughly.
- Protect periwound skin, as appropriate, using a barrier film.
- Apply enough wound filler to cover the wound base and necrotic tissue. Or saturate a sterile gauze pad with wound filler and place it in the wound.
- Cover with an appropriate secondary dressing.

Removal
- Change the dressing if drying occurs and as frequently as needed to ensure a moist wound environment.

Hydrogels

TOE-AID Toe and Nail Dressing

Southwest Technologies, Inc.

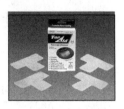

How supplied
Tape: 1¼″ × 1¼″, with ″T″ tape; A6245

Action
Because of its high glycerin content, TOE-AID assists in the natural wound-healing process. The soft gel pad provides a protective cushion to the injury, is highly absorbent, won't dry out, and is bacteriostatic and fungistatic. TOE-AID absorbent dressing is a uniquely formulated glycerin gel pad attached to a hypoallergenic, water-resistant, adhesive T-shaped tape.

Indications
To manage toe conditions ranging from toenail removal to toenail fungus and other toe injuries.

Contraindications
- Contraindicated for highly exudating wounds that may require packing with additional dressing or other highly absorbent material.
- Use cautiously on an infected wound. Consult primary care provider before use.

Application
- Prepare the wound site by cleansing as needed.
    After toenail removal or on an open wound:
- Fold the dressing under the toe first, then overlap the tape to make a waterproof seal.
- Wrap one side of the dressing down around the toe, then repeat with the other side of the dressing.
- *Don't* get the gel wet.
    On intact skin or directly on toenail:
- Be sure to make a waterproof seal to protect the gel from getting wet. The product may be worn in the shower if the tape is properly secured.

Removal
- Change the dressing if leaking occurs or the dressing becomes highly saturated with exudate. When applied to intact skin or directly to the toenail, the dressing may be left in place for up to 7 days.

Hydrogels

Ultrex Gel Wound Dressing with Acemannan Hydrogel
Carrington Laboratories, Inc.

How supplied
Tube: 8 g, 15 g

Action
Ultrex Gel is a sterile, preservative-free, colorless wound dressing containing Acemannan Hydrogel. It is specifically formulated to maintain the moist environment essential to wound healing in patients with painful wounds or sensitivities to other topical dressings.

Indications
To manage pressure ulcers (stages 1, 2, 3, and 4), stasis ulcers, foot ulcers, first- and second-degree burns, postsurgical incisions, and skin conditions associated with peristomal care.

Contraindications
Contraindicated in patients with known hypersensitivity to Acemannan Hydrogel or other components of the dressing.

Application
- Cleanse the wound with a suitable cleanser, such as UltraKlenz, CarraKlenz, or MicroKlenz, by spraying the affected area.
- Gently dry the surrounding skin with soft gauze. No rinsing is required.
- Apply a layer of Ultrex Gel ⅛″ to ¼″ (0.3- to 0.6-cm) thick on areas of ulceration.
- Cover with an appropriate secondary dressing, such as CarraDres, CarraFilm, or CarraSmart Foam.

Removal
- Change dressing according to the wound condition and the amount of exudate, or as directed by the primary care provider.
- Rinse away any remaining gel with gentle irrigation.

Hydrogels

Vigilon Primary Wound Dressing
Bard Medical Division
C.R. Bard, Inc.

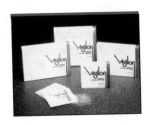

How supplied
Sterile sheet: 4" × 4"; A6242
                     3" × 6", 6" × 8",
                     3" × 8"; A6243
Nonsterile sheet: 4" × 4"; A6242
                    13" × 24"; A6244

Action
Vigilon Primary Wound Dressing provides a moist wound-healing environment and promotes formation of granulation tissue. It relieves pain, burning, itching, and soreness; absorbs wound exudate, odor, and bacteria; and doesn't adhere to tissue. Dressing conforms readily to any wound configuration, cushions and protects the wound, and doesn't interfere with topical medications.

Indications
To prevent skin breakdown and manage skin tears, minor chemical and thermal burns, superficial lacerations, cuts, abrasions, postoperative incisions, and radiation skin reactions. May also be used on pressure ulcers (stages 1, 2, and 3), partial- and full-thickness wounds, lesions and excoriation associated with dermatologic procedures, surgical wounds, tunneling wounds, noninfected wounds, minimally to heavily draining wounds, wounds with serosanguineous or purulent drainage, and red, yellow, or black wounds.

Contraindications
Contraindicated for infected wounds, unless the dressing is used with an appropriate topical antibiotic.

Application
- Cleanse the wound.
- Make sure that both dressing surfaces have a clear film in place.
- Cut dressing to wound size, leaving a 1½" (1.3-cm) overlap if contact with the periwound skin isn't desired.

Hydrogels

- Remove one or both clear film coverings, depending upon desire for occlusion and amount of exudate. (Leaving on one side of the film provides occlusion but offers less absorption.)
- Place the side of the dressing from which the film has been removed onto the wound.
- Apply an appropriate cover dressing, such as roll gauze or a 4″ × 4″ gauze pad.

Removal
- Change dressing as excess exudate accumulates. This may be as frequently as every 24 hours or as infrequently as every 3 days.
- Remove the cover dressing.
- Carefully lift off Vigilon Primary Wound Dressing. If it appears or feels dry, moisten with normal saline solution before removing completely.

Hydrogels

WOUN'DRES Collagen Hydrogel
Coloplast Corporation

How supplied
Tube: 1 oz, 3 oz; A6248

Action
WOUN'DRES Collagen Hydrogel maintains a moist, wound-healing environment, protects new granulation tissue, and promotes autolytic debridement.

Indications
To manage pressure ulcers (stages 2, 3, and 4), venous stasis ulcers, superficial wounds, scrapes, first- and second-degree burns, and partial- and full-thickness wounds. May also be used on tunneling wounds, infected and noninfected wounds, wounds with minimal or moderate drainage, wounds with serosanguineous drainage, and red, yellow, or black wounds.

Contraindications
Contraindicated for third-degree burns.

Application
- Cleanse the wound thoroughly with wound cleanser or normal saline solution.
- Apply WOUN'DRES Collagen Hydrogel directly into the wound.
- Cover with a secondary dressing.

Removal
- Remove the secondary dressing.
- Flush the wound with a wound cleanser or normal saline solution.

Hydrogels

Wound Dressing with ClearSite

Bandage Roll with ClearSite
CONMED Corporation

How supplied
Wound Dressing with ClearSite
Bordered dressing: $3'' \times 4''$, $5'' \times 5''$; A6245
  $7\frac{1}{2}'' \times 9\frac{1}{2}''$; A6246
Borderless dressing: $2'' \times 3''$, $4'' \times 4''$; A6242
  $4\frac{1}{2}'' \times 5''$; A6243
  $8'' \times 8''$, $5'' \times 11\frac{1}{2}''$; A6244
Island dressing: $1\frac{3}{4}'' \times 2\frac{1}{2}''$, $3'' \times 4''$, $5'' \times 5''$; A6245
  $5'' \times 6''$, $4\frac{1}{2}'' \times 9\frac{1}{2}''$; A6246
  $8\frac{1}{2}'' \times 9\frac{1}{2}''$, A6247

Bandage Roll with ClearSite
Bandage roll: $4'' \times 48''$, A6244

Action
Wound Dressing with ClearSite and Bandage Roll with ClearSite contain an absorbent, hydration-balanced hydrogel. Both products promote a moist wound-healing environment and allow continuous wound assessment and charting through transparent dressing and its 1-cm grid pattern.

Indications
To prevent and manage pressure ulcers (stages 1, 2, 3, and 4), partial- and full-thickness wounds, uninfected wounds, first- and second-degree burns, dermal leg ulcers, skin tears, and venous stasis ulcers.

Contraindications
- Contraindicated for infected wounds.
- Contraindicated for use during laser procedures, but may be used as intended following completion of laser procedure.
- Contraindicated for third-degree burns.

Application
- Consult a primary care provider before using these products.
- Cleanse and rinse the wound according to facility policy.
- Dry the wound and surrounding areas because lotions, salves, and moisture will render auxiliary adhesive tapes ineffective.

Hydrogels

- Use scissors to trim the borderless Wound Dressing with ClearSite, if necessary, while the dressing is still on the release liner.

    Wound Dressing with ClearSite bordered, borderless, and island dressings:

- Remove the larger section of the release liner by flexing the dressing and grasping the exposed edge at the split.
- Keep the smaller, unexposed part elevated, and gently position the exposed portion of the gel surface into place on the wound.
- Carefully peel the remaining liner from the dressing, avoiding contact with the exposed gel surface and the wound, then press remaining dressing into place.
- Tape or wrap the dressing to maintain position.

    Bandage Roll with ClearSite:

- Grasp the dressing's leading edge, and unroll a convenient starting length.
- Wrap the limb, starting the leading edge at an undamaged site. Unroll the dressing as needed.
- Cut dressing to desired length.
- Tape or overwrap the dressing to maintain position.

Removal

- Press down, support the skin surrounding the dressing, and carefully lift an edge of the tape.
- Continue slowly around the wound margins until all tape edges are free from the skin surface.
- Lift tape and dressing carefully from the wound.

Hydrogels

Specialty absorptive wound covers

Action
Specialty absorptives are unitized, multilayered dressings that consist of highly absorptive layers of fibers, such as absorbent cellulose, cotton, or rayon. These dressings may or may not have an adhesive border.

Indications
Specialty absorptive dressings may be used as primary or secondary dressings to manage light to heavy drainage from partial- and full-thickness wounds, infected and noninfected wounds, and red, yellow, or black wounds.

Advantages
- Can be used as secondary dressing over most primary dressings
- Are semiadherent or nonadherent
- Are highly absorptive
- Are easy to apply and remove
- May have an adhesive border, making additional tape unnecessary.

Disadvantages
May not be appropriate as a primary dressing for undermining wounds.

HCPCS code overview
The HCPCS codes normally assigned to specialty absorptive wound covers without an adhesive border are:

A6251—pad size ≤16 sq. in.

A6252—pad size >16 sq. in., but ≤48 sq. in.

A6253—pad size >48 sq. in.

The HCPCS codes normally assigned to specialty absorptive wound covers with an adhesive border are:

A6254—pad size ≤16 sq. in.

A6255—pad size >16 sq. in., but ≤48 sq. in.

A6256—pad size >48 sq. in.

Specialty Absorptives

AQUACEL
ConvaTec

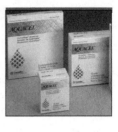

How supplied
Pad: 2″ × 2″, 4″ × 4″; A6196
       6″ × 6″; A6197
Ribbon: ¾″ × 18″; A6199
(Note: Aquacel was recently reassigned to alginate coding.)

Action
AQUACEL hydrofiber wound dressing is a soft, sterile, non-woven pad or ribbon dressing made from sodium carboxymethylcellulose fibers. This conformable and absorbent dressing interacts with wound exudate and forms a soft gel that maintains a moist environment for wound healing, debridement, and easy removal, with little or no damage to healing tissues.

Indications
To manage exuding wounds, pressure ulcers, leg ulcers, abrasions, lacerations, incisions, donor sites, oncology wounds, first- and second-degree burns, and surgical or traumatic wounds that have been left to heal by secondary intent. May be used for wounds that are prone to bleeding, such as mechanically or surgically debrided wounds, donor sites, and traumatic wounds. May also be used to facilitate the control of minor bleeding.

Contraindications
- Contraindicated in patients with known sensitivity to this dressing or its components.
- Contraindicated for use as a surgical sponge.

Application
- Debride the wound prior to application, if necessary.
- Cleanse it with an effective cleansing agent, such as SAF-Clens or normal saline solution.
- Apply wound dressing to the wound site.
- Cover with an appropriate secondary dressing, such as a moisture-retentive dressing.

Specialty Absorptives

Removal

- Change dressing when it becomes saturated with exudate or when good clinical practice dictates. Dressing may be kept in place for up to 7 days.
- Remove the secondary dressing gently, according to the package insert.
- Remove the AQUACEL hydrofiber wound dressing.
- Irrigate the wound with SAF-Clens or normal saline solution if necessary to remove the residual gel without disrupting the delicate granulation tissue.

BAND-AID Brand Island Surgical Dressings

Johnson & Johnson Wound Management
Division of ETHICON, Inc.

How supplied

Island: 4″ × 7″ with 2″ × 5″ pad,
4″ × 10″ with 2″ × 8″
pad; A6254
4″ × 14″ with 2″ × 12″ pad; A6255
Adhesive: 4″ × 6″ with 3″ × 4″ pad; A6254
8″ × 6″ with 3″ × 8″ pad; A6255

Action

BAND-AID Brand Island Surgical Dressings consist of a non-adherent facing, a highly absorbent filler, and tape backing.

Indications

To manage surgical incisions, lacerations, abrasions, and invasive lines.

Contraindications

None provided by the manufacturer.

Application

- Cleanse the wound with normal saline solution or a cleansing agent.
- Apply the dressing over the wound.

Removal

Remove the dressing when it has become soiled.

Specialty Absorptives

BreakAway Wound Dressing
Winfield Laboratories, Inc.

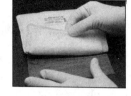

How supplied
Sterile, multilayered pad with releasably attached wound contact layer: 4" × 6"; A6252
6"x 9", 9" × 15", 15"x 18", 15"x 24"; A6253

Action
BreakAway Wound Dressing is a one-piece, multilayered, non-adherent, highly absorbent dressing with the patented releasably attached wound contact layer feature that can be used wet or dry. It protects the wound, supports healing, reduces shearing action and friction, and wicks away drainage. It's the only dressing with a releasably attached N-TERFACE Material wound contact layer that allows observation of the wound surface prior to removal of the wound contact layer, preventing disruption of the healing wound surface. The nonwoven wicking layer draws and contains wound drainage in the rayon and cellulose absorbent layers and helps prevent maceration of periwound area. The air-permeable and absorptive dressing backing is reinforced to provide strength when wet.

Indications
To manage pressure ulcers (stages 2, 3, and 4), partial- and full-thickness wounds, skin graft sites, donor sites, dermatologic conditions, fungating neoplasms, burns, tunneling wounds, and infected and uninfected wounds. May be used for wounds with serosanguineous or purulent drainage, wounds with heavy drainage, minor lacerations, and red, yellow, or black wounds. May also be used as a wet or dry dressing and as a postoperative dressing.

Contraindications
- Contraindicated for preventing skin breakdown.
- Contraindicated for areas needing an occlusive dressing.
- Contraindicated for third-degree burns.

Application
- Use BreakAway Wound Dressing wet or dry.

Specialty Absorptives

- Select a dressing size that covers the wound and periwound area.
- Apply a desired topical agent directly to the wound or dressing.
- If using dressing wet, soak it with normal saline solution or a solution of choice. Squeeze out excess fluid; don't wring.
- Apply dressing with the releasably attached wound contact layer toward the wound.
- Secure the dressing with stretch netting, roll gauze, or tape.

Removal

- Change the dressing daily or more frequently, if needed.
- Lift the dressing gently off the wound.
- If the wound has dried or is overly bloody, hold the wound contact layer in place, and release the absorbent pad component. If the wound contact layer has points of sticking, cleanse it with normal saline solution. Then, remove the wound contact layer. *Note:* Removing the absorbent pad component doesn't damage the sealed construction of the pad.

CombiDERM ACD Absorbent Cover Dressing
ConvaTec

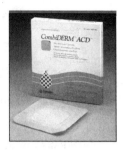

How supplied
Sterile dressing: 4" × 4", 5¼" × 5¼",
6" × 7"; A6237
6" × 10", 8" × 8",
8" × 9"; A6238

Action
CombiDERM ACD Absorbent Cover Dressing is a sterile dressing with a hydrocolloid adhesive and an absorbent pad. This absorbent pad wicks exudate without damaging tissue.

Indications
To manage exuding, chronic dermal ulcers, such as pressure ulcers, leg ulcers, and diabetic ulcers, as well as acute wounds, such as abrasions, lacerations, biopsies, and open and closed surgical wounds.

Contraindications
Contraindicated in patients with a known sensitivity to the dressing or its components.

Application
- Cleanse the wound surface and surrounding skin with an appropriate cleansing solution. Dry the surrounding skin thoroughly. Debride if necessary.
- Determine the ideal dressing size, allowing a minimum 1¼" (3.2 cm) margin beyond the reddened skin.
- If a filler or exudate management product is required, apply AQUACEL Hydrofiber, KALTOSTAT alginate dressing, or another appropriate dressing.
- Remove the release paper from the CombiDERM ACD dressing, and place the pad directly over wound.
- Press and smooth the dressing edges to secure adherence and ensure a seal.

Removal
- Gently press down on the skin and carefully lift the blue tab on the corner of the dressing. Continue until all edges are free.
- Carefully lift away the dressing.

Specialty Absorptives

CombiDERM Non-Adhesive
ConvaTec

How supplied
Sterile dressing: 3″ × 3″; A6234
              5¼″ × 5¼″; A6235
              6″ × 10″; A6236

Action
CombiDERM Non-Adhesive is a sterile nonadhesive wound dressing consisting of absorbent hydrocolloids that provide a moist environment, absorb exudate, and are nondamaging to tissue. It may be used alone or in combination with other primary dressings to manage wound exudate.

Indications
To manage exuding chronic wounds, such as pressure ulcers, leg ulcers, and diabetic ulcers, as well as acute exuding wounds, such as abrasions, lacerations, biopsies, and open and closed surgical wounds.

Contraindications
Contraindicated in patients with a known sensitivity to the dressing or its components.

Application
- Cleanse the wound site, rinse well, and dry the surrounding skin.
- Chose a dressing that extends 1″ (2.5 cm) beyond the wound.
- Apply the dressing white-side-down directly over the wound.
- Secure the dressing with hypoallergenic tape or with a secondary bandage or wrap.
- For highly exuding wounds, the use of Aquacel or Kaltostat in combination with CombiDERM Non-Adhesive is recommended.

Removal
- Change the dressing when clinically indicated or as the softened area approaches the edge of the dressing. The dressing may be left in place for up to 7 days.
- Carefully lift the dressing away from the wound.

Specialty Absorptives

Covaderm Adhesive Wound Dressing

DeRoyal

How supplied

Multilayered pad with fabric tape border: 2½" × 2½" pad with
4" × 4" tape,
2½" × 4" pad with
4" × 6" tape,
2" × 5½" pad with 4" × 8" tape,
2" × 7½" pad with 4" × 10" tape; A6254
2" × 11" pad with 4" × 4" tape; A6255

Action

Covaderm Adhesive Wound Dressing is an absorbent island dressing with a protective, air-permeable, adhesive fabric tape border for aseptic, one-step application. Rounded edges conform to jointed, curved, or irregular wound areas.

Indications

For use as a primary or secondary dressing to manage surgical incisions, superficial lacerations, and abrasions. May also be used as an all-purpose dressing.

Contraindications

None provided by the manufacturer.

Application

- Peel back the edge of the folded release liner.
- Anchor the exposed edge of the tape to the skin, then peel off the remaining release paper.
- Smooth all the tape edges onto the skin.

Removal

Carefully lift the edges of the tape and peel off the dressing.

Specialty Absorptives

CURITY Abdominal Pads
Kendall Health Care Products Company

How supplied
Sterile pad: 5″ × 9″, 7½″ × 8″, 8″ × 10″
Nonsterile pad: 5″ × 9″, 7½″ × 8″, 8″ × 10″, 12″ × 16″, 24″ × 8″,
  12″ × 8″, 12″ × 10″, 24″ × 10″, 10″ × 12″
Nonsterile roll: 8″ × 20 yd

Action
CURITY Abdominal Pads are a secondary dressing that absorb excess wound fluid and protect the wound by cushioning it.

Indications
To prevent skin breakdown and to manage moderately to heavily exuding wounds. May also be used as part of a decreasing system for virtually any wound requiring fluid retention and cushioning.

Contraindications
Contraindicated for tunneling wounds.

Application
- Choose a primary dressing based on wound type and apply it.
- Cover the primary dressing with a CURITY Abdominal Pad.
- Secure the abdominal pad with tape, bandage roll, or another appropriate product.

Removal
- Carefully remove the securing product.
- Remove the CURITY Abdominal Pad from the primary dressing.

NEW PRODUCT
DuPad Abdominal Pads, Open End
Dumex Medical

How supplied
Pad, open end,
sterile: 5″ × 9″, 8″ × 8″, 8″ × 10″, 8″ × 24″
Pad, open end,
nonsterile: 5″ × 9″, 8″ × 8″, 8″ × 10″, 8″ × 12″, 10″ × 12″,
                   8″ × 24″, 10″ × 24″, 12″ × 16″, 8″ × 20 yds

Action
These highly absorbent cotton-filled sterile and non-sterile pads
provide protection for heavily exudating wounds.

Indications
For use as a secondary dressing for highly exudating wounds.

Contraindications
None provided by the manufacturer.

Application
- Cleanse the wound with PrimaDerm Dermal Cleanser or saline
  solution. Dry the periwound skin.
- Apply an appropriate primary dressing.
- Cover the primary dressing with DuPad Abdominal Pad, and
  secure with tape, gauze roll, or other appropriate dressing.

Removal
Gently remove all layers.

NEW PRODUCT
DuPad Abdominal Pads, Sealed End
Dumex Medical

How supplied
Pad, sterile: 5″ × 9″, 8″ × 8″, 8″ × 10″
Pad, nonsterile: 5″ × 9″, 8″ × 8″, 8″ × 10″

Action
These highly aborbent cotton filled pads provide cushioning to protect heavily exudating wounds. Sterile and nonsterile pads are available.

Indications
For use as a secondary dressing for highly exudating wounds.

Contraindications
None provided by the manufacturer.

Application
- Cleanse the wound with PrimaDerm Dermal Cleanser or saline solution. Dry the periwound skin.
- Choose an appropriate primary dressing.
- Cover the dressing with DuPad Abdominal Pad, and secure with tape, gauze roll, or other appropriate dressing.

Removal
Gently remove all layers.

Specialty Absorptives

EXU-DRY

Smith & Nephew, Inc.
Wound Management Division

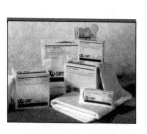

How supplied

Specialty dressing:	Arm 6″ × 9″, Arm 9″ × 15″, Arm/Shoulder; A6253 Scalp/Face, Elbow/Knee/Heel, Boot/Foot L; A6252 Hand, Boot/Foot M/S; A6251 Neck, Buttocks, Leg, Oncology Breast Vest, Burn Jacket/Vest; A6253
Slit disc:	2″, 3″; A6251
Slit tube:	1¾″ × 2½″, 2″ × 3″, 3″ × 4″; A6251 4″ × 6″; A6252
Disc:	2″, 3″, 3″ × 4″; A6251 4″ × 6″; A6252 6″ × 9″, 9″ × 15″, 15″ × 18″, 15″ × 24″, 20″ × 28″; A6253
Incision dressing:	3″ × 9″, 3″ × 12″; A6252
Pad, *nonpermeable:*	24″ × 36″, 36″ × 72″; A6253
Sheet, *permeable:*	36″ × 72″; A6253
Pediatric specialty *dressing:*	Scalp, Infant/Toddler Vest; A6252 Hand, Foot; A6251 Arm, Leg; 6″ × 9″, 9″ × 15″; A6253 Child Vest; A6253
Pad/sheet:	20″ × 28″ Crib Sheet (permeable), 20″ × 28″ Receiving Blanket, 24″ × 36″ Pad (nonpermeable); A6253

Action

EXU-DRY's highly absorptive properties may reduce the need for frequent dressing changes. The dressings are designed to minimize adherence and improve patient comfort. The anti-shear layer helps to minimize friction and shear. May be used wet or dry.

Specialty Absorptives

Indications
To manage exudate in partial- and full-thickness wounds, such as burns and donor or skin graft sites.

Contraindications
None provided by the manufacturer.

Application
- Select a dressing slightly larger than the wound.
- Place the dressing on the wound with the words "Use other side against wound" facing up.
- Secure the dressing with gauze, tape, or netting.

Removal
- Remove the gauze, tape, or netting.
- Lift off the dressing.

MPM Woundgard Bordered Gauze Dressing
MPM Medical, Inc.

How supplied
Nonsterile dressing: 4″ × 4″; A6254
                            6″ × 6″,
                            6″ × 8″; A6255
Sterile dressing: 4″ × 4″, 5″ × 5″, 6″ × 6″; A6254

Action
MPM Woundgard specialty absorptive dressing protects wound from the outside environment and assists the body in maintaining a moist wound environment.

Indications
To manage cuts, burns, abrasions, skin tears, pressure ulcers, and leg ulcers.

Contraindications
None provided by the manufacturer.

Application
- Cleanse the wound of dirt, debris, and necrotic tissue and ensure that periwound skin is dry.
- Remove the dressing's backing and apply the dressing to the wound.

Removal
Gently peel the dressing away from the wound.

Multipad Non-Adherent Wound Dressing
DeRoyal

How supplied
Pad: 2″ × 2″, 4″ × 4″; A6251
4″ × 8″; A6252
7½″ × 7½″

Action
Multipad Non-Adherent Wound Dressing is a thick, multilayered, absorbent wound dressing that won't stick to the wound site or damage fragile granulation tissue. It's comprised of a highly absorptive nonwoven pad between two wound contact layers.

Indications
To manage pressure ulcers (stages 2, 3, and 4), partial- and full-thickness wounds, donor sites, tunneling wounds, infected and noninfected wounds, and red, yellow, or black wounds.

Contraindications
None provided by the manufacturer.

Application
- Position the dressing over the cleansed wound.
- Secure the dressing with tape, roll gauze, or tubular elastic bandages if using it as a primary dressing.
- If using Multipad as a secondary dressing, apply the primary dressing or filler before securing Multipad to the wound.

Removal
- Remove any secondary dressing.
- Gently lift the dressing from the wound.

Primapore Specialty Absorptive Dressing
Smith & Nephew, Inc.
Wound Management Division

How supplied
Pads: 4" × 3⅛"; A6251
6" × 3⅛"; A6252
8" × 4", 11¾" × 4", 13¾" × 4¾"; A6253

Action
Primapore Specialty Absorptive Dressing is a nonadherent pad used to treat various wounds. The thick, absorbent pad minimizes fluid strike-through. Its acrylic adhesive is evenly spread onto a nonwoven backing surface, providing a safe, secure, and comfortable dressing over the wound site. Removal is clean and painless because the nonadherent pad doesn't cause trauma to the underlying tissue.

Indications
For use as a postoperative or secondary dressing. May also be used for cuts, lacerations, and sutured wounds.

Contraindications
None provided by the manufacturer.

Application
- Remove the dressing's backing, and place the dressing over the wound.
- Peel off the remaining backing while smoothing dressing onto skin.

Removal
Carefully lift dressing away from the wound.

Specialty Absorptives

Sofsorb Wound Dressing
DeRoyal

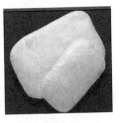

How supplied
Multilayered
pad: 3″ × 3″; A6251
4″ × 6″, 4″ × 6″ with drain
slit, 4″ × 9″; A6252
6″ × 9″, 9″ × 15″, 15″ × 18″, 15″ × 24″; A6253

Action
Sofsorb Wound Dressing is a nonadherent, absorbent, multilayered, one-piece dressing used wet or dry to treat various wounds. The nonwoven layer permits passage of wound drainage into the absorbent pad and prevents it from returning. The center layer absorbs drainage. The cellulose layer wicks drainage horizontally along the pad to increase dressing capacity. The air-permeable backing provides strength and integrity.

Indications
For use as a postoperative dressing and as a primary or secondary dressing to manage burns, minor lacerations, abrasions, and heavily draining skin ulcers. May also be used on pressure ulcers (stages 2, 3, and 4), partial- and full-thickness wounds, tunneling wounds, infected and noninfected wounds, wounds with heavy drainage, wounds with serosanguineous or purulent drainage, and red, yellow, or black wounds.

Contraindications
None provided by the manufacturer.

Application
- Apply dry dressing with the wound contact layer toward the wound surface.
- Alternatively, soak the dressing with normal saline solution or another topical solution. Squeeze out excess fluid, then apply the dressing with the wound contact layer toward the wound surface.
- Secure with a stretch net dressing, roll gauze, or tape.

Removal
- Moisten with normal saline solution, if necessary.
- Carefully lift the dressing off the wound.

Specialty Absorptives

SURGI-PAD Combine Dressing

Johnson & Johnson Wound Management
Division of ETHICON, Inc.

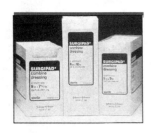

How supplied
Pad: 8″ × 7½″, 8″ × 10″; A6253
        5″ × 9″; A6252

Action
SURGI-PAD Combine Dressing provides protection and padding for major surgical wounds and maximizes absorbency, wicking, and dispersal of wound exudate.

Indications
To manage pressure ulcers (stages 3 and 4), partial- and full-thickness wounds, chronic or acute wounds, and nondraining or minimally draining wounds. May also be used to protect or pad the wound, or to absorb exudate.

Contraindications
None provided by the manufacturer.

Application
- Cleanse the wound with normal saline solution or other cleansing agent.
- Apply the dressing over the wound.
- Secure with tape as appropriate.

Removal
Gently remove the dressing.

Specialty Absorptives

NEW PRODUCT

TENDERSORB WET-PRUF Abdominal Pads

Kendall Health Care Products Company

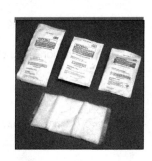

How supplied

Sterile Pad: 5″ × 9″; A6252
7½″ × 8″,
8″ × 10″; A6253

Nonsterile Bulk: 5″ × 9″; A6252
7½″ × 8″, 8″ × 10″; A6253

Action

TENDERSORB WET-PRUF Abdominal Pads can be used as secondary dressings to absorb excess wound fluid. They also protect the wound by cushioning it.

Indications

For use as part of a dressing system for virtually any wound requiring fluid retention and cushioning. May also be used to prevent skin breakdown and to manage wounds with moderate to heavy drainage.

Contraindications

Contraindicated for tunneling wounds.

Application

- Apply a primary dressing based on wound type.
- Cover the primary dressing with a TENDERSORB WET-PRUF Abdominal Pad.
- Secure the pad with tape, bandage roll, or another appropriate product.

Removal

- Remove the securing tape or bandage roll.
- Remove the TENDERSORB WET-PRUF Abdominal Pad from the primary dressing.

Specialty Absorptives

Surgical supplies, miscellaneous

When the Statistical Analysis Durable Medical Equipment Regional Carrier (SADMERC) and the four Durable Medical Equipment Regional Carriers (DMERCs) perform a Coding Verification Review and do not reach a consensus coding decision, they sometimes assign the product or procedure to a general category. Therefore, a variety of dissimilar products and procedures are usually assigned to this category. These products in this category do not have a universal definition, utilization guidelines, or a rate on the DMERC Fee Schedule. Yet, each product listed under this category has an individual action, indication, contraindication, and application and removal process. It remains the clinician's responsibility to understand each product prior to utilization.

When submitting claims for products or procedures in this category, the provider and supplier must check with the payer for the supporting documentation that's required.

HCPCS code overview

The HCPCS code normally assigned to miscellaneous surgical supplies is:

A4649 — surgical supplies, miscellaneous.

Biafine RE (Radiodermatitis Emulsion)

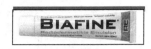

Medix Pharmaceuticals Americas, Inc.

How supplied
Tube: 1.65 oz(46 g), 3.3 oz (93 g); A6250

Action
Biafine RE Radiodermatitis Emulsion is a versatile, oil-in-water emulsion dressing that provides deep dermal hydration and reduces the frequency and severity of radiation-induced skin reactions. It provides macrophage recruitment (up to 10 times the norm), autolytic debridement, a moist healing environment, exudate absorption, and odor removal.

Indications
To protect against or manage radiation dermatitis.

Contraindications
Contraindicated for rashes due to food or medicine allergies.

Application
For protection against reactions:
- Gently massage a generous amount of Biafine RE into the irradiated area, three times daily.
- Begin applications immediately after the first radiation session.
- Don't apply within 4 hours of the next radiation session.
    To manage moist desquamation:
- After radiation treatment, apply a thick (1/4″ to ½″ [0.6 to 1.3 cm]) layer of Biafine RE on and around the affected area.
- Cover with moist or petrolatum gauze; secure if necessary.
- Immediately before the next radiation treatment, remove the dressing and rinse and dry the area.
- Reapply Biafine RE dressing after each radiation treatment.
    To manage desquamation and erythema:
- Gently massage a generous amount of Biafine RE on and around the affected area, three times daily.
- Do not apply 4 hours prior to a radiation session.

Removal
Biafine RE is water soluble. Remove it with normal saline solution, sterile water, or any wound cleanser.

Biafine WDE (Wound Dressing Emulsion)

Medix Pharmaceuticals
Americas, Inc.

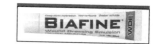

How supplied

Tube: 1.65 oz (46 g), 3.3 oz (93 g); A6250

Action

Biafine WDE Wound Dressing Emulsion is a versatile and effective oil-in-water dressing that positively stimulates the patients' own healing mechanisms through the selective macrophage recruitment (up to 10 times the norm), leading to the proliferation of fibroblasts and the promotion of granulation tissue. Also assists in autolytic debridement, provides a moist healing environment, absorbs exudate, and removes odors throughout all phases of the healing process.

Indications

To manage partial- and full-thickness wounds, including pressure, diabetic, arterial, and venous ulcers; first- and second-degree burns, including sunburn; minor abrasions; and superficial wounds.

Contraindications

Contraindicated for skin rashes related to food or medicine allergies.

Application

- Apply a thick (¼″ to ½″ [0.6 cm to 1.3 cm]) layer of Biafine WDE on and around the affected area.
- For undermined and tunneling areas, apply Biafine WDE using a needleless syringe.
- Cover with gauze moistened with saline solution. An occlusive dressing is acceptable instead of moistened gauze. Forty percent of the demineralized water in Biafine's formula penetrates to the dermal level within 1 hour of application. *Note:* Never use a dry cover dressing as it will absorb Biafine's water and prevent deep dermal hydration.
- Apply an appropriate secondary dressing, if necessary, and secure it with tape. Use a transparent dressing on black necrotic wounds, and change it every 12 to 24 hours to maximize tissue hydration and autolytic debridement.

Removal

- Change dressing every 24 hours to maintain peak macrophage recruitment.
- Remove Biafine WDE with normal saline solution, sterile water, or any wound cleanser. (Biafine WDE is water soluble.)

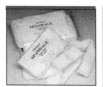

NEW PRODUCT
MTSPANDAGE (Latex-Free)

NEW PRODUCT
MTSPANDAGE PRE-CUTS (Latex-Free)

Mtspandage
Pre-cuts

NEW PRODUCT
SPANDAGE (Latex-Free)

NEW PRODUCT
SPANDAGE CUSTOM PRE-CUTS (Latex-Free)
MEDI-TECH INTERNATIONAL, CORP.

Spandage

How supplied
MTSPANDAGE (Latex-Free) and SPANDAGE (Latex-Free)
Tube: Uncut
MTSPANDAGE CUSTOM PRE-CUTS (Latex-Free) and SPANDAGE
CUSTOM PRE-CUTS (Latex-Free)
Tube: Individual precuts in sizes to fit a wide range of body
    areas from head to toes; A4649

Action
These secondary dressing retainers hold a dressing in place,
eliminating the use of adhesive tape as well as the discomfort
of tape removal, tape excoriation problems, tape residue on
the skin, and the need for hypoallergenic tapes. They provide
freedom of movement and allow aeration to the wound, which
promotes healing.

Indications
To hold firmly and comfortably any wet or dry dressing or compress on almost any part of the body.

Contraindications
None provided by the manufacturer.

Application
■ Usually, place both hands into the appropriate size
  MTSPANDAGE tube and stretch it over the dressing.

- Withdraw your hands from the tube, allowing MTSPANDAGE to fit the contour of the dressed area.

  Head:
- Cut 10″ to 12″ of tubing, or use precut size.
- Stretch tube over the head from the top of the head to under the chin, creating a face mask.
- Cut the tube away from the face, from the midforehead to under the chin. If face is to remain covered, don't cut.

  Skull cap:
- Cut 12″ to 14″ of tubing, or use precut size.
- Stretch one end of the tube over the cranium to just above the eyebrows.
- Make one full twist of the remaining tube, place both of your hands into the opening, and restretch the remainder down over the cranium.

  Finger/Toe (using applicator):
- Push a length of tubing onto applicator equal to twice the applicator's length, and place the applicator over the entire dressed appendage.
- Pull a small amount of tubing off the applicator, hold it with thumb and forefinger at the base of the appendage, and pull the applicator off. Cut tubing at the tip of the appendage.
- Repeat process if additional pressure is required to secure the dressing, but never apply more than two layers.

  Hand:
- Cut 14″ of tubing, or use precut size.
- Stretch one end of the tube over the hand.
- Make one full twist in the remaining tube at the fingertip, and restretch the remainder back over the hand as far as the wrist.
- Uninjured fingers may be left free by cutting finger holes.

  Shoulder/Axilla/Breast/Mastectomy:
- Cut 20″ of tubing, or use precut size.
- Make a 3″ vertical cut in the tube's fold approximately 6″ from one end. This cut will be a neck hole.
- Insert the affected arm into the long piece of net and bring the net up to the neck.
- Pass the head through the 3″ cut so that the net fits like a sling.

  Chest/Upper abdomen:
- Cut 20″ of tubing, or use precut size.

- Approximately 3″ from the top of the tube, make two identical 3″ vertical cuts in the opposite folds.
- Place both hands into the tube at the end farthest from the 3″ cuts. Then, stretch the tube over the patient's head and raised arms, pulling each arm through one of the 3″ cuts, as if putting on a sweater.
- Draw the stretched tube down over the shoulders to the waist.
- This "sweater" can also serve to secure electrodes for ECG monitoring.

Elbow/Forearm/Leg/Knee:

- Cut 8″ of tubing, or use precut size.
- Allow tube to extend approximately 2″ beyond the dressing at each end.

Genital/Anal/Perineal areas:

- Cut 20″ of tubing, or use precut size.
- Make a 4″ vertical cut directly in the center of the fold.
- With both hands in the top part of the tube, stretch the panty-like tube up the legs and over the hips to the waist, while keeping the lower length of the tube (or tail) hanging in the rear.
- With the tail hanging in the rear and below, pass the legs through the indicated side leg cuts and bring the tail up to the waist, passing over the first layer.

Gluteus/Lower Abdomen/Hip/Groin/Buttocks/Thigh:

- Cut 14″ of tubing, or use precut size.
- At a point 2″ from the top of the tube, make a 2″ cut through one side of the net.
- For bandaging the right side of the affected areas: With the 2″ cut on the left side of the tube, pass the affected right leg through the long part of the tube, and the left leg through the 2″ cut.
- For bandaging the left side of the affected areas: With the 2″ cut on the right side of the tube, draw the legs through the two stretched openings and pull the panty upward to above the waist.

Amputation:

- Cut 12″ of tubing, or use precut size.
- Apply one end of tube over the stump.
- Make one full twist in the remaining tube at the stump tip, and restretch the remainder back over the stump.

Foot:
- Cut 10″ of tubing, or use precut size.
- Extend the tube from ankle to toes.

Removal
- If not soiled, MTSPANDAGE may remain in place for 3 days or more. For examination or dressing change, lift or roll it back over the dressed area.
- Lift one end of MTSPANDAGE, raise the lower end of the tube, and remove. Because the dressing retainer molds itself to the contours of the body without adhesion, removing it from hairy skin doesn't cause pain.

OsmoCyte Island Wound Dressing
Bard Medical Division
C.R. Bard, Inc.

How supplied
Pad: 2″ × 2½″, 4½″ × 4½″; A4649

Action
A sterile, highly absorptive dressing used to manage exuding wounds. Its unique hydropolymer pad captures moisture for easy and complete removal of wound drainage.

Indications
To manage exuding wounds, including infected and noninfected wounds, pressure ulcers, diabetic ulcers, venous stasis ulcers, arterial ulcers, first- and second-degree burns, donor sites, postoperative incisions, other bleeding surface wounds, dermal lesions, trauma injuries, and incisions.

Contraindications
- Contraindicated for third-degree burns.
- Contraindicated for surgical implantation.

Application
- Cleanse wound using normal saline solution or other appropriate wound cleanser.
- Apply dressing directly to the wound.

Removal
- Change the dressing according to the amount of exudate. Dressing may remain in place up to 7 days.
- Remove the dressing by gently lifting it from each corner. Flushing the wound with sterile saline solution prior to removal may facilitate removal.

OsmoCyte Pillow Wound Dressing

OsmoCyte PCA Pillow Wound Dressing
Bard Medical Division, C.R. Bard, Inc.

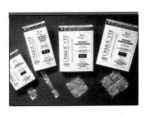

How supplied
OsmoCyte
Sterile Pillow: ¾″ × 6″, 1½″ × 3″, 3″ × 3″, 4″ × 4″; A4649
OsmoCyte
PCA Pillow: ¾″ × 6″, 1½″ × 3″, 3″ × 3″, 4″ × 4″; A4649

Action
OsmoCyte Pillow Wound Dressing and OsmoCyte PCA Pillow Wound Dressing are sterile, highly absorptive pillow dressings for the management of exuding wounds. The unique hydropolymer beads are encased in a gentle mesh for easy and complete removal. The granules absorb wound fluid over time via continuous hydrophilic attraction, offering exudate management while providing a cushioning, moist wound environment. OsmoCyte PCA Pillow Wound Dressing contains a patented copper peptide that is released into the wound as it absorbs exudate.

Indications
To manage infected and noninfected exuding wounds, including pressure ulcers (stages 2, 3, and 4), partial- and full-thickness wounds, tunneling wounds, diabetic ulcers, venous stasis ulcers, arterial ulcers, first- and second-degree burns, donor sites, postoperative incisions, other bleeding surface wounds, dermal lesions, trauma injuries, and incisions.

Contraindications
- Contraindicated for third-degree burns.
- Contraindicated for surgical implantation.

Application
- Irrigate the wound site with normal saline solution or another appropriate wound cleanser.
- Apply the dressing to the moist wound surface.

- Cover with an appropriate secondary dressing, and secure it in place.

Removal

- Time dressing changes to the amount of exudate and the condition of the wound. Change the dressing when saturated or at least every 7 days, with more frequent changes for infected wounds.
- Remove the dressing by gently lifting it from each corner. Flushing the wound with sterile saline solution prior to removal may facilitate removal.

Transparent films

Action
Transparent films are adhesive, semipermeable, polyurethane membrane dressings that vary in thickness and size. They are waterproof and impermeable to bacteria and contaminants, yet they permit water vapor to cross the barrier. These dressings maintain a moist environment, promoting formation of granulation tissue and autolysis of necrotic tissue.

Indications
Transparent films may be used as a primary or secondary dressing to prevent and manage stage 1 pressure ulcers, partial-thickness wounds with little or no exudate, and wounds with necrotic tissue or slough.

Advantages
- Retain moisture
- Are impermeable to bacteria and other contaminants
- Facilitate autolytic debridement
- Allow wound observation
- Don't require secondary dressings

Disadvantages
- May not be recommended for infected wounds
- Not recommended for wounds with moderate to heavy drainage because they don't absorb
- Not recommended for use on fragile skin
- Require a border of intact skin for adhesive edge of dressing
- May be difficult to apply and handle
- May dislodge in high-friction areas

HCPCS code overview
The HCPCS codes normally assigned to transparent film dressings are:
A6257—pad size ≤16 sq. in.
A6258—pad size more than >16 sq. in., ≤48 sq. in.
A6259—pad size >48 sq. in.

BIOCLUSIVE Select Transparent Dressing

Johnson & Johnson Wound Management
Division of ETHICON, Inc.

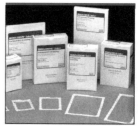

How supplied
Film: 1¾" × 2¾", 2¾" × 2⅜",
3" × 4"; A6257
4" × 5", 5" × 7", 4" × 10"; A6258

Action
BIOCLUSIVE Select Transparent Dressing is a semiocclusive bacterial and viral barrier that protects skin from exogenous fluid and contaminants and minimizes scar formation. It allows evaporation, promotes gas and water vapor exchange, and creates a moist wound-healing environment.

Indications
To manage access devices, peripheral I.V. sites, central venous catheters, and total parental nutrition, central venous pressure, and neonatal I.V. sites. May also be used for care of endoscopy incisions, small surgical incisions, skin biopsies, donor sites, and second-degree burns.

Contraindications
None provided by the manufacturer.

Application
- Peel away the middle section of the dressing's frame.
- Place the window frame over the wound area or I.V. site.
- Gently smooth and secure the dressing to skin.
- Remove the frame using a circular motion. Perforation will release with gentle pressure.

Removal
- Gently pick up a corner of the dressing. Stretch the dressing away from the center of the wound, partially lifting it.
- Peel the dressing back until you feel resistance.
- Repeatedly stretch and peel the dressing as necessary until it's removed.

Transparent Films

BIOCLUSIVE Transparent Dressing

Johnson & Johnson Wound Management
Division of ETHICON, Inc.

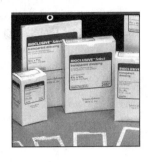

How supplied
Film: 1½" × 1½", 2" × 3"; A6257
4" × 5", 5" × 7", 4" × 10";
A6258
8" × 10"; A6259

Action
BIOCLUSIVE Transparent Dressing is a semiocclusive bacterial and viral barrier that protects skin from exogenous fluid and contaminants and minimizes scar formation. It allows evaporation, promotes gas and water vapor exchange, and creates a moist wound-healing environment.

Indications
To manage I.V. sites, total parenteral nutrition sites, pressure ulcers (stages 1 and 2), second-degree burns, donor sites, minimally draining or nondraining clean surgical wounds, lacerations, and abrasions, and to prevent skin breakdown. May also be used on partial-thickness wounds, noninfected wounds, red wounds, and for autolytic debridement.

Contraindications
Contraindicated for infected wounds.

Application
- Cleanse the wound with an appropriate topical antiseptic, such as hydrogen peroxide or normal saline solution.
- Remove oil from the surrounding skin with alcohol or acetone alcohol, and dry the skin thoroughly. To ensure proper adhesion of the dressing, maintain a 1" (2.5 cm) margin of dry periwound skin.
- Hold the dressing with the center paper tab face-up, and remove the center backing paper.
- Grasp the side paper tabs, position the dressing over the wound site, and smooth the center portion into place.

- Peel away the side backing papers one at a time while smoothing the film onto the skin.

Removal

- Gently pick up a corner of the dressing. Stretch the dressing away from the center of the wound, partially lifting it.
- Peel the dressing back until you feel resistance.
- Repeatedly stretch and peel the dressing as necessary until it's removed.

Blisterfilm
Kendall Health Care Products
Company

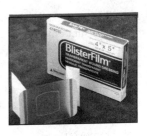

How supplied
Film sheet: 2″ × 3″ with 1″ × 1″
window, 3½″ × 4″ with
2″ × 2″ window; A6257
4″ × 5″ with 2″ × 2″
window, 5½″ × 6″ with 3″ × 3″ window; A6258

Transparent Films

Action
BlisterFilm Transparent Dressing is a flexible, semipermeable polyurethane film that provides a nonadherent, adhesive-free wound covering. The dressing is held in place with a perimeter adhesive system that doesn't touch the wound. It permits gas exchange; provides a bacterial barrier, covering and protecting wounds against environmental contamination; maintains a moist wound-healing environment; and reduces pain.

Indications
To manage a wide range of nondraining wounds and catheter exit sites and to prevent skin breakdown. May be used on pressure ulcers (stages 1 and 2), stage 3 pressure ulcers (nondraining or with packing), partial-thickness wounds, noninfected wounds, wounds with minimal drainage (with packing), wounds with serosanguineous drainage (with packing), and red, yellow, or black wounds.

Contraindications
Contraindicated for wounds with copious drainage or for infected wounds.

Application
- Cleanse and thoroughly dry the wound area.
- Peel back the dressing's release paper, position the dressing, and apply it to the wound.
- Smooth the edges of the dressing.

Removal
- Lift and slowly pull the dressing in the direction of hair growth.
- Alternatively, affix a small piece of surgical tape to the edge of the dressing and peel back.

CarraFilm Transparent Film Dressing
Carrington Laboratories, Inc.

How supplied
Film
sheet: 2¾" × 2⅜"; A6257
4" × 5½", 6" × 6"; A6258
8" × 10"

Action
CarraFilm Transparent Film Dressing is an adhesive, semipermeable membrane dressing that is sterile and impervious to moisture and bacteria but permeable to moisture vapor and oxygen.

Indications
For use as a protective wound dressing on minor abrasions, closed surgical wounds, superficial pressure ulcers, skin grafts, and donor sites, or as a secondary cover dressing over other types of primary dressings. May also be used on superficial, partial-thickness wounds; wounds with necrosis or slough; wounds with low, medium, or high exudate; and red, yellow, or black wounds.

Contraindications
Contraindicated for infected wounds.

Application
- Cleanse the wound and periwound tissue. Dry the periwound skin.
- Clip or shave excess hair at site, if desired. A skin barrier wipe may be used on intact skin.
- Gently pull the dressing's paper tabs away from the center to partially expose the dressing.
- Apply the exposed dressing to the wound site without tension, to prevent skin shear. Press and smooth it into place.
- Pull the tabs at an angle with even pressure to release them from the dressing.

Removal
- Change the dressing as needed according to the wound condition and amount of exudate or as directed by the primary care provider.
- CarraFilm may remain in place up to 7 days.

Transparent Films

CarraSmart Film Transparent Film Dressing
Carrington Laboratories, Inc.

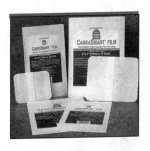

How supplied
Film sheet: 4" × 5", 6" × 7"; A6258

Action
CarraSmart Film Transparent Film Dressing has the same properties as CarraFilm, an adhesive semipermeable membrane dressing, but also allows selective drainage evaporation through the film and thus may be used as a primary or secondary dressing over highly exuding wounds. It has an extremely high moisture vapor transport rate (MVTR)—the measure of a surface's "breathability," its ability to allow evaporation of moisture. MVTR is measured in grams/meters squared/day ($g/m^2/d$). Normal skin releases 240 to 1,800 $g/m^2/d$, while burn patients lose 3,000 to 5,200 $g/m^2/d$. Wound care products with high MVTR maintain an optimal wound care environment by venting and retaining moisture as needed. On wounds with high exudate levels, these products can reduce the frequency of dressing changes and can prevent maceration under the film.

Indications
For use as a protective wound dressing on minor abrasions, closed surgical wounds, superficial pressure ulcers, skin grafts, and donor sites, and as a secondary cover dressing over other types of primary dressings. May also be used on superficial, partial-thickness wounds; wounds with necrosis or slough; wounds with low, medium, or high exudate; and red, yellow, or black wounds.

Contraindications
Contraindicated for infected wounds.

Application
- Cleanse wound and periwound tissue. Dry periwound skin. Clip or shave excess hair at site, if desired. A skin barrier wipe may be used on intact skin.
- Gently pull the dressing's paper tabs away from the center to partially expose the dressing.

Transparent Films

- Apply the exposed dressing to the wound site without tension, to prevent skin shear. Press and smooth it into place.
- Pull the tabs at an angle with even pressure to release them from the dressing.

Removal

- Change the dressing as needed according to the wound condition and amount of exudate or as directed by the primary care provider.
- Dressing may stay in place up to 7 days.

NEW PRODUCT
ClearCell Transparent Film Dressing
Dumex Medical

How supplied
Sterile film: 2″ × 3″, 4″ × 5″, 5″ × 7″, 6″ × 8″
Sterile film: 8″ × 10″
Nonsterile film: 4″ × 5″

Action
ClearCell Transparent Film Dressing is a transparent polyurethane film that provides a warm, moist wound-healing environment, allowing the transmission of moisture vapor to reduce the risk of maceration.

Indications
For use as a primary or secondary dressing. May be used to fix I.V. catheter sites and to prevent friction and shear on intact skin.

Contraindications
None provided by the manufacturer.

Application
- Cleanse the wound with PrimaDerm Dermal Cleanser or saline. Dry the adjacent skin.
- Peel off the dressing's release paper while positioning the dressing over the wound.
- Press the dressing in place, avoiding wrinkling the dressing and skin.
- Remove the release liner and confirm full seal integrity around the perimeter of the dressing.

Removal
- Gently grasp one edge of the dressing and stretch it along the surface of the skin.
- Continue around the entire dressing until it's easily lifted off.

Transparent Films

ClearSite Transparent Membrane
CONMED Corporation

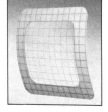

How supplied
Film: 2″ × 3″, 4″ × 5″, 6″ × 8″

Action
ClearSite TM Transparent Membrane is a latex-free, semipermeable polyurethane adhesive film that provides a moist wound healing environment and allows transmission of moisture to reduce the risk of maceration.

Indications
To cover and protect wounds and minor skin irritations.

Contraindications
Contraindicated for infected wounds.

Application
- Gently clean and dry the wound and surrounding area. Remove excessive hair at site, if necessary.
- Holding the dressing's tabs, remove the printed liner.
- Apply the dressing to the wound.
- Remove the dressing's clear liner, then pull to remove the white tab.

Removal
- Change the dressing according to facility policy.
- While supporting the skin, firmly grasp an edge of the dressing and pull or stretch it parallel with the skin surface. This will release the adhesive film from the skin.

NEW PRODUCT
DERMAVIEW
DermaRite Industries

How supplied
Film: 4" × 5"

Action
DermaView is a semiocclusive bacterial
and viral barrier that protects skin from urine and fecal breakdown. This semipermeable dressing maintains a moist wound
environment.

Indications
May be used as a primary or secondary dressing, to secure other dressings, or for infected wounds that need autolytic debridement.

Contraindications
- Contraindicated for infected areas or for patients with deep
  systemic infections.
- Contraindicated for full-thickness wounds involving muscle,
  tendon or bone.

Application
- Cleanse the wound area.
- Consulting the dressing instructions, peel off area surface
  labeled #1.
- Position the dressing over the wound, and press it down gen-
  tly and around the wound's perimeter.
- Pull out tab #2 and discard it. Peel back tab #3.
- Smooth the dressing out firmly from the center toward the
  edges.

Removal
- Lift and slowly stretch one corner of the dressing in the direction of the hair growth.
- Continue stretching or pulling around the perimeter of the
  dressing, then remove remaining film.

Mefilm
Mölnlycke Health Care

How supplied
Pad: 2.4″ × 2.6″; A6257
4″ × 5″, 4″ × 10″; A6258
6″ × 8.5″; A6259

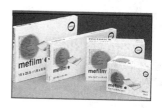

Action
Mefilm is a flexible, transparent, breathable polyurethane film dressing coated with a polyacrylic adhesive. It's moisture- and vapor-permeable and allows excess moisture from exudate and skin transpiration to be vented. Mefilm acts as a barrier to bacteria and fluid strike-through and prevents external contamination.

Indications
To manage superficial pressure ulcers, closed surgical wound sites, I.V. sites, abrasions, lacerations, superficial burns, and donor sites with low exudate. Also used to prevent skin breakdown.

Contraindications
Contraindicated for full-thickness wounds and third-degree burns.

Application
- Cleanse the application area and dry the healthy surrounding skin.
- Choose a dressing size that allows a margin to adhere to dry healthy skin around the wound or catheter site.
- Remove the white backing paper marked number "1."
- Apply Mefilm and remove the small white side tab marked number "2."
- Remove the supporting transparent sheet marked number "3."

Removal
- The dressing may be left in place for several days, depending on the condition of the wound and surrounding skin.
- Gently press down on the surrounding skin and carefully lift an edge of the dressing. Carefully stretch the dressing tangentially to the skin surface.

Transparent Films

OpSite

OpSite FLEXIGRID
Smith & Nephew, Inc.
Wound Management Division

How supplied
OpSite
Film sheet: $5\frac{1}{2}'' \times 4''$, $11'' \times 4''$; A6258
$\qquad$ $5\frac{1}{2}'' \times 10''$, $11'' \times 6''$, $11'' \times 11\frac{3}{4}''$, $11'' \times 17\frac{3}{4}''$,
$\qquad$ $17\frac{3}{4}'' \times 2\frac{5}{8}''$; A6259

OpSite FLEXIGRID
Film sheet: $2\frac{3}{8}'' \times 2\frac{3}{4}''$; A6257
$\qquad$ $4'' \times 4\frac{3}{4}''$, $6'' \times 8''$, $4\frac{3}{4}'' \times 10''$; A6258

Action
OpSite consists of a polyurethane membrane that creates a moist environment by trapping the wound exudate. It's waterproof and aids in preventing bacterial contamination. OpSite FLEXIGRID dressings provide a unique wound measurement grid that can be written on to provide a record of the change in wound size.

Indications
To protect skin from friction and for use as secondary dressings to secure foams, alginates, and gauzes while protecting the wound.

Contraindications
None provided by the manufacturer.

Application
- Remove the dressing's backing paper and expose the adhesive surface.
- Place the dressing gently over the wound, allowing the film to cover at least 1″ (2.5 cm) of undamaged skin around the wound.
- If using OpSite FLEXIGRID, remove the flexible plastic grid.

Removal
- Lift a corner of the dressing and begin stretching it horizontally along the skin surface, breaking the adhesive bond.
- Continue stretching from the edges toward the center. When two sides of the dressing are partially removed, grasp both sides and stretch horizontally, parallel to the skin, until the entire dressing can be removed.

Transparent Films

OpSite PLUS

OpSite Post-Op
Smith & Nephew, Inc.
Wound Management Division

How supplied
OpSite PLUS:
Pad: 4″ × 4¾″ with 2″ × 3″ pad, 6″ × 6″ with 4″ × 4″ pad;
    A6203
OpSite Post-Op:
Pad: 2″ × 2″ with 1″ × 1″ pad, 2½″ × 2″ with 1½″ × 1″ pad,
    3¾″ × 3⅜″ with 3″ × 1½″ pad, 6⅛″ × 3⅜″ with
    5″ × 1½″ pad, 9¼″ × 3⅜″ with 7½″ × 1½″ pad; A6203

Action
OpSite PLUS and OpSite Post-Op Dressings combine OpSite transparent film with an absorbent, nonadherent pad. Drainage can be monitored without disturbing the dressing. Moisture vapor permeability combined with nonsensitizing adhesive allows the wound and the skin under the dressing to breathe. The dressing stays in place, reducing the risk of maceration. The OpSite film is impermeable to water and body fluids. The pad is highly absorbent, minimizing the number of dressing changes. Its nonadherent surface leaves the wound site undisturbed, reducing pain and wound trauma during dressing changes.

Indications
For use as primary dressings for skin tears, pressure ulcers (stages 1, 2, and 3), postoperative and arthroscopic wounds, minor cuts, and lacerations. May also be used as secondary dressings over gels and alginates.

Contraindications
None provided by the manufacturer.

Application
- Remove one backing tab and place the dressing over the wound.
- Peel off the remaining backing while smoothing the dressing onto the skin.
- Remove the film carrier.

Transparent Films

Removal

- Grasp a corner of the dressing's clear film and pull it parallel to the skin. This stretching action releases the adhesive for gentle removal.
- Continue stretching around the circumference of the dressing, then lift it off.

Transparent Films

Polyskin MR Moisture Responsive Transparent Dressing

Kendall Health Care Products Company

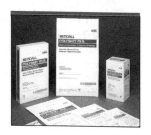

How supplied

Sterile film sheet: 2" × 2¾"; A6257
4" × 4¾"; A6258

Action

POLYSKIN MR Moisture Responsive Transparent Dressing responds to fluid by increasing or decreasing its moisture vapor transfer rate and provides an optimal wound-healing environment.

Indications

To manage pressure ulcers (stages 1, 2, 3, and 4), partial- and full-thickness wounds, infected and uninfected wounds, wounds with light drainage, and red wounds.

Contraindications

None provided by the manufacturer.

Application

- Check that the wound has a margin of intact skin to ensure successful application.
- Peel tab #1 from the dressing's backing to expose the adhesive surface.
- Apply the dressing to the wound and smooth it into place.
- Remove tab #2.

Removal

- Lift one corner of the dressing.
- Pull or stretch the dressing gently in the direction of hair growth.

Transparent Films

Polyskin II Transparent Dressing
Kendall Health Care Products Company

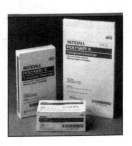

How supplied
Sterile film sheet: 1½″ × 1½″,
2″ × 2¾″; A6257
4″ × 4¾″, 4″ × 8″,
6″ × 8″; A6258
8″ × 10″; A6259

Action
Polyskin II Transparent Dressing supports autolytic debridement of wounds with eschar by maintaining a moist wound environment and acting as a barrier against bacteria.

Indications
To manage partial-thickness wounds or dry necrotic wounds that require debridement and to prevent skin breakdown. May be used to dress I.V. sites, donor sites, ulcers, and surgical sites. May also be used to help manage pressure ulcers (stages 1 and 2), noninfected wounds, and wounds with minimal drainage.

Contraindications
Contraindicated for exuding wounds, friable skin around wounds, and wounds with sinus tracts.

Application
- Check that the wound has a margin of intact skin to ensure successful application.
- Peel tab #1 from the dressing's backing to expose the adhesive surface.
- Apply the dressing to the wound and smooth it into place.
- Remove tab #2.

Removal
- Change the dressing based on the amount of accumulated exudate.
- Lift and slowly pull the dressing in the direction of hair growth.
- Alternatively, affix a small piece of surgical tape to the edge of the dressing and peel back.

ProCyte Transparent Film Dressing
Bard Medical Division
C.R. Bard, Inc.

How supplied
Pad: 2¼″ × 2¾″; A6257
4″ × 5½″, 6″ × 6″; A6258
8″ × 10″; A6259

Action
ProCyte Transparent Film Dressing consists of a thin, transparent polyurethane film coated with a nonsensitizing adhesive. The dressing is sterile and acts as an impervious barrier to moisture and bacteria, while remaining permeable to moisture vapor and oxygen.

Indications
To secure intravascular catheters and other devices to the skin. May also be used as a protective dressing on minor abrasions, superficial pressure ulcers, skin grafts, donor sites, and closed surgical wounds.

Contraindications
Not intended to replace primary wound-closure methods.

Application
- According to facility policy, cleanse the skin and the catheter or wound site thoroughly. Allow the skin to dry completely. Clip or shave excess hair.
- Gently pull the dressing's paper tabs away from center to partially expose dressing.
- Apply the exposed dressing to wound, pulling the tabs with even pressure to release the dressing.
- Smooth the dressing edges onto the skin.

Removal
Grasp the edge of the dressing, and gently pull in the direction of hair growth.

Transparent Films

Suresite
Medline Industries, Inc.

How supplied
Film: 2″ × 3″; 2⅜″ × 2¾″ window
 style; A6257
 4″ × 5″, 4″ × 4½″ with
 Matrix, 4″ × 4½″ window
 style ; A6258

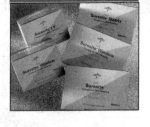

Action
Suresite is a sterile, hypoallergenic film dressing that acts as a
barrier to bacteria and water while creating a moist wound environment. It's permeable to oxygen and vapor.

Indications
To manage peripheral and central I.V. catheter sites and minor
abrasions and skin tears, and to help prevent skin breakdown.
May also be used for pressure ulcers (stages 1 and 2), partial-
thickness wounds, noninfected wounds, and wounds with minimal drainage.

Contraindications
Contraindicated for use as a primary dressing on moderately to
heavily draining wounds.

Application
- Cleanse the wound with normal saline solution or another appropriate cleanser, such as Skintegrity Wound Cleanser. Dry the
 surrounding area. Allow any skin preparation to dry completely.
- Remove the dressing's backing paper, exposing the adhesive.
- Gently place the dressing over the wound and apply it, leaving at least 1¼″ to 1½″ (2.5 cm) of healthy periwound skin.
- Remove the flexible plastic grid or paper window frame, if
 applicable.

Removal
- Suresite can be worn during showering to protect the wound
 or the I.V. hub. If exudate accumulates under the dressing,
 change the dressing immediately.
- Lift a corner of the dressing and begin stretching it horizontally along the skin surface. When two sides are partially removed, grasp both sides and stretch parallel to the skin.

Transparent Films

3M Tegaderm Transparent Dressing

3M Tegaderm HP Transparent Dressing
3M Health Care

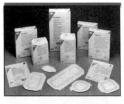

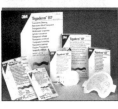

How supplied
3M Tegaderm HP Transparent
Dressing
Film sheet: $2^{3}/8'' \times 2^{3}/4''$; A6257
$4'' \times 4^{3}/4''$; A6258
Film sheet (sacral):
$4^{1}/2'' \times 4^{3}/4''$; A6258
Oval: $2^{1}/8'' \times 2^{1}/2''$, $4'' \times 4^{1}/2''$; A6257
$5^{1}/2'' \times 6^{1}/2''$; A6258
3M Tegaderm Transparent Dressing
Film sheet (picture frame): $1^{3}/4'' \times 1^{3}/4''$; A6257
$2^{3}/8'' \times 2^{3}/4''$; A6257
$4'' \times 4^{3}/4''$; A6258
Film sheet (original frame): $2^{3}/8'' \times 2^{3}/4''$; A6257
$4'' \times 4^{3}/4''$, $4'' \times 10''$, $6'' \times 8''$; A6258
$8'' \times 12''$; A6259
Film sheet (oval frame): $4'' \times 4^{1}/2''$; A6258
Film sheet (I.V. frame): $2^{3}/4'' \times 3^{1}/4''$, $3^{1}/2'' \times 4^{1}/4''$; A6257
Film sheet (first aid style): $2^{3}/8'' \times 2^{3}/4''$; A6257
$4'' \times 5^{1}/2''$; A6258

Action
3M Tegaderm Transparent Dressing is a sterile, waterproof, clear, thin film dressing. Designed to be applied over I.V. devices and clean skin or wounds, it provides a breathable bacterial and viral barrier to outside contaminants. 3M Tegaderm HP Transparent Dressing is specially formulated to provide greater staying power in the presence of moderate amounts of moisture.

Indications
3M Tegaderm Transparent Dressing: To cover and protect catheter sites and wounds, to maintain a moist environment for wound healing, and to facilitate autolytic debridement. Suitable for use as a secondary dressing, protective eye covering, and protective cover over at-risk skin. May also be used to secure devices to the skin.

Transparent Films

3M Tegaderm HP Transparent Dressing: For use with I.V. catheters and other intravascular catheters and percutaneous devices.

Contraindications
- Contraindicated for infected wounds and infected catheter sites.
- Not intended to replace sutures or other primary wound closure methods.

Application
- Peel the liner from the dressing, exposing the adhesive surface.
  3M Tegaderm HP Dressing:
- Center the dressing over the catheter site or wound.
  3M Tegaderm HP Dressing with Secure Strip:
- Position the dressing so the notch fits over the catheter hub and the insertion site is centered in the transparent film.
- Slowly remove the frame while smoothing down the dressing edges.
- Then, smooth the dressing from the center toward the edges, using firm pressure to enhance adhesion.

Removal
- Gently grasp an edge and slowly peel the dressing from the skin in the direction of hair growth. Avoid skin trauma by peeling the dressing back, rather than pulling it up from the skin.
- Alternatively, for removal from I.V. sites or other devices, grasp one edge of the dressing and gently pull it straight out to stretch it and release the adhesion. A medical solvent can also facilitate removal.
- Take care not to dislodge catheters or other devices or to disrupt the wound surface while removing the dressing. Support the skin and the catheter while removing the dressing.
- If the dressing adheres to the wound surface where epithelialization has taken place, gently soak it off.

Transparent Films

Transeal Transparent Wound Dressing
DeRoyal

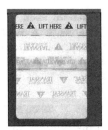

How supplied
Film: 1¾″ × 1¾″, 2½″ × 2¾″; A6257
4″ × 4¾″, 4″ × 10″, 6″ × 8″; A6258
8″ × 12″; A6259

Action
Transeal is a transparent, breathable polyurethane wound dressing coated with an acrylic, pressure-sensitive adhesive that acts as a second skin. Transeal has the highest vapor transmission rate available, yet it's impermeable to external contaminants, such as water, dirt, debris, and bacteria.

Indications
To prevent skin breakdown and to manage pressure ulcers (stages 1, 2, 3, and 4), partial- and full-thickness wounds, tunneling wounds, donor sites, I.V. sites, first- and second-degree burns, acute wounds, infected and noninfected wounds, draining wounds, and red, yellow, or black wounds. May be used as a primary or secondary dressing depending on wound type.

Contraindications
Contraindicated as a primary dressing for heavily draining wounds.

Application
- Cleanse and thoroughly dry the wound and surrounding skin.
- Peel off the dressing's backing layer to expose the adhesive side of the dressing.
- Position the dressing over the wound and press it gently into place.
- Peel off the clear carrier film to leave the dressing in place.

Removal
Remove the dressing by gently peeling away in the direction of hair growth.

Transparent Films

UniFlex
Smith & Nephew, Inc.
Wound Management Division

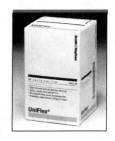

How supplied
Film sheet: 4" × 5½"; A6258

Action
UniFlex is a permeable film dressing that helps prevent bacterial contamination and water entry.

Indications
To cover wounds and damaged skin. May be used as a secondary dressing to secure foams, alginates, and gauzes in place while protecting the wound. May also be used to anchor I.V. tubing.

Contraindications
None provided by the manufacturer.

Application
- Grasp the two tails of the dressing's backing paper and pull them away from the film.
- Place the film dressing over the wound, other dressing, or I.V. tubing to be secured, and gently press it into place.
- Separate the backing paper from the film on the sides.

Removal
- Gently lift one corner of the film dressing.
- Stretch the dressing horizontally, parallel to the skin surface, thus breaking the adhesive bond.

Wound fillers

Action
Wound fillers are agents manufactured in a variety of forms, including pastes, granules, powders, beads, and gels. They provide a moist wound-healing environment, absorb exudate, and help debride the wound bed by softening the necrotic tissue.

Indications
Wound fillers may be used as primary dressings to manage partial- and full-thickness wounds, minimally to moderately exuding wounds, infected and noninfected wounds, and wounds requiring packing to fill dead space.

Advantages
- May be absorbent
- Promote autolytic debridement
- Are easy to apply and remove
- May be used in combination with other products
- Fill dead space.

Disadvantages
- Most dry wound fillers aren't recommended for use in dry wounds
- Require secondary dressing.

HCPCS code overview
The HCPCS codes normally assigned to wound fillers not elsewhere classified are:
A6261 — gel/paste, per fluid ounce
A6262 — dry form, per gram.

Wound Fillers

AcryDerm STRANDS Absorbent Wound Filler
AcryMed, Inc.

How Supplied
Strands: 6 g; A6262

Action
AcryDerm STRANDS Absorbent Wound Filler absorbs excess exudate and maintains a moist environment to promote wound healing. It maintains intimate wound contact without drying out, facilitating autolytic debridement.

Indications
To manage pressure ulcers (stages 2, 3, and 4), partial- and full-thickness wounds, tunneling wounds, infected wounds along with appropriate antibiotic treatment, and uninfected wounds. May also be used on wounds with moderate or heavy drainage, and red, yellow, or black wounds.

Contraindications
- Contraindicated for preventing skin breakdown.
- Contraindicated for stage 1 pressure ulcers.

Application
- Cut product to desired size.
- Place loosely in the wound cavity.
- Secure with an appropriate nonocclusive cover dressing.

Removal
- Gently remove cover dressing.
- Remove soiled AcryDerm STRANDS Absorbent Wound Filler.

Wound Fillers

Bard Absorption Dressing
Bard Medical Division
C.R. Bard, Inc.

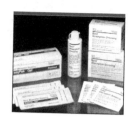

How supplied
Sterile bottle: 60 g; A6262
Sterile packet: 3 g; A6262
EasyPak Gel
(premixed): 28.3 g; A6261

Action
Bard Absorption Dressing is nonadherent, molds to the wound, and absorbs exudate and particulate matter. It provides a moist wound environment to help remove slough and absorb odors.

Indications
To clean, deodorize, and protect all secreting lesions, including pressure ulcers, partial- and full-thickness wounds, dehiscent wounds, tunneling and undermined wounds, infected and noninfected wounds, and all wounds with heavy drainage.

Contraindications
None provided by the manufacturer.

Application
- Prepare dressing. Mix 3 g of dry flake with 30 ml (1 oz) of sterile water at a 1:10 ratio, or use EasyPak Gel.
- Cleanse the wound.
- Apply the dressing to the wound, using an applicator such as a tongue blade. For deep, narrow wounds, use a large-volume syringe.
- Fill the wound approximately ⅜" (1 cm) deep.
- Cover with an appropriate cover dressing.

Removal
- Change when strike-through occurs or the dressing changes consistency and liquefies.
- Remove the cover dressing.
- Remove Bard Absorption Dressing by irrigating or using a gloved hand or sponge.

Wound Fillers

CarraSorb M Freeze Dried Gel Wound Dressing with Acemannan Hydrogel
Carrington Laboratories, Inc.

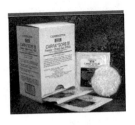

How supplied
Wafer: 4″ diameter; A4649

Action
CarraSorb M Freeze Dried Gel Wound Dressing is pure aloe vera gel containing Acemannan Hydrogel with all water extracted in freeze-drying. It's a sterile, preservative-free primary dressing, nonirritating and nontoxic, that returns to a moldable hydrogel as it absorbs exudate (up to 20 times its weight) without fiber residue. The gel maintains a moist wound environment.

Indications
To manage and dress pressure ulcers (stages 1, 2, 3, and 4), venous stasis ulcers, first- and second-degree burns, cuts, abrasions, skin irritations, radiation dermatitis, diabetic ulcers, foot ulcers, postsurgical incisions, and skin conditions associated with peristomal care. May also be used on partial- and full-thickness wounds, tunneling wounds, infected and noninfected wounds, wounds with moderate exudate, wounds with serosanguineous drainage, and red, yellow, or black wounds.

Contraindications
Contraindicated for patients with a known sensitivity to Acemannan Hydrogel or any other component of the dressing.

Application
- Flush wound with a suitable cleanser, such as UltraKlenz, CarraKlenz, or MicroKlenz.
- Apply the dressing to the wound bed by folding it into the wound or tearing it to pack into undermined areas.
- Cover with a secondary dressing, such as CarraFilm or CarraSmart Film.

Removal
- Change dressing as needed according to wound condition and amount of exudate or as directed by the primary care provider. Generally, a daily change is indicated.
- Rinse away any remaining gel residue with gentle irrigation.

Catrix 5 Rejuvenation Cream
Lescarden Inc.

How supplied
Tube: 1.25 oz

Action
Catrix 5 Rejuvenation Cream, a 5% concentration of Catrix Wound Dressing in a moisture-rich cream base, is formulated to accelerate the skin's natural rejuvenation process. Created to ease the discomfort of dermatologic procedures, it reduces the effects of aging, stress, and exposure to the elements, reduces redness and irritation, soothes, and moisturizes. The mineral oil- and fragrance-free cream offers UVA and UVB protection.

Indications
To counteract the irritating adverse effects often associated with topical retinoids, glycolic acid peels, alpha-hydroxy acid, and fluouroplex. Used primarily in cosmetic dermatology and plastic surgery patients.

Contraindications
For external use only. Avoid contact with eyes.

Application
- Smooth the cream onto cleansed skin morning and night.
- If also using a dermatologic therapy, cleanse the skin, then apply therapy as instructed by the primary care provider, followed by Catrix 5 Rejuvenation Cream.
- For 1 week before a dermatologic procedure, apply Catrix 5 Rejuvenation Cream daily, then follow the directions above.
- Ten days following a dermatologic procedure such as laser resurfacing, Catrix 5 Rejuvenation Cream may be used in place of Catrix 10 Ointment. Apply according to directions above.
- Continued daily use after healing will keep the skin healthy and supple.

Wound Fillers

Catrix 10 Ointment
Lescarden Inc.

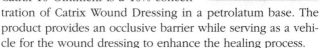

How supplied
Tube: 2 oz

Action
Catrix 10 Ointment is a 10% concentration of Catrix Wound Dressing in a petrolatum base. The product provides an occlusive barrier while serving as a vehicle for the wound dressing to enhance the healing process.

Indications
To manage wounds following laser resurfacing and deep dermabrasion. Also useful for mild psoriasis. Used primarily in cosmetic dermatology and plastic surgery patients.

Contraindications
For external use only. Avoid contact with eyes.

Application
- Following laser resurfacing, apply a liberal layer of Catrix 10 Ointment every 2 to 5 hours or as often as needed to keep the treated area moist.
- Apply enough to fully coat and occlude the treated area.
- Continue using for 7 days or as directed by the primary care provider.

Removal
- In the unlikely event of crust formation, gently soak off ointment using water or another solution, as directed.
- Reapply the ointment.

Wound Fillers

Catrix Wound Dressing
Lescarden Inc.

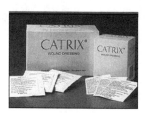

How supplied
Topical powder: 1-g packet; A6262

Action
Topically applied powder made from bovine tracheal cartilage containing micronized collagen, mucopolysaccharides, and growth factors that accelerate the healing of cutaneous wounds. The dressing maintains a moist wound environment, promotes angiogenesis, promotes the proliferation and migration of fibroblasts, stimulates the growth of keratinocytes, and creates a protective barrier against bacterial infections and other agents.

Indications
To manage pressure ulcers (stages 1, 2, 3, and 4), stasis ulcers, first- and second-degree burns, diabetic ulcers, foot ulcers, post-surgical incisions, radiation dermatitis, cuts and abrasions, partial-thickness wounds, and skin conditions associated with peristomal care. Also useful for wound exudate absorption.

Contraindications
Contraindicated in patients with a documented adverse reaction to bovine products.

Application
- Debride and cleanse the wound. Treat with medication, if needed.
- Apply Catrix Wound Dressing to the wound in an even manner to a thickness of no more than ¹⁄₁₆″.
- In hard-to-reach wounds, mix Catrix Wound Dressing with 2 to 5 cc glyceride or 4 to 10 ml saline solution to form a paste that can be applied directly to the wound, completely covering it.
- If needed, apply a nonocclusive dressing, such as Telfa.
- Apply one or two times a day, as needed.

Wound Fillers

FlexiGel Strands Absorbent Wound Dressing

Smith & Nephew, Inc.
Wound Management Division

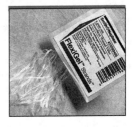

How supplied
Packet: 6 g; A6262

Action

FlexiGel Strands Absorbent Wound Dressing is a moist wound-healing gel sheet cut into attached strips (strands) with 20% glycerin added. The sheet is made of a polyacrylamide matrix with embedded hydrophilic polysaccharide particles to absorb excess exudate while maintaining a moist wound-healing environment that supports autolytic debridement.

Indications

To manage wounds with moderate or heavy exudate, cavity wounds, or shallow wounds. May also be used for venous ulcers, arterial ulcers, diabetic ulcers, pressure ulcers (stages 1, 2, 3, and 4), skin graft and donor sites, abrasions, lacerations, and surgical wounds.

Contraindications

Contraindicated for third-degree burns.

Application

- Cleanse wound with normal saline solution or other appropriate wound cleanser.
- Fill wound cavity approximately 50% to allow for absorptive swelling of the strands.
- Cover strands with an appropriate nonocclusive dressing.

Removal

- Change dressings when strike-through is observed on the cover dressing.
- Strands will fall out onto the cover dressing when removed. The dressing will come out in one piece. If strands separate, they can be flushed out of the wound bed.

Wound Fillers

*hy*CURE
The Hymed Group Corporation

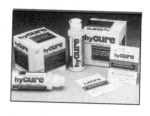

How supplied
Packets: 1g (24 packets/box);
A6262
Bottle: 40g; A6262

Action
A medical hydrolysate of type I collagen, *hy*CURE interacts with the wound site, forming a gel when it mixes with wound exudate and providing a moist healing environment. Naturally absorbent, *hy*CURE protects the wound bed and newly formed granulation tissue by forming an occlusive gelatinous barrier, controls the evaporation of fluid, reduces pain, and soothes and deodorizes. The product conforms to any wound site and is biocompatible and biodegradable.

Indications
To manage chronic and acute wounds and skin ulcers, including pressure ulcers (stages 1, 2, 3, and 4), venous stasis ulcers, diabetic ulcers, first- and second-degree burns, ulcers resulting from arterial insufficiency, surgical wounds, traumatic wounds, and superficial wounds.

Contraindications
None provided by the manufacturer.

Application
- Cleanse the wound site, leaving the wound moist.
- Apply *hy*CURE directly to the wound site to approximately ¼″ (6 mm) thickness.
- Cover the wound with a nonadherent dressing, such as Telfa.

Removal
- Change the secondary dressing and reapply *hy*CURE every 24 hours or as needed.
- *hy*CURE doesn't need to be removed with subsequent dressing changes.

Wound Fillers

*hy*CURE SMART GEL
The Hymed Group Corporation

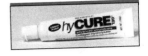

How supplied
Tube: 1 oz (28.4 g); A6261

Action
*hy*CURE SMART GEL—an all-natural product containing no preservatives, alcohol, or synthetic substances—interacts with the wound site to provide a moist environment that encourages healing. It protects the wound bed and newly formed granulation tissue by the formation of an occlusive gelatinous barrier, absorbs wound exudate, and promotes natural autolysis by rehydrating and softening necrotic tissue and eschar, which encourages autolytic debridement. It also reduces pain, soothes, and deodorizes. The product conforms to any wound site and is biocompatible and biodegradable.

Indications
To manage chronic and acute wounds and skin ulcers, such as pressure ulcers (stages 1, 2, 3, and 4), venous stasis ulcers, ulcers resulting from arterial insufficiency, surgical wounds, diabetic ulcers, traumatic wounds, superficial wounds, first- and second-degree burns, and other general dermatologic conditions.

Contraindications
None provided by manufacturer.

Application
- Cleanse the wound.
- Apply *hy*CURE SMART GEL directly into the wound and onto the surrounding area.
- Cover the wound with a nonadherent dressing.

Removal
- Remove the secondary dressing and reapply gel every 24 hours or as needed.
- To ease removal, soak the dressing in warm water

IODOFLEX PAD
Healthpoint

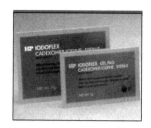

How supplied
Sterile pad: 5 g (4 cm × 6 cm),
10 g (8 cm × 6 cm);
A6262

Action
IODOFLEX PAD cleanses the wound by absorbing fluid, pus, exudate, and bacteria. It actively fights infection by reducing the bacterial load through a time-released antimicrobial.

Indications
To manage draining wounds, such as pressure ulcers, venous stasis ulcers, and infected traumatic and surgical wounds.

Contraindications
- Contraindicated in patients with a known sensitivity to iodine.
- Contraindicated in patients with Hashimoto's thyroiditis, Graves' disease, or nontoxic nodular goiter. Use cautiously in patients with a history of thyroid disorder; such patients are more susceptible to an alteration in thyroid metabolism with chronic use.
- Contraindicated in pregnant or breast-feeding patients.
- Contraindicated for internal use and use in eyes.

Application
- Cleanse the wound with ALLCLENZ Wound Cleanser.
- Remove carrier gauze from one or both sides of the pad, and lay the pad into the wound.
- Cover with a secondary dressing.

Removal
- Change the pad when its color changes from brown to yellow-gray.
- Flush the pad from the wound with ALLCLENZ Wound Cleanser during each dressing change.

Wound Fillers

IODOSORB GEL
Healthpoint

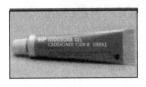

How supplied
Sterile tube: 40 g; A6261

Action
IODOSORB GEL cleanses the wound by absorbing fluid, pus, exudate, bacteria, enzymes, and cellular residue. It actively fights infection by reducing the bacterial load through a time-released antimicrobial.

Indications
To manage draining wounds, such as pressure ulcers, venous stasis ulcers, and infected traumatic and surgical wounds.

Contraindications
- Contraindicated in patients with a known sensitivity to iodine.
- Contraindicated in patients with Hashimoto's thyroiditis, Graves' disease, or nontoxic nodular goiter. Use cautiously in patients with a history of thyroid disorder; such patients are more susceptible to an alteration in thyroid metabolism with chronic use.
- Contraindicated in pregnant or breast-feeding patients.
- Contraindicated for internal use and use in eyes.

Application
- Cleanse the wound with ALLCLENZ Wound Cleanser.
- Apply ⅛″ to ¼″ (0.3 to 0.6 cm) IODOSORB GEL onto dry gauze and then place onto wound bed.
- Cover with a secondary dressing.

Removal
- Change gel when color changes from brown to a yellow-gray.
- Flush IODOSORB GEL from the wound with ALLCLENZ Wound Cleanser during each dressing change.

Wound Fillers

Kollagen-Medifil II Gel
BioCore Medical Technologies, Inc.

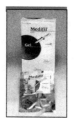

How supplied
Syringe: 3 ml (0.1 fl oz), 9 ml (0.33 fl oz);
A6261

Action
Kollagen-Medifil II Gel consists of type I bovine
collagen particles suspended in a solution. The product becomes fluid at body temperature to fill in all surface irregular-
ities in the wound, and creates an environment conducive to
wound healing. The applicator allows easy access to tunneling
or undermined wound areas.

Indications
To manage chronic wounds, such as pressure ulcers (stage 2,
3, and 4); venous, arterial, and diabetic ulcers; surgical wounds
(including donor sites and grafts and wounds resulting from
Mohs', laser, or podiatric surgery); surgical wound dehiscence;
and traumatic wounds (including abrasions, lacerations, partial-thickness wounds, burns, and skin tears).

Contraindications
Contraindicated in patients sensitive to products of bovine origin.

Application
- For minimally draining or dehydrated wounds, apply gel ¼"
  (0.6 cm) thick.
- For tunneling or undermined wounds, apply gel directly into
  tunneling or undermined areas.
- If dead space is present, gently pack the wound with saline-
  moistened gauze or a dressing of choice. Don't pack tightly.
  Apply the gel to the packing material before placing it in the
  wound.
- Cover with a nonadherent secondary dressing, such as impregnated gauze, hydrocolloid, hydrogel sheet, semipermeable film or foam, or other appropriate dressing.

Wound Fillers

Removal

- Reapply every 24 hours for moderately to heavily exudating wounds, according to instructions for the wound type.
- Change the secondary dressing daily or as indicated by the amount of drainage.
- Remove the secondary dressing. If it adheres to the wound, irrigate with sterile normal saline solution until the dressing loosens. Lift gently.
- Irrigate the wound with sterile normal saline solution to cleanse it thoroughly. If specialty dressings or wound fillers have been used, irrigate the wound thoroughly to remove all traces of these materials and any foreign bodies present in the wound bed.
- If the gel has been used for an undermined or tunneled wound, gently flush the area with sterile normal saline solution to remove old drainage and debris.

Kollagen-Medifil II Particles
BioCore Medical Technologies, Inc.

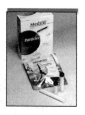

How supplied
Sterile vial: 2.5ml (0.25 g), 5 ml (0.5 g), 10 ml
(1.0 g), 15 ml (1.5 g); A6262

Action
Kollagen-Medifil II Particles are made of type I bovine collagen that's similar in molecular structure to the collagen found
in human skin. The particles lay down a collagen matrix in the
wound bed, attracting the cellular components necessary to
stimulate the healing process. Of all BioCore's Kollagen products, Kollagen-Medifil II Particles cover the largest surface area.

Indications
To manage pressure ulcers (stages 2, 3, and 4), partial- and full-
thickness wounds (except third-degree burns), podiatric surgical wounds, infected and noninfected wounds, wounds with
drainage, red or yellow wound beds, and scattered areas of
slough or necrosis.

Contraindications
- Contraindicated in patients sensitive to products of bovine
  origin.
- Contraindicated for third-degree burns.

Application
- Apply Kollagen-Medifil II Particles to cover the wound surface, using the appropriate amount for the type of wound, as
  follows: For minimal drainage, completely cover the surface
  of the wound bed. For moderate drainage, cover with ⅛" to
  ¼" (0.3 to 0.6 cm). For heavy drainage, cover with ¼" (0.6 cm).
- Don't pack the wound tightly; particles are highly absorbent
  and will expand.
- Gently fill dead space with a dressing to prevent premature
  wound closure.
- Apply a secondary dressing, choosing the appropriate dressing for the type of wound, as follows: For minimal drainage,
  use nonadherent, impregnated gauze; hydrocolloid; hydrogel; semipermeable film; or foam. Check the dressing at least
  daily (or as recommended by the manufacturer or based on
  clinical indications), and rehydrate as necessary. For moder-

ate or heavy drainage, cover the site with an absorbent dressing, such as conventional gauze, abdominal pads, or a specialty absorptive dressing.

- Dress infected wounds as follows: If a topical medication is ordered, apply the topical agent to the wound first; then cover the topical agent with Kollagen-Medifil II Particles. Change particles daily (or more often, depending on drainage) until the infection is resolved. Flush with sterile normal saline solution. When the infection is resolved, change the particles once every 2 or 3 days until the wound closes.
- Dress tunneling or undermined wounds as follows: Make a thick liquid of 5 ml Kollagen-Medifil II Particles and 10 ml sterile normal saline solution in a sterile receptacle. Use a syringe (without needle) to apply to tunneling or undermined areas. Gently fill the wound with gauze or another appropriate dressing to eliminate dead space. Apply Medifil mixture to the packing material before applying it to the wound.
- To provide more moisture to a dry wound or to dress a difficult area such as the bottom of the foot or the toes, make a paste of 5 ml of Kollagen-Medifil II Particles and 5 ml of sterile normal saline solution in a sterile receptacle. Apply to the wound dressing or directly to the wound surface with a sterile tongue blade or cotton-tipped applicator. Cover the wound with a sterile nonadherent dressing or hydrocolloid (noninfected wounds only), hydrogel, semipermeable film or foam, or impregnated gauze.

Removal

- Change the secondary dressing every 1 to 3 days or as indicated by the amount of drainage.
- If the secondary dressing adheres to the wound, irrigate with sterile normal saline solution until the dressing is loosened. Lift it gently.
- Irrigate the wound with sterile normal saline solution to cleanse thoroughly.
- If Kollagen-Medifil II Particles adhere to the wound after irrigation with sterile normal saline solution, don't remove them.

Multidex Maltodextrin Wound Dressing Gel or Powder
DeRoyal

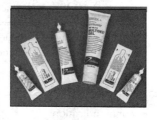

How supplied
Powder: 6 g tube, 12 g tube, 25 g tube, 45 g tube; A6262
Gel: ⅐-oz packet, ¼-oz tube, ½-oz tube, 3-oz tube; A6261

Action
Multidex Maltodextrin Wound Dressing establishes and maintains a moist environment for tissue granulation by mixing with wound exudate, thus controlling dehydration, drainage, and odor.

Indications
To be used as a primary or secondary dressing to manage pressure ulcers (stages 2, 3, and 4), venous stasis ulcers, diabetic ulcers, neuropathic ulcers, and poorly healing wounds. May also be used on tunneling wounds, partial- and full-thickness wounds, infected and noninfected wounds, wounds with heavy or purulent drainage, and red, yellow, or black wounds.

Contraindications
None provided by the manufacturer.

Application
- Irrigate the wound with normal saline solution.
- Apply the dressing over the entire wound to a minimum thickness of ⅛″ to ¼″ (0.3 to 0.6 cm). For deep wounds, fill to the skin surface.
- Cover with a nonadherent dressing.

Removal
- Remove the secondary dressing.
- Irrigate the wound with normal saline solution. Any remaining dressing may be left in the wound.

Wound Fillers

Other products

The "Other products" category comprises a wide variety of products used to facilitate wound management. Each product details its:

- action
- indications
- contraindications
- application process
- removal process.

Please refer to each product listing for further information regarding these products.

In this section, the manufacturer has either received a HCPCS code or hasn't yet received or applied for one.

NEW PRODUCT

AcryDerm Silver Antimicrobial Hydrophilic Wound Dressings
AcryMed, Inc.

How supplied
Sheet dressing (low to moderate exudate):
   $2'' \times 2''$, $4'' \times 4''$, $4'' \times 8''$, $8'' \times 8''$
Perforated sheet dressing (moderate to high exudate):
   $4'' \times 4''$, $4'' \times 8''$, $8'' \times 8''$

Action
AcryDerm Silver Antimicrobial Hydrophilic Wound Dressings create an optimal environment to manage wound moisture levels, promote moist wound healing and debridement, and protect new granulation and epithelial tissue. They contain a proprietary broad-spectrum silver-cascade antimicrobial, which may reduce the bioburden in wounds for up to 7 days.

Indications
To manage full- and partial-thickness wounds, including decubitus ulcers, venous stasis ulcers, diabetic ulcers, first-and second-degree burns, abrasions and lacerations, donor sites, and surgical wounds. May also be used over debrided and grafted partial-thickness wounds.

Contraindications
None provided by the manufacturer.

Application
Sheet dressing:
- Cleanse the wound according to facility policy.
- Cut the dressing to size, if necessary. Ensure that dressing extends at least $1''$ (2.5 cm) beyond wound edges.
- Apply the dressing using a rolling motion.
- Secure with hypoallergenic tape, nonwoven breathable tape, or transparent film, or roll gauze for extra fragile skin.
   Perforated dressing:
- Cover with a secondary absorbent dressing, which may be replaced as it becomes saturated.

Removal
Carefully lift the edge of the dressing and peel it off the skin.

Other Products

NEW PRODUCT
AcryDerm Silver Antimicrobial Absorbent Wound Filler
AcryMed, Inc.

How supplied
Wound filler (stranded): 6 grams

Action
AcryDerm Silver Antimicrobial Absorbent Wound Filler absorbs up to 30 cc of wound fluid, promotes moist wound healing and debridement, and prevents the wound from drying out. It contains a proprietary broad-spectrum silver-cascade antimicrobial, which may reduce the bioburden in wounds for up to 7 days.

Indications
To manage full- and partial-thickness wounds, including decubitis ulcers, venous stasis ulcers, diabetic ulcers, first- and second-degree burns, abrasions and lacerations, donor sites and surgical wounds, and over-debrided and grafted partial-thickness wounds. May also be used for cavity wounds and heavy-exudate wounds.

Contraindications
None provided by the manufacturer.

Application
- Cut the wound filler to the desired size.
- Place it loosely in the wound cavity, filling only half the cavity depth to allow for swelling, or spread it out over a flat wound.
- Secure with an appropriate absorbent cover dressing.

Removal
- Change the wound filler when evidence of strike-through appears on the cover dressing.
- Gently remove the cover dressing, then remove the soiled wound filler.

Other Products

Acticoat
Smith & Nephew, Inc.
Wound Management Division

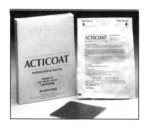

How supplied
Pad: Wide variety of sizes; A4649

Action
Acticoat is a nonadherent, antimicrobial barrier that protects against pathogens without delaying wound healing. The immediate and controlled release of ionic silver allows the dressing to remain in place for an extended period.

Indications
To help reduce the risk of infection in partial- and full-thickness wounds, including pressure ulcers, venous ulcers, diabetic ulcers, first- and second-degree burns, and donor sites. May also be used over debrided and grafted partial-thickness wounds.

Contraindications
- Contraindicated in patients with a known sensitivity to silver.
- Use on third-degree burns hasn't been evaluated.

Application
- Cleanse the wound according to facility policy. Avoid using oil-based cleansing agents.
- Cut the dressing to fit the wound size.
- Place the silver side of the dressing against the wound.
- If the wound is draining, apply the dressing dry. If the wound is dry, moisten the dressing with water and apply it to the wound. Don't use topical antimicrobials with Acticoat.
- Secure the dressing with an appropriate secondary dressing.

Removal
- Remove the secondary dressing.
- Remove Acticoat from the wound bed. Ensure that the dressing is moist before removing it.

Other Products

Acticoat Absorbent
Smith & Nephew, Inc.
Wound Management Division

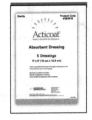

How supplied
Pad: 4" × 5"
Rope: ¾" × 12"

Action
Acticoat Absorbent absorbs excess wound fluid to form a gel that maintains a moist environment for optimal wound healing. The sustained release of broad-spectrum ionic silver actively protects the dressing from bacterial contamination.

Indications
To protect wounds from bacterial penetration. The dressing's barrier function may help reduce infection in partial- and full-thickness wounds with moderate to heavy exudate, including pressure ulcers, venous ulcers, diabetic ulcers, and surgical and traumatic wounds.

Contraindications
- Contraindicated in patients with a known sensitivity to silver.
- Use on third-degree burns hasn't been evaluated.

Application
- Cleanse the wound using conventional, non-oil-based techniques, and leave the wound moist.
- Cut the dressing to fit the wound size.
- Apply the dressing to the wound and secure it with a secondary dressing that will maintain the moist environment.

Removal
- Change the dressing depending on the amount of exudate present and the condition of the wound.
- Remove the secondary dressing, then remove Acticoat Absorbent from the wound bed. Ensure that the dressing is moist before removing it.
- If the dressing dries and adheres to the wound, moisten or soak the dressing before removing it.

Other Products

Acticoat 7
Smith & Nephew, Inc.
Wound Management
Division

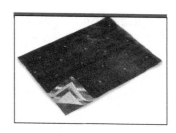

How supplied
Pad: 4″ × 5″, 6″ × 6″

Action
Acticoat consists of two layers of absorbent, rayon/polyester inner core sandwiched between three layers of silver-coated, polyethylene netting. The sustained release of broad-spectrum ionic silver actively protects the dressing from bacterial contamination, while the inner core maintains the moist environment needed for wound healing. Acticoat 7 delivers seven days of uninterrupted antimicrobial activity.

Indications
To prevent infection in partial- and full-thickness wounds, including pressure ulcers, venous ulcers, diabetic ulcers, first-and second-degree burns, grafts, and donor sites. May also be used over debrided and grafted wounds.

Contraindications
- Contraindicated in patients with a known sensitivity to silver.
- Use on third-degree burns hasn't been evaluated.

Application
- Moisten the dressing with sterile water.
- Cut the dressing to fit the wound size.
- Place the blue side of the dressing against the wound.
- Secure the dressing with an appropriate secondary dressing that will maintain moisture.

Removal
- Change the dressing depending on the amount of exudate present and the condition of the wound. The dressing may be worn for up to 7 days.
- Remove the secondary dressing; then remove Acticoat 7 from the wound bed. Ensure that the dressing is moist before removing it.

Other Products

Arglaes Antimicrobial Barrier

Medline Industries, Inc.

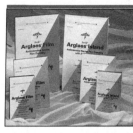

How supplied

Film dressing: 2⅜″ × 3⅛″,
　　　　　　 4″ × 4¾″,
　　　　　　 4¾″ × 10″
　　　　　　 3¼″ × 14″ (postop)
Alginate pad:: 2⅜″ × 3⅛″, 4″ × 4¾″, 6″ × 10″

Action

Arglaes Antimicrobial Barrier applies the principle of moist wound healing and also serves as a potent antimicrobial barrier that remains effective for 7 days. Arglaes technology utilizes sustained release of ionic silver that's antibacterial and antifungal but remains completely noncytotoxic. Arglaes Antimicrobial Barrier has a high moisture vapor transfer rate and is available as a transparent film dressing, with or without an alginate pad.

Indications

To manage superficial wounds, lacerations, cuts and abrasions, leg ulcers, pressure ulcers (stages 2, 3, and 4), donor sites, partial- and full-thickness wounds, infected and noninfected wounds, wounds with light to heavy drainage, wounds with serosanguineous or purulent drainage, and red, yellow, or black wounds.

Contraindications

- Contraindicated for third-degree burns.
- Contraindicated in patients with known hypersensitivity to silver or heavy metals.

Application

- Cleanse the application site with normal saline solution or another appropriate cleanser, such as Skintegrity Wound Cleanser. Dry the surrounding skin to ensure it's free from any greasy substance. Allow any skin preparation to dry completely.
- Select an appropriate-sized dressing that allows 1¼″ to 1½″ (3.2 to 3.8 cm) of attachment to healthy periwound skin.

- With one hand, hold the dressing's white tab with the printed side facing up. With the other hand, take hold of the loose film flap and gently peel off the release sheet.
- Hold the dressing on both ends, then turn it over so the adhesive surface is facing the wound. Ensure that both edges of the white tab are held together.
- Apply the dressing, pressing firmly and smoothing down. Make sure the edges of the dressing are firmly fixed in place.
- Take hold of the second release sheet at the end of the dressing opposite the white tab and gently peel away and discard.
- For moderately to heavily draining wounds, use the O-Technique. It involves cutting small openings into the dressing prior to removing the carrier sheet. Excess drainage is allowed to pass through the dressing onto an absorbent secondary dressing. The technique is also helpful when using Arglaes under a compression dressing.

Removal

- Gently lift up one corner of the dressing and begin stretching it horizontally along the skin surface to break the adhesive bond.
- When two sides of the dressing are partially removed, grasp both sides and stretch the dressing horizontally, parallel to the skin.

Other Products

BIOBRANE Temporary Wound Dressing

Bertek (Dow Hickam)
Pharmaceuticals

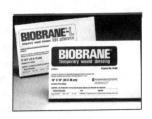

How supplied
Pieces: 5″ × 5″, 5″ × 15″, 10″ × 15″;
  A9270

Action
BIOBRANE is an adherent, flexible, temporary wound dressing. It's a biocomposite of an ultrathin, semipermeable silicone membrane bonded to a flexible knitted nylon fabric and purified collagen peptides. The dressing controls water vapor loss at rates comparable to those of normal skin and provides a flexible, adherent covering for the wound surface.

Indications
To manage donor sites and clean, debrided, or excised superficial and medium-depth partial-thickness wounds. May also be used as a protective covering over meshed autografts.

Contraindications
Contraindicated in patients showing allergic reactions to BIOBRANE (rare). If a patient shows evidence of an allergic reaction, remove the dressing and discontinue its use.

Application
- Debride and clean the wound completely. Remove blisters, debris, and loose tissue. BIOBRANE won't adhere to dirty, infected, or nonviable tissue. Wounds may be cleaned with a germicidal soap and rinsed with normal saline solution.
- Establish hemostasis before applying the dressing.
- Apply BIOBRANE dull side down. Place the fabric (dull side) against the wound and apply with slight tension.
- Stretch the dressing slightly over the wound bed to remove wrinkles. Wrinkles may prevent uniform adherence or create pockets in which fluid can accumulate.
- Secure the dressing in place. Under slight tension, immobilize the dressing using tape, skin closure strips, staples, or sutures. Apply liquid adhesives to undamaged skin to improve the adherence of skin closure strips or tape.

Other Products

- Wrap the area with a gauze dressing or another stenting device to hold BIOBRANE firmly in contact with the wound surface for 24 to 36 hours.

Removal

- Remove the gauze dressing after 24 to 36 hours. Avoid dislodging the adherent BIOBRANE.
- If BIOBRANE is adherent and no fluid has accumulated, leave the site open to the air or rewrap it with a light, dry dressing. When appropriate, begin promoting movement of the body part associated with the burn, and bathe the patient according to standard burn protocol.
- If BIOBRANE is loose and covers viable nonpurulent tissue, aspirate any accumulated fluid or air. Wrinkles, air, or fluid may also be rolled out to the edge. Reapply the outer gauze dressing, and reinspect in 24 to 36 hours for adherence.
- If the loose BIOBRANE covers purulent tissue, remove the dressing from the affected area. Institute appropriate therapeutic treatment.
- Remove staples, tape, sutures, or skin closure strips 3 to 4 days after application or when adherence is achieved.
- Trim BIOBRANE away from the edges of the wound as healing progresses.
- Peel BIOBRANE from its site when the wound is healed (usually 7 to 14 days). BIOBRANE will peel off healed tissue relatively easily. If bleeding occurs or the patient complains of significant pain, stop removal of the dressing and wait 1 or 2 additional days.
- Either soak the dressing in water or apply a petroleum-based product before removal. This will make removal easier and more comfortable for the patient.

CHONDROPROTEC
The Hymed Group Corporation

How supplied
Vial: 1000 mg/10 ml

Action
CHONDROPROTEC, a polysulfated glycosamino-
glycan, is a unique topical wound management
dressing. CHONDROPROTEC creates a moist wound-healing
environment, protects new granulation tissue, conforms to any
wound site, is easy to apply and redress, and promotes natural autolysis by rehydrating and softening necrotic tissue and
eschar, thereby encouraging autolytic debridement.

Indications
To manage pressure ulcers (stages 1, 2, 3, and 4), venous stasis ulcers, first- and second-degree burns, secreting and bleeding dermal lesions, trauma injuries, partial- and full-thickness
wounds, surgical incisions, and donor sites.

Contraindications
Not indicated for use as a long-term or permanent dressing.

Application
- Debride wounds that are contaminated or infected prior to
  using CHONDROPROTEC.
- Irrigate wound with normal saline solution.
- Apply CHONDROPROTEC liberally to the wound surface.
- Cover with extra gauze or an abdominal pad for the first 24
  to 96 hours, if the wound has heavy drainage.
- Cover with a nonadherent dressing, such as Telfa dressing,
  when the drainage stops or becomes light.

Removal
- Change the dressing as needed.
- Irrigate the wound site with saline solution, then reapply
  CHONDROPROTEC.

Hyalofill Biopolymeric Wound Dressing
ConvaTec

How supplied
Dressing: 2″ × 2″, 4″ × 4″
Ribbon: 0.5 g

Action
Hyalofill Biopolymeric Dressing is
absorbent and conformable fibrous fleece (F) or ribbon (R)
composed of Hyaff, an ester of hyaluronic acid. As it absorbs
wound exudate, it forms a soft, cohesive gel that provides a
moist wound environment, aiding autolytic debridement and
allowing nontraumatic removal without damaging newly formed
tissue.

Indications
To manage leg ulcers, pressure ulcers (stages 1, 2, 3, and 4),
diabetic ulcers, surgical wounds, second-degree burns, and
wounds prone to bleeding, such as mechanically or surgically
debrided wounds, donor sites, and traumatic wounds. May also
be used on abrasions, lacerations, and minor cuts. Hyalofill R
also suitable for deep exuding wounds, sinuses, and fistulae.

Contraindications
Contraindicated in patients with known hypersensitivity to this
product or to avian proteins.

Application
- Cleanse the wound, rinse well, and dry the surrounding skin.
- Place the Hyalofill Biopolymeric Wound Dressing onto the
  surface of the lesion. If using Hyalofill R, gently place the rib-
  bon in position inside the cavity; don't pack too tightly.
- Cover with a sterile secondary dressing.

Removal
- Dressings applied to heavily exuding or sloughy wounds may
  need daily replacement initially, then every 3 or 3 days as
  exudate decreases.
- Thoroughly irrigating the wound with sterile saline solution
  or using forceps or gloved fingers may aid removal.

Other Products

HYCOAT
The Hymed Group Corporation

How supplied
Vial: 30 mg/6 ml, 50 mg/10 ml

Action
HYCOAT is a sterile solution of sodium
hyaluronate. As a protective tissue coating,
it plays an important role in several aspects

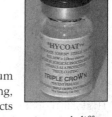

of wound healing. It enhances epithelial migration and differentiation and accelerates wound healing with reduced tissue fibrosis. HYCOAT also favors tissue hydration and improves the microcirculatory perfusion of healing tissue. There is some evidence that hyaluronate influences scarless tissue repair.

Indications
To manage pressure ulcers (stages 1, 2, 3, and 4), acute wounds, first- and second-degree burns, surgical wounds, venous stasis ulcers, and autograft procedures.

Contraindications
Not indicated for use as a long-term or permanent dressing.

Application
- Before using HYCOAT, debride wounds that are contaminated or infected.
- Cleanse the wound or surgical site.
- Either pour the HYCOAT solution directly from the vial onto the wound, or draw it up into a syringe to apply it.
- Cover treated area with a nonadherent dressing, such as Telfa.

Removal
- Change dressing as needed, repeating application of HYCOAT.
- Irrigate the wound with saline solution.

NEW PRODUCT
Kerlix A.M.D. Antimicrobial Bandage Roll

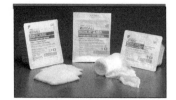

NEW PRODUCT
Kerlix Antimicrobial Super Sponge
Kendall Health Care Products Company

How supplied
Bandage roll: 4.5″ × 4.1 yds. (1 per tray)
Super sponge: Medium (2, 5, or 10 per tray)

Action
Kerlix A.M.D. bandage rolls and super sponges resist bacterial colonization within the dressing and reduce bacterial penetration through the dressing as well. Broad-spectrum effectiveness provides protection against gram-positive and gram-negative microorganisms, including methicillin-resistant *Staphylococcus aureus* and vancomycin-resistant enterrococcus infections, and fungi and yeasts. Kerlix A.M.D. also limits cross-contamination from patient to patient, patient to clinician, and patient to the environment.

Indications
To manage pressure ulcers (stages 1, 2, 3, and 4), partial- and full-thickness wounds, tunneling wounds, infected and noninfected wounds, draining wounds, and red, yellow, or black wounds.

Contraindications
Contraindicated for third-and fourth-degree burns.

Application
Apply Kerlix A.M.D. as a primary dressing or as a secondary dressing.

Removal
Gently remove the dressing.

Other Products

Mepiform Self-Adherent Silicone Dressing
Mölnlycke Health Care

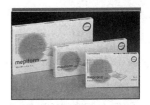

How supplied
Sterile sheet: 2″ × 3″, 4″ × 7″, 1.6″ × 10″

Action
Mepiform is a thin, flexible, self-adherent silicone gel sheet. It features Safetac technology, a unique hydrophobic silicone-coating that allows the dressing to be applied, removed, and reapplied with minimal discomfort to the patient and no disturbance to the area. Because of its high moistur-vapor transfer rate, Mepiform helps prevent moisture buildup under the dressing and reduces uncomfortable itching.

Indications
To manage old and new hypertrophic and keloid scars and closed wounds. May prevent the formation of hypertrophic and keloid scarring.

Contraindications
None provided by the manufacturer.

Application
- Cleanse the scar tissue or closed wound with mild soap and water. Rinse and pat dry. Ensure that the scar and surrounding skin are dry.
- If necessary, cut the dressing to the appropriate shape.
- Remove the release film and apply the dressing to the scar without stretching the dressing.

Removal
- Optimally, Mepiform should be worn 24 hours per day. It may be removed once daily, when showering or bathing, and reapplied.
- Change the dressing when it begins to lose its adherent properties. Dressing wear time varies by person and averages 7 days.
- To remove the dressing, peel it back.

Provant Wound Closure System
Regenesis Biomedical, Inc.

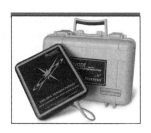

How supplied
Power unit, treatment applicator pad, and disposable treatment applicator pad covers.

Action
The Provant Wound Closure System, based upon cell proliferation induction (CPI) technology, is a medical device that induces proliferation of fibroblasts and epithelial cells for wound healing. Fibroblasts initiate wound healing and trigger the biochemical cascade that leads to granulation in the wound bed and overall healing. Epithelial cells complete the healing and closure process. This medical device also stimulates the secretion of multiple growth factors within the first 30-minute treatment through a calcium-dependent cellular mechanism. The CPI treatment signal administered by the Provant Wound Closure System penetrates 7 to 8 cm through dressings and damaged tissue layers to initiate these critical events in the wound healing process.

Indications
To treat symptoms associated with the inflammatory phase of wound healing in soft tissues. Also used to induce granulation, epithelialization, and angiogenesis through the regeneration of human soft tissue during the wound healing process.

Contraindications
- Contraindicated for treatment of bone or deep internal organs and for use over joints of patients with immature bone development.
- Contraindicated in patients who have metallic implants in the area of application or who have cardiac pacemakers.
- Contraindicated in pregnant patients.

Application
- Connect the base unit of the Provant Wound Closure System to a power outlet.

Other Products

- Place a single-use, disposable, treatment applicator pad cover over the treatment applicator pad before each use. This cover serves as an infection control barrier and aids in directing the treatment dose to the wound site. It also enhances the dosage regulation circuitry, ensuring the most accurate dosing to the wound site.
- Place the covered treatment applicator pad over any standard wound dressing which has been applied to the wound site, and push the start/stop button. Removal of the dressing is not necessary or required for Provant treatment.
- The device automatically delivers a preset therapeutic dose to the treatment area through the treatment applicator pad. The length of treatment is 30 minutes, administered twice daily. An internal countdown timer in the base unit automatically regulates the length of treatment and turns off the system when the dosing is complete. A visible timer display indicates the total treatment time remaining. Treatment dosing and time are preset by the manufacturer to maximize the proliferation of fibroblasts and epithelial cells for wound closure. No adjustments by the patient or caregiver are necessary or possible.
- In hospitals and long-term care facilities, a wound care nurse or a physical therapist typically administers the therapy. In outpatient settings, the primary care provider typically prescribes the Provant Wound Closure System for administration by the patient, family member, or other caregiver twice daily at home.

Removal

Discard the single-use disposable applicator cover after each 30-minute treatment.

Other Products

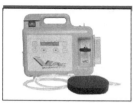

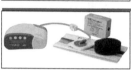

`NEW PRODUCT`
V.A.C. Device

`NEW PRODUCT`
MiniV.A.C. Device
KCI

How supplied
V.A.C. Unit and MiniV.A.C. unit;
K0538
Dressing kit (small, medium, large);
K0539
Other dressing kit components; K0539
V.A.C. canister with or without Isolyser; K0540

Action
The V.A.C. (Vacuum Assisted Closure) device assists in wound closure by applying localized negative pressure to the wound. V.A.C. negative pressure is applied to a special porous dressing positioned in the wound cavity or over a flap or graft. This porous dressing distributes negative pressure throughout the wound and helps remove interstitial fluids from the wound. The MiniV.A.C. provides adjustable negative-pressure therapy in a convenient, battery-powered, ambulatory device.

Indications
To manage chronic, acute, traumatic, and subacute wounds; dehisced wounds; diabetic ulcers; pressure ulcers; flaps; and grafts.

Contraindications
- Contraindicated for necrotic tissue with eschar, wounds with malignancy, untreated osteomyelitis, and fistulas to organs or body cavities.
- Contraindicated for use over exposed arteries or veins.
- Precautions indicated for patients with active bleeding or difficult wound hemostasis or who are using anticoagulants.

Application
- Follow universal precautions. Use gloves, gown, and goggles if splashing or exposure to body fluids is likely.

Other Products

- Aggressively cleanse the wound, according to facility policy. Debride any necrotic tissue or eschar, achieve hemostasis (avoiding use of bone wax, which blocks the negative pressure needed to initiate the healing response), and shave hair at the borders of the wound, if applicable.

- Irrigate the wound with normal saline or other prescribed solution.

- Dry and prepare periwound tissue as appropriate. (*Note:* If skin is moist due to perspiration, oil, or body fluids, use a degreasing medical cleansing agent. You may need to apply a skin preparation agent, such as Mastisol or No-Sting, around the wound, if achieving an airtight seal proves difficult.)

- Select a V.A.C. dressing size to fill the entire wound cavity. Cut the V.A.C. foam to fit the size and shape of the wound, including tunneling and undermined areas. (*Note:* Avoid cutting the foam directly over the wound to prevent loose particles from falling into the wound.)

- When placing a V.A.C. dressing near blood vessels, ensure that all vessels are adequately protected with overlying fascia, tissue, or other protective barriers. Weakened, irradiated, or sutured blood vessels require greater care.

- Size and trim the transparent occlusive drape that will cover the foam dressing as well as a 1″ to 2″ (2.5- to 5-cm) border of intact skin. Don't discard excess drape; you may need it later as a patch.

- Gently place the foam into the wound cavity, covering the entire wound base and sides, including tunneling and undermined areas. (*Note:* If the wound is larger than the largest foam dressing, use more than one dressing. Make sure that the edges of the foam dressings touch each other.)

- Apply tubing to the foam in the wound. Tubing can be laid on top of the foam, or inserted into a hole in the foam dressing. The tubing should be positioned away from bony prominences. (*Note:* If using more than one dressing for a single wound, apply V.A.C. tubing to only one dressing. For deeper wounds, regularly reposition tubing to minimize pressure on wound edges. Cushion skin under the tubing with excess foam.)

- Cover the foam and 3 to 5 cm of surrounding healthy tissue with drape to ensure an occlusive seal. (*Note:* For fragile periwound skin, use a skin preparation prior to drape application, or frame the wound with a skin barrier or Duoderm. Cut the drape to a size large enough to cover the foam dressing and the skin barrier layer only.)

- Lift the tubing and pinch 1 to 3 cm of drape together under the tubing to help hold the tubing away from the skin, to cushion the tubing, and to help prevent leaks. (*Note:* Don't stretch the drape and don't compress the foam into the wound with transparent occlusive drape. Simply cover and seal around the foam. This helps minimize tension and shearing forces on periwound tissue.)
- Secure the tubing with an additional piece of drape or tape several centimeters away from the dressing. This prevents pull on the primary dressing area, which can cause leaks.
- Use excess drape to patch leaks and secure borders as needed.

    V.A.C. device:

- Remove the canister from the sterile packaging and push it into the V.A.C. unit until it clicks into place. (*Note:* If the canister is not engaged properly, the V.A.C. alarm will sound.)
- Connect the dressing tubing to the canister tubing. Make sure both clamps are open.
- Place the V.A.C. unit on a level surface or hang from the foot board. (*Note:* The V.A.C. unit will sound an alarm and deactivate therapy if the unit is tilted beyond 45 degrees.)
- Depress the green-lit power button. Adjust the V.A.C. unit settings. Press the THERAPY ON/OFF button to activate subatmospheric pressure therapy. In less than 1 minute of operation, the V.A.C. dressing should collapse, unless leaks are present.
- If you hear or suspect a leak (small leaks may create a whistling noise), check areas around the tubing for the source. Air leaks most often occur around the tubing. You can often fix a leak by gently pressing around the tubing and wrinkles to better seal the drape. You can also use excess drape to patch over leaks.

Removal

- Keep therapy on. Never leave subatmospheric pressure therapy off for more than 2 hours per day.
- Change the V.A.C. dressing every 48 hours or, if infection is present, every 12 hours.

- To remove the dressing, raise the tubing connector above the level of the pump unit.
- Tighten clamps on the dressing tubing.
- Separate the canister tubing and dressing tubing by disconnecting the connector.
- Allow the pump unit to pull the exudate in the canister tubing into the canister. Then, tighten the clamps on the canister tubing.
- Press the THERAPY ON/OFF button to deactivate the pump.
- Gently stretch the drape horizontally and slowly pull up from the skin. Don't peel.
- Gently remove the foam from the wound. (*Note:* If the dressing adheres to the wound base, consider imposing a single layer of nonadherent, porous material [for example, Mepitel, Adaptic, N-terface, or wide-meshed Vaseline-impregnated gauze] between the dressing and the wound when reapplying the dressing. The nonadherent material must have wide enough pores to allow unrestricted passage of air and fluid. Because tissue growth into the V.A.C. dressing may cause adherence, also consider more frequent dressing changes.)
- *Note:* If previous dressings were difficult to remove, make sure the dressing tubing is unclamped, then introduce 10 to 30 cc of normal saline solution into the tubing to soak underneath the foam. For best results, let sit for 15 to 30 minutes. Saline solution can also be injected directly into the foam while low vacuum (50 mm Hg) is applied to the dressing. Clamp the tubing once the saline solution starts to flow into the dressing tubing. Wait 15 to 30 minutes then gently remove the dressing.
- *Note:* If the patient experiences pain during a dressing change, the primary care provider may consider ordering 1% lidocaine solution to be introduced down the tubing or injected into the foam with the pump turned on at a lower pressure (50 mmHg). After instilling the lidocaine, clamp the tube and wait 15 to 20 minutes before gently removing the dressing. Also, the primary care provider may consider lowering the target pressure.
- Use the V.A.C. dressings only with the V.A.C. device. Remove V.A.C. dressings if subatmospheric pressure therapy is terminated.

Other Products

Warm-Up Wound Therapy
Augustine Medical, Inc.

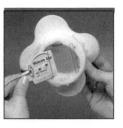

How supplied
Temperature control unit, AC adapter, sterile wound cover, warming card

Action
Warm-Up therapy is a wound management system that warms wounds toward normothermia. Most wounds are hypothermic, averaging 5.6° F cooler than core body temperature. Hypothermia causes vasoconstriction, depresses neutrophil activity, and lowers collagen deposition—all of which delay wound healing. Warm-Up therapy increases blood flow to the wound, which in turn increases subcutaneous oxygen tension and delivery of growth factors to the wound bed. The Warm-Up therapy system maintains physiologically appropriate levels of temperature and moisture in and around the wound, providing a beneficial healing environment.

The Warm-Up system's sterile, noncontact wound cover is placed over the wound to protect it from contamination and trauma. The wound cover consists of a water-resistant thin shell with an adhesive border, a clear window for wound observation, and a foam frame to absorb exudate and keep the cover from contacting the wound. A pocket in the window holds the warming card over the wound.

Indications
For local management of partial- and full-thickness wounds including venous, arterial, diabetic/neuropathic, and pressure ulcers (stages 2, 3, and 4). May be used on an infected wound as long as concurrent antibiotic treatment is used to treat the infection.

Contraindications
Contraindicated for third-degree burns.

Application
- Thoroughly cleanse the wound and surrounding skin, and dry the periwound skin.
- Choose the appropriate size wound cover, allowing for adequate healthy periwound skin between the edge of the foam

frame and the wound. Make sure there are no holes in the wound cover or wrinkling and folding of its edges, which could defeat its use as a barrier.

- Peel away half of the wound cover's adhesive liner, and press the cover's adhesive side to the skin.
- Peel away the other half of the adhesive liner and finish pressing the cover to the skin. To avoid damaging the skin, don't stretch the wound cover or the skin while applying the wound cover.
- Gently smooth the edges of the wound cover.
- Plug the warming card into the temperature control unit, and insert the warming card into the pocket on the wound cover.
- Turn the temperature control unit on. The warming card will warm to a preset temperature of 100.4°F (38°C).
- After 1 hour of warming therapy, turn the temperature control unit off and remove the warming card. The recommended protocol for warming therapy is 1 hour, three times per day.

Removal

- The wound cover may remain in place for 72 hours, or as clinically indicated.
- Change the wound cover if it leaks or no longer stays on the skin. Determine the frequency of wound cover changes by evaluating the wound and periwound condition and the amount of exudate. (*Note:* Within the first 10 days of initiating Warm-Up therapy, wound exudate may temporarily increase, a normal consequence of the wound healing process.)
- For removal, gently press down on the skin along one edge of the wound cover. Carefully lift the edge of the wound cover. Slowly peel away the wound cover until all edges are free.

Drugs

Overview

In this section, you'll find a list of products that are considered drugs because their administration provokes a series of physio-chemical events within the body. The drugs listed in this section each have unique actions, indications, and contraindications specific to the individual product. This information can also be found on the product's package insert. The clinician holds responsibility for understanding how each of these products affects the cascade of wound-healing events.

Products listed in this section are reimbursed as prescription drugs. The clinician must contact the appropriate payor regarding specific payment information for a given drug.

Drugs

ACCUZYME
Healthpoint

How supplied
Tube: 30 g

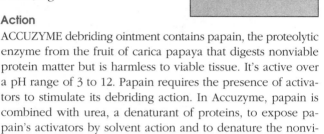

Action
ACCUZYME debriding ointment contains papain, the proteolytic enzyme from the fruit of carica papaya that digests nonviable protein matter but is harmless to viable tissue. It's active over a pH range of 3 to 12. Papain requires the presence of activators to stimulate its debriding action. In Accuzyme, papain is combined with urea, a denaturant of proteins, to expose papain's activators by solvent action and to denature the nonviable protein matter in lesions and render it more susceptible to enzymatic digestion.

Indications
To debride necrotic tissue and liquefy slough in acute and chronic lesions, such as pressure ulcers, varicose and diabetic ulcers, burns, postoperative wounds, pilonidal cyst wounds, carbuncles and miscellaneous traumatic or infected wounds.

Contraindications
Contraindicated in patients with known sensitivity to papain or any other components of this preparation.

Application
- Cleanse the wound with AllClenz Wound Cleanser or normal saline solution. Avoid cleansing with hydrogen peroxide solution as it may inactivate the papain.
- Apply Accuzyme directly to the wound.
- Cover with an appropriate dressing and secure into place.
- *Note:* Papain may also be inactivated by the salts of heavy metals such as lead, silver, and mercury. Avoid contact with medications containing these metals.

Removal
- Reapply one or two times a day.
- Flush the wound with ALLCLENZ Wound Cleanser or normal saline solution to remove any accumulation of liquefied necrotic material.

CLODERM Cream (clocortolone pivalate, 0.1%)
Healthpoint

How supplied
Cream: 15 g, 45g

Action
The mechanism of anti-inflammatory activity of topical steroids, such as Cloderm Cream, is unclear.

Indications
To relieve inflammation and pruritus caused by corticosteroid dermatoses, especially stasis and contact dermatitis. May be used under compression dressings.

Contraindications
Contraindicated in patients with known sensitivity to any components of the preparation.

Application
- Apply sparingly to affected area three times daily.
- Rub in gently.

Drugs

Collagenase SANTYL Ointment

Smith & Nephew, Inc.
Wound Management Division

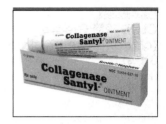

How supplied
Tube: 15 g, 30 g

Action
Collagenase Santyl Ointment is a sterile enzymatic debriding agent that digests collagen in necrotic tissue. Because collagen accounts for 75% of the dry weight of skin tissue, the product is particularly effective for removing necrotic tissue without destroying healthy granulation tissue, thus encouraging epithelization of dermal ulcers and severly burned areas.

Indications
To debride chronic dermal ulcers and severely burned areas.

Contraindications
Contraindicated in patients with known local or systemic hypersensitivity to collagenase.

Application
- Gently cleanse the wound with a gauze pad saturated with normal saline or another cleansing agent.
- For infected wounds, use a topical antibiotic powder before applying the ointment; use together until infection subsides.
- When clinically indicated, cross-hatch thick eschar with a #10 blade before applying ointment.
- Apply the ointment directly to the wound, or place on a gauze pad before applying. Apply carefully within the wound area.
- If appropriate, cover the wound according to facility policy.
- Cease application when debridement of necrotic tissue is complete and granulation tissue is well established.

Removal
Irrigate the wound with normal saline solution to flush out necrotic tissue.

Granulex Spray
Bertek (Dow Hickam)
Pharmaceuticals

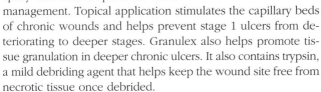

How supplied
Spray: 2 oz, 4 oz; A9270

Action
Granulex is a topical aerosol wound
spray that aids in pressure ulcer
management. Topical application stimulates the capillary beds
of chronic wounds and helps prevent stage 1 ulcers from de-
teriorating to deeper stages. Granulex also helps promote tissue granulation in deeper chronic ulcers. It also contains trypsin,
a mild debriding agent that helps keep the wound site free from
necrotic tissue once debrided.

Indications
To prevent skin breakdown and aid management of pressure
ulcers (stages 1, 2, 3, and 4), partial- and full-thickness wounds,
tunneling wounds, infected and noninfected wounds, wounds
with minimal drainage or those with serosanguineous drainage,
and red wounds.

Contraindications
Contraindicated for use on fresh arterial clots.

Application
- Gently cleanse the affected area.
- For stage 1 pressure ulcers, spray lightly into a gloved hand
  and gently apply it to the area three times a day. For stage
  2, 3, and 4 pressure ulcers, spray directly on the wound.

Removal
Cleanse the affected area gently with a wound cleanser.

Drugs

PANAFIL
Healthpoint

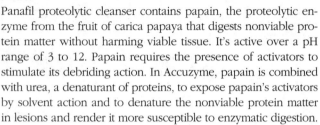

How supplied
Tube: 30 g

Action
Panafil proteolytic cleanser contains papain, the proteolytic enzyme from the fruit of carica papaya that digests nonviable protein matter without harming viable tissue. It's active over a pH range of 3 to 12. Papain requires the presence of activators to stimulate its debriding action. In Accuzyme, papain is combined with urea, a denaturant of proteins, to expose papain's activators by solvent action and to denature the nonviable protein matter in lesions and render it more susceptible to enzymatic digestion.

Panafil's chlorophyllin-copper-sodium complex adds healing action to the cleansing action of the proteolytic papain-urea combination. Its basic wound-healing properties are promotion of healthy granulation, control of local inflammation, reduction of wound odor, and promotion of wound healing.

Indications
To treat acute and chronic lesions, such as varicose, diabetic, and decubitus ulcers; burns; postoperative wounds; pilonidal cyst wounds; carbuncles; and traumatic or infected wounds.

Contraindications
None provided by the manufacturer.

Application
- Cleanse the wound with ALLCLENZ Wound Cleanser or saline solution but not hydrogen peroxide; it may inactivate papain.
- Apply Panafil directly to the wound.
- Cover with appropriate dressing and secure into place. Panafil Ointment may be applied under pressure dressings.
- *Note:* Papain may be inactivated by the salts of heavy metals, such as lead, silver, and mercury. Avoid contact with medications containing these metals.

PRUDOXIN Cream (doxepin hydrochloride, 5%)
Healthpoint

Drugs

How supplied
Cream: 45g

Action
Prudoxin Cream's exact mechanism of action is unknown. A histamine blocking drug, it appears to compete at histamine-1 and histamine-2 receptor sites and inhibit their biological activation.

Indications
For short-term management (up to 8 days) of moderate pruritus in adult patients with the following forms of ecxzematous dermatitis: atopic dermatitis and lichen simplex chronicus.

Contraindications
- Contraindicated in patients with untreated narrow angle glaucoma.
- Contraindicated in patients with a tendency to urinary retention.

Application
- Apply a thin film of the cream to affected areas 3 or 4 times daily.
- Allow at least 3 to 4 hours between applications.

REGRANEX (becaplermin) Gel 0.01%

Ortho-McNeil Pharmaceutical, Inc.

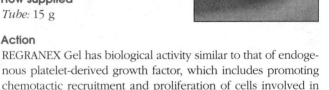

How supplied
Tube: 15 g

Action
REGRANEX Gel has biological activity similar to that of endogenous platelet-derived growth factor, which includes promoting chemotactic recruitment and proliferation of cells involved in wound repair and enhancing formation of granulation tissue.

Indications
To treat lower-extremity diabetic neuropathic ulcers that extend into subcutaneous tissue or beyond and which have an adequate blood supply. Along with good ulcer care practices, increases incidence of complete healing by 43% over placebo gel.

Contraindications
- Contraindicated in patients with known hypersensitivity to any of its components (such as parabens) or with neoplasms at the site of application.
- Not for use in wounds that close by primary intention because it's a nonsterile, low bioburden, preserved product.

Application
- Debride the wound.
- Apply the gel once daily in a carefully measured quantity. The daily dose should be recalculated weekly or biweekly by the primary care provider.
- Squeeze the calculated length of gel onto a clean, firm, nonabsorbent surface, such as waxed paper. Don't allow the tip of the tube to touch the wound or any other surface.
- Using a clean cotton swab, tongue depressor, or similar tool, spread the measured gel evenly over the wound in a continuous layer approximately 1/16" (0.2 cm) thick.
- Cover with a saline-moistened gauze dressing.

Removal
- After approximately 12 hours, gently rinse the ulcer with normal saline solution or water to remove residual gel.
- Cover with saline-moistened gauze; don't reapply the gel.

Part Three

ADDITIONAL DRESSINGS AND PRODUCTS

Overview

This section contains general dressings and products that may be used for wound management. Due to the high volume of general products that are manufactured, the section groups similar products into tables. The table headings closely follow the categories outlined by the Medicare Part B Surgical Dressing Policy. Each table may include more than one category. In that case, each representative category and its respective Health Care Financing Administration Common Procedure Coding System (HCPCS) code are identified above the table.

> *NOTE:* Inclusion in these tables does not mean that the manufacturers have applied for and/or received the HCPCS code identified above the tables. The provider and supplier are responsible for verifying the correct HCPCS codes before submitting claims to any payer.

To ensure uniform Medicare claim coding by all suppliers of wound care dressings, the Statistical Analysis Durable Medical Equipment Regional Carrier (SADMERC) performs a Coding Verification Review. If manufacturers wish to have a HCPCS code assigned to their products, they must submit a formal application to the SADMERC.

SADMERC and the four Durable Medical Equipment Regional Carriers (DMERCs) review the applications to determine the correct HCPCS codes for Medicare billing. These reviews result in a consensus coding decision. The assignment of a HCPCS code to a product should not be construed as an approval or endorsement of the product by SADMERC or Medicare and does not imply or guarantee reimbursement or coverage.

Many other payers also require the assigned HCPCS codes on their claim forms.

Abdominal dressing holders/binders

Abdominal dressing holder/binder products are hypoallergenic adhesive straps used in place of regular surgical tapes to avoid removing and reapplying tape during dressing changes.

The HCPCS code normally assigned abdominal dressing holder/binder is: A4462 — each.

Product	Manufacturer
DERMICEL Montgomery Straps	Johnson & Johnson Wound Management, Division of ETHICON, Inc.

Compression bandage systems

Compression therapy products are used to manage edema and promote the return of venous blood flow to the heart. Conventional management with a zinc oxide-impregnated bandaging system, such as an Unna Boot, provides inelastic compression. Multilayered, sustained, graduated high-compression bandages aid in the management of wounds caused by venous insufficiency.

The HCPCS code(s) normally assigned compression bandage systems are:

A4460 – elastic bandage

A4649 – surgical supplies, miscellaneous.

Product	Manufacturer or distributor	Type of compression	Subcategory
* AltoPress	Dumex Medical	Elastic	Single-layer compression system
CircAid Compression System Circ-Plus with Foot-piece	Coloplast	Inelastic	Interlocking bands
CircAid Compression System Thera-Boot	Coloplast	Inelastic	Interlocking bands with pre-attached foot-piece

(continued)

* Asterisk denotes a new product.

Product	Manufacturer or distributor	Type of compression	Subcategory
*Duboot Two-Layer Paste Bandage System	Dumex Medical	Elastic/Inelastic	Cohesive wrap/Unna boot
*Dufore Four-Layer Compression Bandaging System	Dumex Medical	Elastic	Multilayer compression system
DYNA-FLEX Multi-Layer Compression System	Johnson & Johnson Wound Management, Division of ETHICON, Inc.	Elastic	Multilayer compression system
Primer Modified Unna Boot	Western Medical, Ltd.	Inelastic	Unna boot/paste bandage
Primer Unna Boot	Western Medical, Ltd.	Inelastic	Unna boot/paste bandage
Profore Four Layer Bandaging System	Smith & Nephew, Inc., Wound Management Division	Elastic	Multilayer compression system
Profore Latex Free Four Layer Bandage System	Smith & Nephew, Inc., Wound Management Division	Elastic	Multilayer compression system
Profore Lite Multi-Layer Compression Bandage System	Smith & Nephew, Inc., Wound Management Division	Elastic	Multilayer compression system
Tenderwrap Unna Boot Bandage	Kendall Health Care Products Co.	Inelastic	Unna boot/paste bandage
*Tresflex Three-Layer Compression Bandaging System	Dumex Medical	Elastic	Multilayer compression system
UNNA-FLEX Elastic Unna Boot	ConvaTec	Inelastic	Unna boot
*UnnaPress Paste Bandage	Dumex Medical	Inelastic	Unna boot/paste bandage

* Asterisk denotes a new product.

Elastic bandages

The HCPCS code normally assigned elastic bandage rolls is: A4460 — per roll.

Product	Manufacturer
*Compriband	Dumex Medical
Comprilan	Beiersdorf-Jobst, Inc.
CURITY Elastic Bandage	Kendall Health Care Products Co.
*Duban Cohesive Elastic Bandage	Dumex Medical
*Duflex Synthetic Conforming Bandage	Dumex Medical
*DuGrip Tubular Bandage	Dumex Medical
*DuSor Elastic Bandage – With Clips	Dumex Medical
DYNA-FLEX Cohesive Compression Bandage	Johnson & Johnson Wound Management, Division of ETHICON, Inc.
DYNA-FLEX Elastic Bandages	Johnson & Johnson Wound Management, Division of ETHICON, Inc.
*Elastive Adhesive Bandage – Nonlatex	Dumex Medical
FLEX-WRAP Self Adherent Wrap	Kendall Health Care Products Co.
Matrix Latex Free Elastic Bandage with Double Velcro	Medline Industries, Inc.
SetoPress High Compression Bandage	ConvaTec
Soft Wrap Elastic Bandage	Medline Industries, Inc.
SurePress High Compression Bandage	ConvaTec
Sure Wrap Elastic Bandage	Medline Industries, Inc.
SurgiGrip Tubular Elastic Support Bandage	Western Medical, Ltd.

(continued)

* Asterisk denotes a new product.

Product	Manufacturer
Swift Wrap Elastic Bandage with Single Velcro	Medline Industries, Inc.
TENSOR Elastic Bandage	Kendall Health Care Products Co.
3M Coban Self-Adherent Wrap	3M Health Care
Tubigrip Shaped Support Bandage	ConvaTec

Gauze, elastic rolls

The HCPCS codes normally assigned to gauze, elastic rolls are:
A6263 — nonsterile, per linear yard
A6405 — sterile, per linear yard.

Product	Manufacturer
CONFORM Elastic Bandage	Kendall Health Care Products Co.
* Netfix Retention Dressing	Dumex Medical
Sof-Form Conforming Stretch Bandage	Medline Industries, Inc.
Surgilast Latex-Free Tubular Elastic Dressing Retainer	Western Medical, Ltd.
Surgilast Tubular Elastic Dressing Retainer	Western Medical, Ltd.

Gauze, impregnated with other than water, normal saline, or hydrogel, without adhesive border

Impregnated gauze dressings are woven or nonwoven materials in which substances such as iodinated agents, petrolatum, zinc compounds, crystalline sodium chloride, chlorhexadine gluconate, bismuth tribromophenate, aqueous saline, or other agents have been incorporated into the dressing material by the manufacturer.

The HCPCS codes normally assigned to gauze, impregnated with other than water, normal saline, or hydrogel, without an adhesive border are:

* Asterisk denotes a new product.

A6222—pad size 16 sq. in. or less

A6223—pad size more than 16 sq. in., but less than or equal to 48 sq. in.

A6224—pad size more than 48 sq. in.

A6266—any width roll, per linear yard.

Product	Manufacturer
ADAPTIC Non-Adhering Dressing	Johnson & Johnson Wound Management, Division of ETHICON, Inc.
ADAPTIC PG Petrolatum Gauze Non-Adherent Dressing	Johnson & Johnson Wound Management, Division of ETHICON, Inc.
ADAPTIC X Xeroform Gauze Non-Adherent Dressing	Johnson & Johnson Wound Management, Division of ETHICON, Inc.
Aquaphor Gauze Non-Adhering Dressing	Beiersdorf-Jobst
CURASALT Sodium Chloride Dressing	Kendall Health Care Products Co.
Curity Oil Emulsion Dressing	Kendall Health Care Products Co.
DERMAGRAN (Zinc-Saline) Wet Dressing	Derma Sciences, Inc.
Kerlix/Curity Saline Dressing	Kendall Health Care Products Co.
Medline Oil Emulsion	Medline Industries, Inc.
Medline Petrolatum Gauze	Medline Industries, Inc.
Medline Xeroform Gauze	Medline Industries, Inc.
* Medi-Tech Hydrophilic Gauze	Medi-Tech International Corporation
Mesalt	Mölnlycke Health Care
Mesalt Ribbon	Mölnlycke Health Care
NUGAUZE Packing Strips-Iodoform	Johnson & Johnson Wound Management, Division of ETHICON, Inc.
* Pak-Its Gauze Packing Strips – Iodoform	Dumex Medical
Scarlet Red Ointment Dressing	Kendall Health Care Products Co.

(continued)

* Asterisk denotes a new product.

Product	Manufacturer
Vaseline Petrolatum Gauze	Kendall Health Care Products Co.
Xeroflo Gauze Dressing	Kendall Health Care Products Co.
Xeroform Petrolatum Gauze	Kendall Health Care Products Co.

Gauze, impregnated with water or normal saline, without adhesive border

The HCPCS codes normally assigned to gauze, impregnated with water or normal saline dressings, without an adhesive border are:
A6228—pad size 16 sq. in. or less
A6229—pad size more than 16 sq. in., but less than or equal to 48 sq. in.
A6230—pad size more than 48 sq. in.

Product	Manufacturer
CURITY Saline Dressing	Kendall Health Care Products Co.
*Dumex Wet Dressings	Dumex Medical
MPM Gauze Impregnated Saline Dressing	MPM Medical, Inc.
*Pak-Its Saline Impregnated Gauze	Dumex Medical

Gauze, nonelastic rolls

The HCPCS codes normally assigned to gauze, nonelastic rolls are:
A6264—nonsterile, per linear yard
A6406—sterile, per linear yard.

Product	Manufacturer
Bulkee II	Medline Industries, Inc.
Cotton Plain Packing	Dumex Medical Surgical Products Ltd.
CURITY Packing Strips	Kendall Health Care Products Co.
*Duform Synthetic Conforming Bandage	Dumex Medical

(continued)

* Asterisk denotes a new product.

Product	Manufacturer
KERLIX LITE	Kendall Health Care Products Co.
Kerlix Rolls	Kendall Health Care Products Co.
KLING Fluff Rolls	Johnson & Johnson Wound Management, Division of ETHICON, Inc.
FLUFTEX Rolls	DeRoyal
Medline Plain Packing Strips	Medline Industries, Inc.
NUGAUZE Packing Strips	Johnson & Johnson Wound Management, Division of ETHICON, Inc.
Pak-Its Gauze Packing Strips – Plain	Dumex Medical
SOF-BAND Bulky Bandage	Johnson & Johnson Wound Management, Division of ETHICON, Inc.
Surgitube Tubular Gauze	Western Medical, Ltd.

Gauze, nonimpregnated, with adhesive border

The HCPCS codes normally assigned to gauze, nonimpregnated, with an adhesive border are:

A6219 — pad size 16 sq. in. or less

A6220 — pad size more than 16 sq. in., but less than or equal to 48 sq. in.

A6221 — pad size more than 48 sq. in.

Product	Manufacturer
Bordered Gauze Dressing	Carrington Laboratories
CovRSite CovRSite Plus	Smith & Nephew, Inc., Wound Management Division
DermaRite Bordered Gauze	DermaRite Industries
GENTELL BORDERED GAUZE	Gentell, Inc.
Hyperion Bordered Gauze	Hyperion Medical Inc.
Medline Bordered Gauze	Medline Industries, Inc.
Mepore Absorbent Island Dressing	Mölnlycke Health Care

* Asterisk denotes a new product.

Gauze, nonimpregnated, without adhesive border

The HCPCS codes normally assigned to gauze, nonimpregnated, nonsterile dressings without an adhesive border are:

A6216—pad size 16 sq. in. or less

A6217—pad size more than 16 sq. in., but less than or equal to 48 sq. in.

A6218—pad size more than 48 sq. in.

The HCPCS codes normally assigned to gauze, nonimpregnated, sterile dressings without an adhesive border are:

A6402—pad size 16 sq. in. or less

A6403—pad size more than 16 sq. in., but less than or equal to 48 sq. in.

A6404—pad size more than 48 sq. in.

Product	Manufacturer
Avant Gauze – Nonsterile	Medline Industries, Inc.
Avant Gauze Drain Sponge	Medline Industries, Inc.
Bulkee Super Fluff Sponges	Medline Industries, Inc.
Curity Cover Sponges	Kendall Health Care Products Co.
Curity Gauze Pads	Kendall Health Care Products Co.
CURITY Gauze Sponges	Kendall Health Care Products Co.
* Ducare Gauze Dressings/Sponges	Dumex Medical
* Dulix 6-ply Fluff Sponge	Dumex Medical
* Dusoft Non-Woven Dressings/Sponges	Dumex Medical
EXCILON Drain Sponge	Kendall Health Care Products Co.
FLUFTEX Sponges	DeRoyal
Johnson & Johnson Gauze Sponges	Johnson & Johnson Wound Management, Division of ETHICON, Inc.
Kerlix 4x4 Sponges	Kendall Health Care Products Co.
Kerlix Packing Sponges	Kendall Health Care Products Co.
Medline Gauze Pads – Bulk, nonsterile	Medline Industries, Inc.

(continued)

---

* Asterisk denotes a new product.

Product	Manufacturer
Medline Gauze Pads – Sterile	Medline Industries, Inc.
*PrimaPad Nonadherent Absorbent Pad	Dumex Medical
Sof-Form	Medline Industries, Inc.

Tapes

Securing a dressing is an essential step in dressing management. One way to secure dressings is with the use of tapes. Each product is manufactured using various materials, widths, adhesives, and hypoallergenic properties.

The HCPCS code normally assigned tapes and closures is: A6265—all types, per 18 sq. in.

Product	Manufacturer
CONFORM Elastic Tape	Kendall Health Care Products Co.
Coverlet Adhesive Dressing	Beiersdorf-Jobst
Cover-Strip Sterile Wound Closure Strip	Beiersdorf-Jobst
CURASILK	Kendall Health Care Products Co.
CURITY Clear	Kendall Health Care Products Co.
CURITY Standard Porous	Kendall Health Care Products Co.
DERMICEL Hypo-Allergenic Cloth Tape	Johnson & Johnson Wound Management, Division of ETHICON, Inc.
DERMIFORM Hypo-Allergenic Knitted Tape	Johnson & Johnson Wound Management, Division of ETHICON, Inc.
DERMIVIEW Hypo-Allergenic Transparent Tape	Johnson & Johnson Wound Management, Division of ETHICON, Inc.
ELASTIKON Elastic Tape	Johnson & Johnson Wound Management, Division of ETHICON, Inc.
Episeal	DeRoyal
Hypafix Dressing Retention Rolls	Smith & Nephew, Inc., Wound Management Division
Hy-Tape, The Original Pink Tape	Hy-Tape Corporation

(continued)

* Asterisk denotes a new product.

Product	Manufacturer
JOHNSON & JOHNSON Waterproof Tape	Johnson & Johnson Wound Management, Division of ETHICON, Inc.
Medfix Dressing Retention Bandage	Medline Industries, Inc.
Medfix Cloth Tape	Medline Industries, Inc.
Medfix Ortho-Porous Sports Tape	Medline Industries, Inc.
Medfix Paper Tape	Medline Industries, Inc.
Medfix Transparent Tape	Medline Industries, Inc.
* Mefix Megazinc Pink Adhesive Tape	Mölnlycke Health Care
Scanpor Non-Woven Tape	Bard Medical Division, C.R. Bard, Inc.
Sta-Fix Tape	Southwest Technologies, Inc.
TENDERSKIN	Kendall Health Care Products Co.
3M Blenderm Surgical Tape	3M Health Care
3M Cloth Adhesive Tape	3M Health Care
3M Durapore Surgical Tape	3M Health Care
3M Medipore H Soft Cloth Surgical Tape	3M Health Care
3M Medipore Pre-cut Dressing Covers	3M Health Care
3M Medipore Soft Cloth Surgical Tape	3M Health Care
3M Microfoam Surgical Tape	3M Health Care
3M Microfoam Surgical Tape Patch	3M Health Care
* 3M Micropore Plus Surgical Tape	3M Health Care
3M Micropore Surgical Tape	3M Health Care
3M Transpore Surgical Tape	3M Health Care
* 3M Transpore White Dressing Tape	3M Health Care
* Ultraclear Transparent Tape	Dumex Medical
* Ultrafix Adhesive Dressing	Dumex Medical
* Ultrapore Paper Tape	Dumex Medical

(continued)

* Asterisk denotes a new product.

Product	Manufacturer
* Ultraproof Waterproof Tape	Dumex Medical
* Ultrasilk Cloth Tape	Dumex Medical
WET-PRUF	Kendall Health Care Products Co.
* Woundstrip Wound Closure Strips	Dumex Medical
ZONAS Porous Tape	Johnson & Johnson Wound Management, Division of ETHICON, Inc.

Wound cleansers

Wound cleansers are an essential step in wound management. These solutions are used to remove debris or foreign materials from the wound. Each cleanser listed provides the health care professional with proactive products for positive outcomes.

The HCPCS code normally assigned wound cleansers is: A6260—any type, any size.

Product	Manufacturer
ALLCLENZ Wound Cleanser	Healthpoint
Biolex Wound Cleanser	Bard Medical Division, C.R. Bard, Inc.
CarraKlenz Wound and Skin Cleanser	Carrington Laboratories
ClinsWound Wound Cleanser	SAGE Pharmaceuticals, Inc.
Comfeel Sea-Clens	Coloplast
CONSTANT-CLENS	Kendall Health Care Products Co.
Dermagran Wound Cleanser with Zinc	Derma Sciences, Inc.
* DermaKlenz	DermaRite Industries
* DermaMed	DermaRite Industries
DiaB Klenz Wound Cleanser	Carrington Laboratories
Gentell Wound Cleanser	Gentell, Inc.
Hyperion Wound Cleanser	Hyperion Medical Inc.

(continued)

* Asterisk denotes a new product.

Product	Manufacturer
*Hypertonic Seasalt Dermal Solution	Dumex Medical
Iamin Wound Cleanser	Bard Medical Division, C.R. Bard, Inc.
Lobana Saline Wound Cleanser	Ulmer Pharmacal Company
*MEDI-TECH Wound Cleanser	Medi-Tech International Corporation
MicroKlenz Antiseptic Wound Cleanser	Carrington Laboratories
MPM Antimicrobial Wound Cleanser	MPM Medical, Inc.
MPM Wound and Skin Cleanser	MPM Medical, Inc.
*PrimaDerm Dermal Cleanser – Preservative Free	Dumex Medical
*PrimaDerm Dermal Cleanser – Preserved	Dumex Medical
RadiaKlenz	Carrington Laboratories
Restore Wound Cleanser	Hollister
SeptiCare	Sage Pharmaceuticals
Skintegrity Wound Cleanser	Medline Industries, Inc.
UltraKlenz Wound Cleanser	Carrington Laboratories

Wound pouches

Wound pouches collect and contain drainage as well as protect the skin around the wound from corrosive discharge.

The HCPCS code normally assigned wound pouch is: A6154—each.

Product	Manufacturer
Hollister Wound Drainage Collector	Hollister Incorporated

* Asterisk denotes a new product.

Appendices

Manufacturer resource guide

Selected references

Index

Appendix A
Body mass index

The body mass index (BMI) is the relationship between height and weight. Use this chart as an indicator for determining optimal weight for health and as a resource to assess obesity.

HEIGHT (inches)

WEIGHT (lbs)	58	59	60	61	62	63	64	65	66	67	68	69	70	71	72	73	74	75	76
	4'10"	4'11"	5'0"	5'1"	5'2"	5'3"	5'4"	5'5"	5'6"	5'7"	5'8"	5'9"	5'10"	5'11"	6'0"	6'1"	6'2"	6'3"	6'4"
100	21	20	20	19	18	18	17	17	16	16	15	15	14	14	14	13	13	13	13
105	22	21	21	20	19	19	18	18	17	16	16	16	15	15	14	14	14	13	13
110	23	22	22	21	20	20	19	18	18	17	17	16	16	15	15	15	14	14	13
115	24	23	23	22	21	20	20	19	19	18	18	17	17	16	16	15	15	14	14
120	25	24	23	23	22	21	21	20	19	19	18	18	17	17	16	16	15	15	15
125	26	25	24	24	23	22	22	20	20	20	19	18	18	17	17	17	16	16	15
130	27	26	25	25	24	23	22	22	21	20	20	19	19	18	18	17	17	16	16
135	28	27	26	26	25	24	23	23	22	21	21	20	19	19	18	18	17	17	16
140	29	28	27	27	26	25	24	23	23	22	21	21	20	20	19	19	18	18	17
145	30	29	28	27	27	26	25	24	23	23	22	21	21	20	20	19	19	18	18
150	31	30	29	28	27	27	26	26	24	24	23	22	22	21	20	20	19	19	18
155	32	31	30	29	28	28	27	26	25	24	24	23	22	22	21	20	20	19	19
160	34	32	31	30	29	28	28	27	26	25	24	24	23	22	22	21	21	20	20
165	35	33	32	31	30	29	28	28	27	26	25	24	24	23	22	22	21	21	20
170	36	34	33	32	31	30	29	28	27	27	26	25	24	24	23	22	22	21	21
175	37	35	34	33	32	31	30	29	28	27	27	26	25	24	24	23	23	22	21
180	38	36	35	34	33	32	31	30	29	28	27	27	26	25	24	24	23	23	22
185	39	37	36	35	34	33	32	31	30	29	28	27	27	26	25	24	24	23	23
190	40	38	37	36	35	34	33	32	31	30	29	28	27	27	26	25	24	24	23
195	41	39	38	37	36	35	34	33	32	31	30	29	28	27	27	26	25	24	24
200	42	40	39	38	37	36	34	33	32	31	30	30	29	28	27	26	26	25	24
205	43	41	40	39	38	36	35	34	33	32	31	30	29	29	28	27	26	26	25
210	44	43	41	40	38	37	36	35	34	33	32	31	30	29	29	28	27	26	26
215	45	44	42	41	39	38	37	36	35	34	33	32	31	30	29	28	28	27	26
220	46	45	43	42	40	39	38	37	36	35	34	33	32	31	30	29	28	28	27
225	47	46	44	43	41	40	39	38	36	35	34	33	32	31	31	30	29	28	27
230	48	47	45	44	42	41	40	38	37	36	35	34	33	32	31	30	30	29	28
235	49	48	46	44	43	42	40	39	38	37	36	35	34	33	32	31	30	29	29
240	50	49	47	45	44	43	41	40	39	38	37	36	35	34	33	32	31	30	29
245	51	50	48	46	45	43	42	41	40	38	37	36	35	34	33	32	32	31	30

(continued)

HEIGHT (inches)

WEIGHT (lbs)	58	59	60	61	62	63	64	65	66	67	68	69	70	71	72	73	74	75	76
	4'10"	4'11"	5'0"	5'1"	5'2"	5'3"	5'4"	5'5"	5'6"	5'7"	5'8"	5'9"	5'10"	5'11"	6'0"	6'1"	6'2"	6'3"	6'4"
250	52	51	49	47	46	44	43	42	40	39	38	37	36	35	34	33	32	31	30
255	53	52	50	48	47	45	44	43	41	40	39	38	37	36	35	34	33	32	31
260	54	53	51	49	48	46	45	43	42	41	40	38	37	36	35	34	33	33	32
265	56	54	52	50	49	47	46	44	43	42	40	39	38	37	36	35	34	33	32
270	57	55	53	51	49	48	46	45	44	42	41	40	39	38	37	36	35	34	33
275	58	56	54	52	50	49	47	46	44	43	42	41	40	38	37	36	35	34	34
280	59	57	55	53	51	50	48	47	45	44	43	41	40	39	38	37	36	35	34
285	60	58	56	54	52	51	49	48	46	45	43	42	41	40	39	38	37	36	35
290	61	59	57	55	53	51	50	48	47	46	44	43	42	41	39	38	37	36	35
295	62	60	58	56	54	52	51	49	48	46	45	44	42	41	40	39	38	37	36
300	63	61	59	57	55	53	52	50	49	47	46	44	43	42	41	40	39	38	37

KEY:

Underweight   Healthy weight   Hefty   Overweight   Obese

Excerpted from Hess, C.T. Clinical Wound Manager Manual Series for the Wound Care Department. © Wound Care Strategies, Inc., 2001.

Appendix B
Braden scale

To use this scale, assess the patient for each category, assign a score of 1 to 4, and then calculate the total score. If the patient's score is 16 or less, consider him at high risk for pressure ulcer development.

SENSORY PERCEPTION Ability to respond appropriately to pressure-related discomfort	**1. Completely limited** Patient is unresponsive to painful stimuli (doesn't moan, flinch, or grasp) or has limited ability to feel pain over most of body surface due to diminished level of consciousness or sedation.	**2. Very limited** Patient responds only to painful stimuli, can't communicate discomfort except by moaning or restlessness, or has a sensory impairment that limits the ability to feel pain or discomfort over half of body.
MOISTURE Degree to which skin is exposed to moisture	**1. Constantly moist** Skin is moistened almost constantly by perspiration, urine, and so on. Dampness is detected every time patient is moved or turned.	**2. Moist** Skin is usually but not always moist. A linen change is required at least once each shift.
ACTIVITY Degree of physical activity	**1. Bedbound** Patient is confined to bed.	**2. Chairbound** Patient's ability to walk is severely limited or nonexistent. Patient can't bear his own weight or must be assisted into a chair or wheelchair.
MOBILITY Ability to change and control body position	**1. Completely immobile** Patient doesn't make even slight changes in body or extremity position without assistance.	**2. Very limited** Patient makes occasional slight changes in body or extremity position but is unable to make frequent or significant changes independently.

	DATE OF ASSESSMENT			

3. Slightly limited
Patient responds to verbal commands but can't always communicate discomfort or need to be turned or has some sensory impairment that limits his ability to feel pain or discomfort in one or two extremities.

4. No impairment
Patient responds to verbal commands and has no sensory deficit that would limit his ability to feel or voice pain or discomfort.

3. Occasionally moist
Skin is occasionally moist, and an extra linen change is required approximately once per day.

4. Rarely moist
Skin is usually dry and linen requires changing only at routine intervals.

3. Walks occasionally
Patient walks occasionally during the day but only for very short distances, with or without assistance. Patient spends most of each shift in a bed or chair.

4. Walks frequently
Patient walks outside the room at least twice per day and inside the room at least once every 2 hours during waking hours.

3. Slightly limited
Patient independently makes frequent though slight changes in body or extremity position.

4. No limitations
Patient makes major and frequent changes in position without assistance.

(continued)

NUTRITION Usual food in- take pattern	**1. Very poor** Patient never eats a com- plete meal and rarely eats more than one-third of any food offered. Patient eats two servings or less of protein (meat or dairy products) per day, takes fluids poorly, does- n't take a liquid dietary sup- plement, or is NPO or main- tained on clear liquids or I.V. fluids for more than 5 days.	**2. Probably inadequate** Patient rarely eats a com- plete meal and generally eats only about one-half of any food offered. Patient eats three servings of pro- tein (meat or dairy prod- ucts) per day, occasionally will take a dietary supple- ment, or receives less than an optimum amount of liq- uid diet or tube feeding.
FRICTION AND SHEAR	**1. Problem** Patient requires moderate to maximum assistance in mov- ing. Complete lifting without sliding against sheets is im- possible and he frequently slides down in the bed or chair, requiring repositioning with maximum assistance. Spasticity, contractures, or agitation lead to almost con- stant friction.	**2. Potential problem** Patient moves feebly or re- quires minimum assistance. During a move, skin slides to some extent against sheets, the chair, restraints, or other devices. Patient maintains relatively good position in a chair or bed most of the time but occa- sionally slides down.

	DATE OF ASSESSMENT			

3. Adequate
Patient eats over one-half of most meals and eats a total of four servings of protein (meat or dairy products) each day. Occasionally, patient will refuse a meal but will usually take a supplement if offered or is on a tube feeding or total parenteral nutrition regimen.

4. Excellent
Patient eats most of every meal and never refuses a meal. Patient usually eats a total of four or more servings of protein (meat or dairy products) daily. Patient occasionally eats between meals and doesn't require supplementation.

3. No apparent problem
Patient moves in a bed or chair independently and has sufficient muscle strength to lift up completely during the move. Patient maintains good position in a bed or chair at all times.

	TOTAL SCORE			

Appendix C
Wagner ulcer grade classification

This system classifies foot ulcers.

GRADE	CHARACTERISTICS
0	• Preulcer lesion • Healed ulcer • Presence of bony deformity
1	• Superficial ulcer without subcutaneous tissue involvement
2	• Penetration through the subcutaneous tissue; may expose bone, tendon, ligament, or joint capsule
3	• Osteitis, abscess, or osteomyelitis
4	• Gangrene of a digit
5	• Gangrene requiring foot amputation

Reprinted from Glugla, M., and Mulder, G.D., "The Diabetic Foot: Medical Management of Foot Ulcers," in Chronic Wound Care. Edited by Krasner, D. King of Prussia, Pa.: Health Management Publications, Inc., 1990, with permission of the publisher.

Appendix D
Treatment algorithm for pressure ulcers

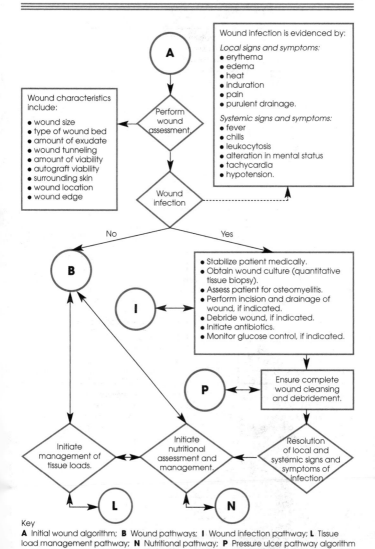

Wound infection is evidenced by:

Local signs and symptoms:
- erythema
- edema
- heat
- induration
- pain
- purulent drainage.

Systemic signs and symptoms:
- fever
- chills
- leukocytosis
- alteration in mental status
- tachycardia
- hypotension.

Wound characteristics include:
- wound size
- type of wound bed
- amount of exudate
- wound tunneling
- amount of viability
- autograft viability
- surrounding skin
- wound location
- wound edge

A

Perform wound assessment.

Wound infection

No — **B**

Yes

I
- Stabilize patient medically.
- Obtain wound culture (quantitative tissue biopsy).
- Assess patient for osteomyelitis.
- Perform incision and drainage of wound, if indicated.
- Debride wound, if indicated.
- Initiate antibiotics.
- Monitor glucose control, if indicated.

P — Ensure complete wound cleansing and debridement.

Resolution of local and systemic signs and symptoms of infection

Initiate management of tissue loads. — **L**

Initiate nutritional assessment and management. — **N**

Key
A Initial wound algorithm; **B** Wound pathways; **I** Wound infection pathway; **L** Tissue load management pathway; **N** Nutritional pathway; **P** Pressure ulcer pathway algorithm

Hess, C.T., *Clinical Wound Manager Manual Series for the Wound Care Department*. © Wound Care Strategies, Inc., 2001.

Appendix E
Treatment algorithm for arterial ulcers

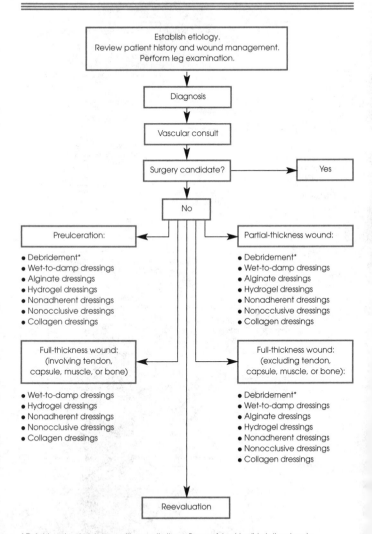

Establish etiology.
Review patient history and wound management.
Perform leg examination.

Diagnosis

Vascular consult

Surgery candidate? ⟶ Yes

No

Preulceration:
- Debridement*
- Wet-to-damp dressings
- Alginate dressings
- Hydrogel dressings
- Nonadherent dressings
- Nonocclusive dressings
- Collagen dressings

Partial-thickness wound:
- Debridement*
- Wet-to-damp dressings
- Alginate dressings
- Hydrogel dressings
- Nonadherent dressings
- Nonocclusive dressings
- Collagen dressings

Full-thickness wound:
(involving tendon, capsule, muscle, or bone)
- Wet-to-damp dressings
- Hydrogel dressings
- Nonadherent dressings
- Nonocclusive dressings
- Collagen dressings

Full-thickness wound:
(excluding tendon, capsule, muscle, or bone):
- Debridement*
- Wet-to-damp dressings
- Alginate dressings
- Hydrogel dressings
- Nonadherent dressings
- Nonocclusive dressings
- Collagen dressings

Reevaluation

* Debride only arterial ulcers with necrotic tissue. Be careful not to disturb the already compromised arteries.

Adapted with permission from Advances in Skin & Wound Care 14(3):147, May/June 2001.

Appendix F
Treatment algorithm for venous ulcers

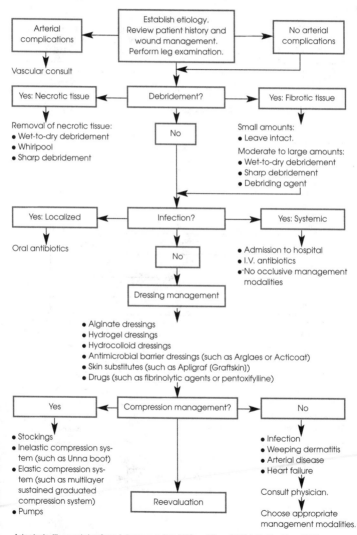

Establish etiology. Review patient history and wound management. Perform leg examination.

- Arterial complications → Vascular consult
- No arterial complications

Debridement?
- Yes: Necrotic tissue → Removal of necrotic tissue:
  - Wet-to-dry debridement
  - Whirlpool
  - Sharp debridement
- No
- Yes: Fibrotic tissue →
  - Small amounts:
    - Leave intact.
  - Moderate to large amounts:
    - Wet-to-dry debridement
    - Sharp debridement
    - Debriding agent

Infection?
- Yes: Localized → Oral antibiotics
- No
- Yes: Systemic →
  - Admission to hospital
  - I.V. antibiotics
  - No occlusive management modalities

Dressing management
- Alginate dressings
- Hydrogel dressings
- Hydrocolloid dressings
- Antimicrobial barrier dressings (such as Arglaes or Acticoat)
- Skin substitutes (such as Apligraf (Graftskin))
- Drugs (such as fibrinolytic agents or pentoxifylline)

Compression management?
- Yes
  - Stockings
  - Inelastic compression system (such as Unna boot)
  - Elastic compression system (such as multilayer sustained graduated compression system)
  - Pumps
- No
  - Infection
  - Weeping dermatitis
  - Arterial disease
  - Heart failure
  - Consult physician.
  - Choose appropriate management modalities.

Reevaluation

Adapted with permission from Advances in Skin & Wound Care 14(3):147, May/June 2001.

Appendix G
Treatment algorithm for diabetic ulcers

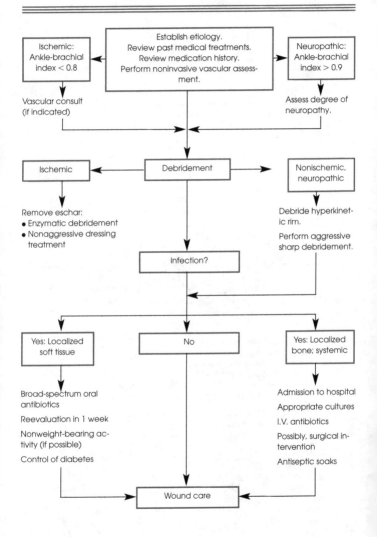

Ischemic:
Ankle-brachial
index < 0.8

Establish etiology.
Review past medical treatments.
Review medication history.
Perform noninvasive vascular assessment.

Neuropathic:
Ankle-brachial
index > 0.9

Vascular consult
(if indicated)

Assess degree of
neuropathy.

Ischemic

Debridement

Nonischemic,
neuropathic

Remove eschar:
• Enzymatic debridement
• Nonaggressive dressing
treatment

Debride hyperkinetic rim.

Perform aggressive
sharp debridement.

Infection?

Yes: Localized
soft tissue

No

Yes: Localized
bone; systemic

Broad-spectrum oral
antibiotics

Reevaluation in 1 week

Nonweight-bearing activity (if possible)

Control of diabetes

Admission to hospital

Appropriate cultures

I.V. antibiotics

Possibly, surgical intervention

Antiseptic soaks

Wound care

Adapted with permission from Advances in Skin & Wound Care 13(1):35, January/February 2000.

Appendix H
Treatment algorithm for diabetic ulcer wound care

Evaluate patient.

Evaluate footwear.

Surgical referral for bony deformities

Grade 0

- Padding and accommodative devices
- Callus debridement

Grade 1

- Follow Grade 1 protocol.
- Topical silver sulfadiazine on highly contaminated wounds
- Nonocclusive dressing
- Weekly evaluation until healed
- Plantar surface — gauze dressing
- Dorsal surface — occlusive or nonocclusive dressing
- Growth factor (rhPDGF-BB) when ankle-brachial index (ABI) is > 0.45

Grade 2

- Follow Grade 1 protocol.
- Rule out osteomyelitis (X-ray, bone scan, bone biopsy)
- Nonweight-bearing activity
- Surgical consult
- Plantar surface — gauze, amorphous hydrogel, alginate, or foam dressing
- Dorsal surface — occlusive dressing
- Topical antimicrobial cream, ointment, or amorphous hydrogel
- Growth factor (rhPDGF-BB) when ABI is < 0.45

Grade 3

- Follow Grade 1 protocol.
- Rule out osteomyelitis (X-ray, bone scan, bone biopsy)
- Plantar surface — gauze, amorphous hydrogel, alginate, or foam dressing
- Dorsal surface — nonocclusive dressing
- Topical antimicrobial cream, ointment, or amorphous hydrogel

Grades 4 and 5

- Surgical consult and intervention

Adapted with permission from *Advances in Skin & Wound Care* 13(1):35, January/February 2000.

Manufacturer resource guide

Name	Address	Web address
Acrymed,Inc.	12232 SW Garden Place Portland, OR 97223	www.acrymed.com
Aloe Life International	4822 Santa Monica Ave. San Diego, CA 92107	www.aloelife.com
Amerx Health Care Corporation	1150 Cleveland Street Suite 410 Clearwater, FL 33755	www.amerigel.com
Augustine Medical, Inc.	10393 West 70th Street Eden Prairie, MN 55344	www.warm-up.com
Bard Medical Division, C.R. Bard, Inc.	8195 Industrial Blvd. Covington, GA 30014	www.bardmedical. com
Bertek (Dow Hickam) Pharmaceuticals	P.O. Box 14149 Research Triangle Park, NC 27709	www.bertek.com
Beiersdorf-Jobst, Inc.	5825 Carnegie Blvd. Charlotte, NC 28209	www.Beiersdorf.com
BioCore Medical Technologies, Inc.	11800 Tech Road Suite 240 Silver Spring, MD 20904	www.biocore.com
Calmoseptine, Inc.	16602 Burke Lane Huntington Beach, CA 92647	www. calmoseptineointment. com
Carrington Laboratories	2001 Walnut Hill Lane Irving, TX 75038	www.carringtonlabs. com
Coloplast Corporation	1955 W. Oak Circle Marietta, GA 30062	www.us.coloplast.com
CONMED Corporation	310 Broad Street Utica, NY 13501	www.conmed.com

Name	Address	Web address
ConvaTec A Bristol-Meyers Squibb Company	100 Headquarters Drive Skillman, NJ 08558	www.convatec.com
Derma Sciences, Inc.	214 Carnegie Center Suite 100 Princeton, NJ 08540	www.DermaSciences.com
DermaRite Industries	3 East 26th Street Paterson, NJ 07513	www.DermaRite.com
DeRoyal	200 DeBusk Lane Powell, TN 37489	www.deroyal.com
Dumex Medical	825 Franklin Court Unit G Marietta, GA 30067	www.dumex.com
Ferris Manufacturing Corporation	16 W. 300 83rd Street Burr Ridge, IL 60521	www.ferrispolymem.com
FNC Medical Corporation	5600 Everglades Units B and C Ventura, CA 93003	www.fncmedical.com
Gentell, Inc.	3600 Boundbrook Ave. Trevose, PA 01953	www.gentell.com
Healthpoint	2600 Airport Freeway Fort Worth, TX 76111	www.healthpoint.com
Hollister Incorporated	2000 Hollister Drive Libertyville, IL 60048	www.hollister.com
The Hymed Group Corporation	1890 Bucknell Drive Bethlehem, PA 18015	www.hymed.com
Hyperion Medical, Inc.	1130 Celebration Blvd. Celebration, FL 34747	www.hyperionmedical.com
Johnson & Johnson Wound Management, Division of ETHICON, Inc.	P.O. Box 151 Somerville, NJ 08876	www.advancedwoundcare.com

Name	Address	Web address
Kendall Health Care Products Company	15 Hampshire Street Mansfield, MA 02048	www.kendallhq.com
KCI	P.O. Box 659508 San Antonio, TX 78265	www.KCI1.com
Lanaseptic Division, Summit Industries, Inc.	P.O. Box 7329 Marietta, GA 30065	www.lanaseptic.com
Lescarden Inc.	420 Lexington Avenue Suite 212 New York, NY 10170	www.catrix.com
Medi-Tech International Corporation	26 Court Street Suite 1301 Brooklyn, NY 11242	www.medi-techintl. com
Medix Pharmaceuticals Americas, Inc.	12505 Starkey Road Suite M Largo, FL 33773	www.biafine.com
Medline Industries, Inc.	1 Medline Place Mundelein, IL 60060	www.medline.com
MedLogic Global Corporation	4815 List Drive Suite 111 Colorado Springs, CO 80919	www.medlogic.com
Merz Pharmaceuticals, LLC	4215 Tudor Lane Greensboro, NC 27310	www.merzusa.com
Mölnlycke Health Care	110 Baldwin Tower Eddystone, PA 19022	www.us.molnlyckehc. com
MPM Medical, Inc.	801 Stadium Drive Suite 109 Arlington, TX 76011	www.diversified-care. com
Omega Medical Products Corporation	494 Saw Mill River Road Yonkers, NY 10701	www.omegamedical products. com
Ormed. Inc.	599 Cardigan Road St. Paul, MN 55126	www.ormedtech.com

Name	Address	Web address
Ortho-McNeil Pharmaceutical, Inc.	1000 Rt. 202 Raritan, NJ 08869	www.regranex.com
Regenesis Biomedical, Inc.	1435 North Hayden Road Scottsdale, AZ 85257	www. RegenesisBiomedical. com
Sage Pharmaceuticals, Inc.	5408 Interstate Drive Shreveport, LA 71109	www.sagepharm. com
Sage Products, Inc.	3909 Three Oaks Road Cary, IL 60013	www.sageproducts. com
Smith & Nephew, Inc., Wound Management Division	11775 Starkey Road P.O. Box 1970 Largo, FL 33779	www.smwmd.com
Southwest Technologies, Inc.	1746 Levee Road North Kansas City, MO 64116	www.elastogel.com
Swiss-American Products, Inc.	4641 Nall Road Dallas, TX 75244	www.Elta.net
3M Health Care	3M Center Bldg 275-4E-01 St. Paul, MN 55144	www.3M. com/healthcare
Ulmer Pharmacal Company	1614 Industry Lane Park Rapids, MN 56470	
Western Medical Ltd.	64 N. Summit Street Tenafly, NJ 07670	www. westernmedical-ltd. com
Winfield Laboratories, Inc.	P.O. Box 832297 Richardson, TX 75083	
Woodward Laboratories, Inc.	11132 Winners Circle Los Alamitos, CA 90720	www.woodwardlabs. com

Selected references

Abu-own, A., et al. "Effect of leg elevation on the skin microcirculation in chronic venous insufficiency," *J Vasc Surg* 20(5):705–710, Nov 1994.

Acute Pain Management Guideline Panel. *Acute Pain Management: Operative or Medical Procedures and Trauma.* Clinical Practice Guideline, No. 1. AHCPR Pub. No. 92-0032. Rockville, Md.: Agency for Health Care Policy and Research, Public Health Service, U.S. Department of Health and Human Services, 1992.

Baumgartner, I., et al. "Constitutive expression of phVEGF165 after intramuscular injection promotes collateral vessel development in patients with critical limb ischemia," *Circulation* 97(12): 114–123, Mar 31, 1998.

Bello, Y.M., and Phillips, T.J. "Chronic leg ulcers: Types and treatments," *Hosp Prac* 35(2):101–108, Feb 15, 2000.

Bergstrom, N., et al. *Pressure Ulcer Treatment.* Clinical Practice Guideline, No. 15. AHCPR Pub. No. 95-0652. Rockville, Md.: Agency for Health Care Policy and Research, Public Health Service, U.S. Department of Health and Human Services, 1994.

Birke, J.A., et al. "A review of causes of foot ulceration in patients with diabetes mellitus," *J Prosthet Orthot* 4(1): 13–22, fall 1991.

Blair, S.D., et al. "Sustained compression and healing of venous ulcers." *BMJ* 297(6657):1159–1161, Nov 5, 1988.

Bollinger, A., and Partsch, H. Wolfe J.H.N., eds. *The initial lymphatics.* New York: Thieme Stratton, 1985.

Bowker, J.H., and Pfiefer, M.A. *Levin and O'Neal's the diabetic foot,* 6th ed. St. Louis: Mosby, 2001.

Brown, P., et al. *Quick reference to wound care.* Gaithersburg, Md.: Aspen, 2001.

Bryant, R.A., ed. *Acute and chronic wounds,* 2nd ed. St. Louis: Mosby, 2000.

Callam, M.J., et al. "Arterial disease in chronic leg ulceration: An underestimated hazard?" Lothian and Forth Valley leg ulcer study. *BMJ* 294(6577): 929–931, Apr 11, 1987.

Carpenter, J.P. "Noninvasive assessment of peripheral vascular occlusive disease," *Adv Skin Wound Care* 13(2):84–85, Mar-Apr 2000.

Catanzariti, A.R. "Prophylactic foot surgery in the diabetic patient," *Adv Wound Care* 12(6):312–317, Jul-Aug 1999.

Chernoff, R. *Geriatric nutrition,* 2nd ed. Gaithersburg, Md.: Aspen, 1999.

Christopoulos, D., et al. "Venous reflux: quantification and correlation with the clinical severity of chronic venous disease," *Br J Surg* 75(4):352–356, Apr 1988.

Collins, N. "Assessment and treatment of involuntary weight loss and protein-calorie malnutrition," *Adv Skin Wound Care* 13(1 Supplement):4–10, Jan-Feb 2000.

Dealey, C. *The care of wounds: A guide for nurses,* 2nd ed. Malden, Mass.: Blackwell Science, 1999.

Erickson, C.A., et al. "Healing of venous ulcers in an ambulatory care program: The role of chronic venous insufficiency and patient compliance," *J Vasc Surg* 22(5):629–636, Nov 1995.

Falabella, A., and Falanga, V. "Uncommon causes of ulcers," *Clin Plast Surg* 25(3):467–479, Jul 1998.

Falanga, V. *Cutaneous wound healing.* London: Martin Dunitz, 2001.

Falanga, V. "Overview of chronic wounds and recent advances," *Dermatol Ther* 9(12):7–17, 1999.

Fronek, H.S. "Vascular studies: Which are indicated and when?" *Dermatol Ther* 1999;9:18–29.

Heng, M.C., et al. "A simplified hyperbaric oxygen technique for leg ulcers," *Arch Dermatol* 120(5):640–645, May 1984.

Himes, D. "Protein-calorie malnutrition and involuntary weight loss: The role of aggressive nutritional intervention in wound healing," *Ostomy Wound Manage* 45(3):46–51, 54–55, Mar 1999.

Inlow, S., et al. "Best practices for the prevention, diagnosis, and treatment of diabetic foot ulcers," *Ostomy Wound Manage* 46(11):55–68, 70–71, Nov 2000.

Kozak, G.P., et al. *Management of diabetic foot problems,* 2nd ed. Philadelphia: W.B. Saunders, 1995.

Krasner, D., and Kane, D., eds. *Chronic wound care: A sourcebook for healthcare professionals,* 2nd ed. Wayne, Pa.: Health Management Publications, 1997.

Kwiecinski, M.G. "Therapeutic value of hyperbaric oxygen in lower extremity ulcerations," *J Foot Surg* 26(5): 394–396, Sep-Oct 1987.

Laing, P. "The development and complications of diabetic foot ulcers," *Am J Surg* 176(2A Supplement): 11S–19S, Aug 1998.

Lopez, A., and Philips, T. "Venous ulcers," *Wounds* 10(5):149–157, Sep-Oct 1998.

Mahan, L.K., and Escott-Stump, S. *Krause's food, nutrition, and diet therapy,* 10th ed. Philadelphia: W.B. Saunders, 2000.

Mayberry, J.C., et al. "Fifteen-year results of ambulatory compression therapy for chronic venous ulcers," *Surgery* 109(5): 575–581, May 1991.

McCaffery, M., and Pasera, C. *Pain Clinical Manual,* 2nd ed. St. Louis: Mosby, 1999.

McCaffery, M. "Overcoming barriers to pain management," *Nursing* 31(4):18, Apr 2001.

McGuckin, M., et al. *Venous leg ulcer guideline.* Philadelphia: Trustees of the University of Pennsylvania, 1997.

Mulder, G.D. "Evaluating and managing the diabetic foot: An overview," *Adv Skin Wound Care* 13(1):33–36, Jan-Feb 2000.

Ongenae, K., and Phillips, T. "Leg ulcer management," *Emerg Med* 25(9):45–53, Jun 30, 1993.

Panel for the prediction and prevention of pressure ulcers in adults. *Pressure ulcers in adults: Prediction and prevention.* Clinical Practice Guideline, No. 3. AHCPR Pub. No. 92-0047. Rockville, Md.: Agency for Health Care Policy and Research, Public Health Service, U.S. Department of Health and Human Services, 1992.

Panel for Urinary Incontinence in Adults. *Urinary incontinence in adults.* Clinical Practice Guideline, AHCPR Pub. No. 92-0038. Rockville, Md.: Agency for Health Care Policy and Research, Public Health Service, U.S. Department of Health and Human Services, 1992.

Reiber, G.E., et al. "The burden of diabetic foot ulcers," *Am J Surg* 176(2A Supplement):5S–10S, Aug 1998.

Rudolph, D.M. "Pathophysiology and management of venous ulcers," *J Wound, Ostomy Continence Nurs* 25(5):248–255, Sep 1998.

Sussman, C., and Bates-Jensen, B., eds. *Wound care: A collaborative practice manual for physical therapists and nurses,* 2nd ed. Gaithersburg, Md.: Aspen Publishers, Inc., 2001.

Tallman, P., et al. "Initial rate of healing predicts complete healing of venous ulcers," *Arch Dermatol* 133(10): 1231–1234, Oct 1997.

University of Texas Treatment Base Diabetic Foot Classification System," *Ostomy Wound Manage* 2000; 46(11): 55-68.

Upson, A.V. "Topical hyperbaric oxygenation in the treatment of recalcitrant open wounds: A clinical report," *Phys Ther* 66(9):1408–1412, Sep 1986.

Valencia, I.C., et al. "Chronic venous insufficiency and venous leg ulceration," *J Am Acad Dermatol* 44(3):401–421, Mar 2001.

Whitney, E.N., and Rolfes, S.R. *Understanding nutrition,* 8th ed. Belmont, Calif.: West/Wadsworth, 1999.

Wunderlich, R.P., et al. "Defining loss of protective sensation in the diabetic foot," *Adv Wound Care* 11(3):123–128, May-Jun 1998.

Zeman, F.J. *Clinical nutrition and dietetics,* 2nd ed. New York: Macmillan, 1991.

Index

t refers to a table; i refers to an illustration

t refers to a table; i refers to an illustration

t refers to a table; i refers to an illustration

t refers to a table; i refers to an illustration

t refers to a table; i refers to an illustration

t refers to a table; i refers to an illustration